Surgery for Complications of Diabetic Retinopathy

Chung-May Yang

Surgery for Complications of Diabetic Retinopathy

Springer

Chung-May Yang
Ophthalmology
National Taiwan University Hospital
Taipei, Taiwan

ISBN 978-981-96-2850-6 ISBN 978-981-96-2848-3 (eBook)
https://doi.org/10.1007/978-981-96-2848-3

This Springer imprint is published by the registered company Springer Nature Singapore Pte Ltd.
The registered company address is: 152 Beach Road, #21-01/04 Gateway East, Singapore 189721, Singapore

Preface

I have had the fortune to witness the tremendous progress in vitreoretinal surgery in the past 30 years. Vitrectomy for complications of diabetic retinopathy is one of the most challenging terrains in vitreoretinal surgery. This book is based on the personal experience and the data collected from a more than 30 years of clinical practice. It has not been intended to be a comprehensive review. In other words, the contents of this book are more of a subjective opinion than a consensus from objective reviews. The readers may not agree with some or many of the contents, but I hope that this book may serve as a stimulus for further studies. Because the contents of the book are derived mostly from personal view or studies, the references I have listed are mostly related to the background information and those authored or co-authored by me.

In the diagnosis and treatment of vitreoretinal diseases, image recording is very important. In this book, I have tried to accommodate as many images as possible from the cases I have treated. I have arranged the images of the case in a way that I used to do in a PowerPoint presentation, and I think that in this arrangement, the images will be more self-explanatory, without the usage of excessive words for explanation in the figure legends. I have put several sets of images together in one figure to show the various presentations of a particular condition. I apologize if such image setup reduces the resolution too much for readers to see the detail or makes readers feel overwhelmed by too many photos.

Each chapter has a main topic. I have arranged the presentation in such a way that one or two cases will be presented first, along with image set, followed by the discussion of that topic. The topics I chose are those that I thought are clinically relevant and that I am familiar with. These topics may not be the ones frequently talked about in the literature or review articles. I hope that they may provide some feeling of freshness for the readers.

I would like to thank my colleagues for case referring and case sharing. A few sets of images came from their file, for which I have made sure to show my courtesy in the figure legends. I would like to especially thank Dr. Po-Ting Yeh, Dr. Yi-Ting Hsieh, and Dr. San-Ni Chen for collaborating with me on several journal articles related to vitrectomy for complications of PDR, which I have included in my reference lists. Special thanks should go to Dr. Yi-Ting Hsieh for the great help to finalize all the details of the book format. Finally, particular thanks go to my wife. Her support and dedication to our family are the main reasons that I can focus on the work that I love.

Taipei, Taiwan Chung-May Yang

Contents

1 Fibrovascular Proliferation and Tractional Retinal Detachment

Abstract

Retinal neovascularization (NV) is the hallmark of proliferative diabetic retinopathy (PDR). The NV complex consists of vessels and fibrous tissue. In the early stage of PDR, when fibrovascular proliferation (FVP) is less prominent, medical treatment may prevent disease progression. Controversy exists as to the best strategy for medical treatment. Panretinal photocoagulation (PRP) was the treatment of choice before anti-vascular endothelial growth factor (VEGF) therapy became available (Group TDRSR, Int Ophthalmol Clin 27:239–253, 1987; Group ETDRSR, Ophthalmology 98:766–785, 1991; Group TDRSR, Am J Ophthalmol 81:383–396, 1976). Studies have shown that repeated intravitreal anti-VEGF injection alone may inhibit NV growth or even improve nonperfusion (Writing Committee for the Diabetic Retinopathy Clinical Research N et al., JAMA 314:2137–2146, 2015). Many investigators prefer the combination of anti-VEGF and PRP to obtain a long-term beneficial effect and to decrease the likelihood of the rebound of FVP when the use of anti-VEGF is stopped or when the follow-up visit becomes difficult for the patient (Gross et al., JAMA Ophthalmol 136:1138–1148, 2018). Nonetheless, a certain proportion of patients still experience progression of FVP, and surgical intervention is needed to restore visual function. The common features of FVP, the evolution of FVP, the surgical technique used to treat eyes with FVP, and the complications associated with FVP are discussed in this chapter.

1.1 Case Report

Patient 1: This 44-year-old man had underlying HT, poorly controlled DM, and dyslipidemia. PRP was applied to both eyes for PDR at an outside hospital. He had been a habitual smoker for 15 years, taking one pack per day. He complained of blurred vision in both eyes for 3 months, with progressive worsening of vision in the left eye in the last 2 weeks. On examination, best-corrected visual acuity (BCVA) was 30 cm in the right eye and 0.08 cm in the left eye. The anterior segment was unremarkable without rubeosis iridis (RI) in both eyes. Fundus examinations revealed a dense FVP over the disc and macular area that extended to the midperiphery in the nasal upper quadrant; macular tractional retinal detachment (TRD), scattered retinal hemorrhage, mild vitreous hemorrhage, and PRP scars in the nasal upper quadrant in the right eye; and a dense FVP over the superior and inferior arcades that extended to the midperiphery in the upper two quadrants, diffuse retinal hemorrhage, preretinal hemorrhage, moderate vitreous hem-

C.-M. Yang, *Surgery for Complications of Diabetic Retinopathy*,
https://doi.org/10.1007/978-981-96-2848-3_1

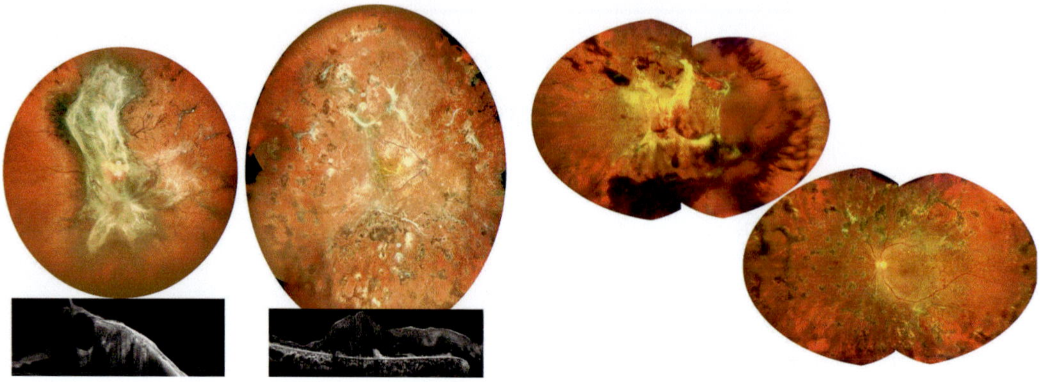

Fig. 1.1 Pre- and postoperative color photos/OCT images of the retina in the two eyes of Patient 1. Both eyes had severe (grade 3 severity) FVP extending from the disc to the arcade and midperiphery. The right eye had evolved to exhibit mainly fibrotic proliferation, while the left eye (the first operated eye) had active FVP. (Courtesy of Dr. Chung-May Yang)

orrhage (VH), and peripheral PRP in the left eye. Two days after IVI, 0.05 mL of Avastin (1.25 mg), 25G pars plana vitrectomy, chandelier light-assisted bimanual FVP removal, internal limiting membrane (ILM) peeling, endolaser, and intravitreal C3F8 infusion were performed in the left eye. The retina reattached after surgery. Eight weeks later, the patient underwent similar procedures in the right eye, except that no ILM peeling was performed. The retina reattached after surgery; however, prominent macular pucker was noted. Phacoemulsification with posterior chamber intraocular lens (PCIOL), epiretinal membrane (ERM) removal and internal limiting membrane removal were performed 16 months later. Her BCVA improved to 0.05 in the right eye and 0.4 in the left eye (Fig. 1.1).

Patient 2: A 51-year-old male with HT and newly diagnosed type 2 DM underwent repeated vitrectomy of the left eye due to progressive FVP and VH. Corneal opacity, neovascular glaucoma (NVG), and no-light perception (NLP) resulted. Progressive VA deterioration subsequently developed in the right eye. He was then referred to our clinic. On examination, BCVA was 0.05 in the right eye, and NLP in the left eye. Fundus examinations revealed an active FVP at the upper and lower arcades, connecting to the disc and extending to the mid-periphery on the nasal side, preretinal hemorrhage around the FVP, and a lower VH. OCT revealed macular thickening without TRD. He underwent vitrectomy, FVP removal, and ILM peeling. After surgery, the retinal structure normalized, and the BCVA improved to 0.6 (Fig. 1.2).

Patient 3: A 51-year-old woman with underlying DM and HT. Her ophthalmic history was significant for PDR in both eyes. PRP was performed on both eyes. The patient complained of blurred vision in the left eye for several months. On examination, BCVA was 0.32 in the right eye and HM/1 M in the left eye. Fundus examinations revealed scattered dot hemorrhage and PRP scarring in the right eye and VH, extensive FVP and TRD in the left eye. A 25G PPV, FVP tissue removal, ICG-assisted foveal-sparing ILM removal, endolaser, and IVI of 0.05 mL of Avastin and 1.2 mL of C3F8 were performed on the left eye. During the operation, FVPs with broad adhesion at more than three sites and extending beyond the equator in two to three quadrants were noted. The retina reattached after surgery. However, a thick premacular membrane causing macular folds developed. Twelve months later, phacoemulsification with PCIOL implantation, ICG-assisted ERM, and ILM removal were performed. Her BCVA was 0.05 in the left eye (Fig. 1.3).

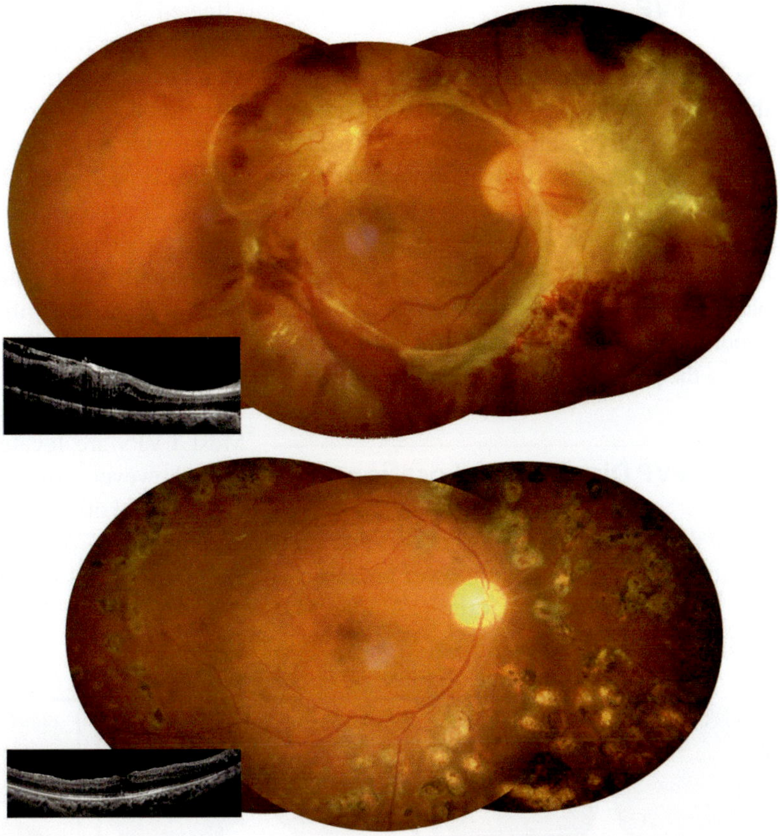

Fig. 1.2 Pre- and postoperative composite color images and OCT images of the retina in Patient 2. The active FVP distributed over the disc, nasal side and around the arcade causing traction thickening of the macula (upper). After surgery, the retina contour improved (lower). (Courtesy of Dr. Chung-May Yang)

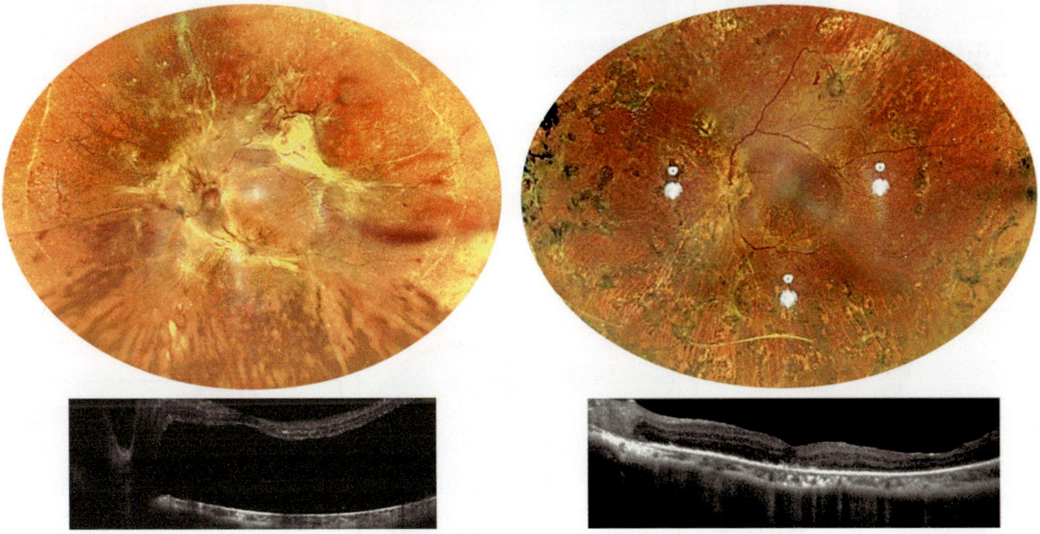

Fig. 1.3 Pre- and postoperative wide angle color photos and OCT images of the retina in Patient 3. The active FVP distributed over the disc, nasal side, and upper and lower arcades and extending to the midperiphery in the upper retina caused TRD (left). After surgery, the retina was reattached (right). (Courtesy of Dr. Chung-May Yang)

1.2 FVP

The FVP is the core lesion in PDR. Abnormal fibrovascular tissues grow from the optic disc or the retinal surface along the posterior hyaloid (PH), causing traction and bleeding. The PDR severity is strongly related to the FVP distribution, the severity of adhesion, and the traction applied to the retina, especially to the central macular area. FVP activity and the degree of hemorrhage are also important factors in determining the progression of PDR.

1.3 FVP Distribution/Location

The FVP usually grows from the disc and extends along the upper and lower arcades. In this distribution pattern, the VA may be affected by traction-induced macular elevation, macular folding, traction schisis, or macular TRD. An active FVP may be complicated by vitreous hemorrhage or preretinal hemorrhage, which may cause a decrease in VA if the macula is obscured. The FVP may be localized around or adjacent to the disc or extend toward the nasal side. In this pattern, traction on the disc, usually from the nasal side, may cause so-called vitreopapillary traction syndrome, resulting in optic disc temporal pallor (please see Chap. 9). The above two patterns may exist at the same time in more severe cases. Most FVPs are located within the equatorial area; however, some may extend beyond the equator, and others may distribute solely in the midperiphery, causing equatorial traction (Figs. 1.4, 1.5, 1.6, 1.7, and 1.8).

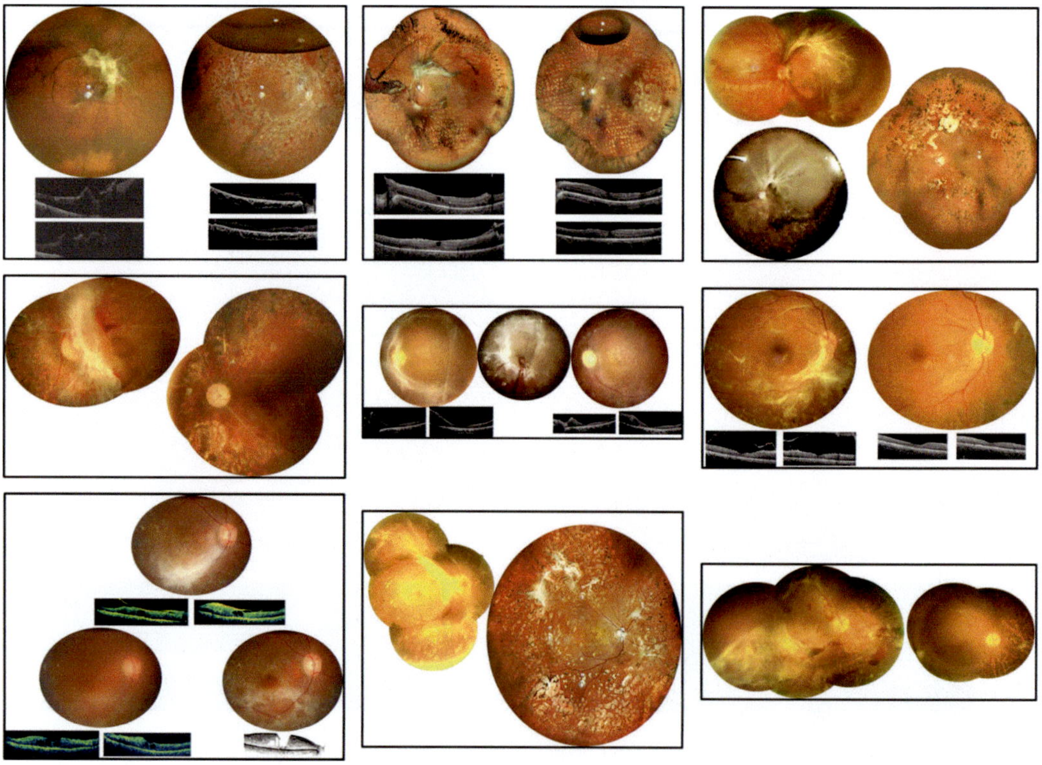

Fig. 1.4 Nine sets of color photos/OCT images showing pre- and postoperative retinal changes in eyes in which the FVP was distributed mainly in the arcade area. The proliferative tissue may be active or predominantly fibrotic (lower left and lower center panels). The FVP severity was mostly moderate (grade 2 severity). In the lower right panel, the FVP extended to the lower temporal midperiphery (left composite color photo). (Courtesy of Dr. Chung-May Yang)

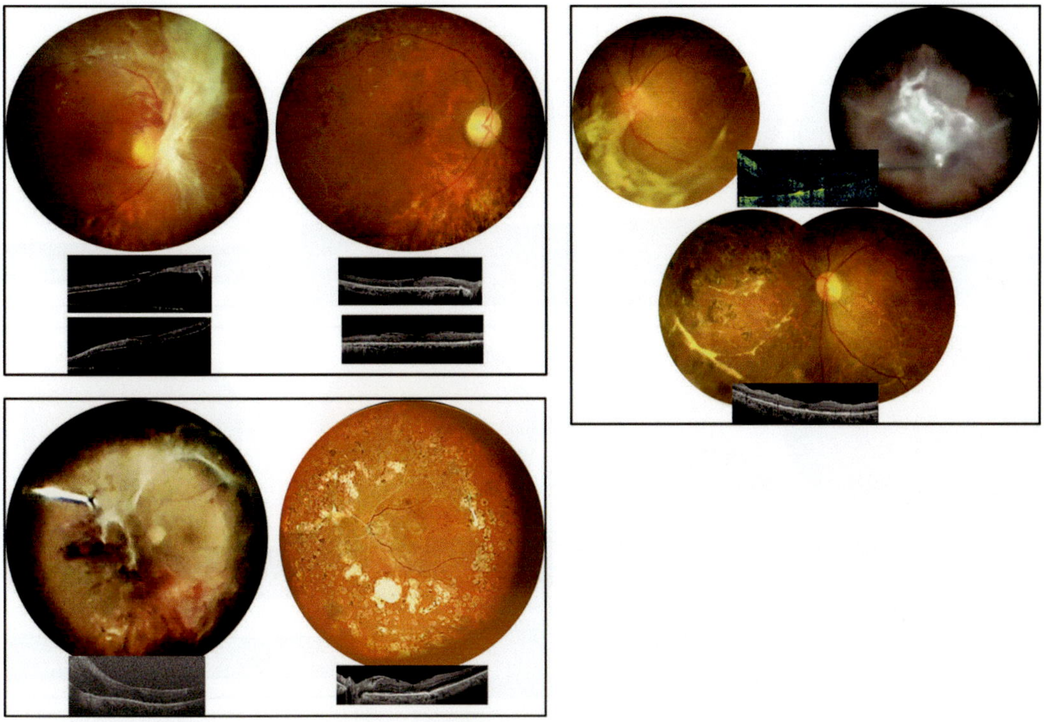

Fig. 1.5 Three sets of pre- and postoperative color photos/OCT images of the FVP were distributed mainly on the disc and nasal sides. TRD was noted preoperatively in the upper two panels. The video image (upper right) in the upper right panel shows the FVP extending from the disc to the lower midperiphery. The anterior edge of this broad adhesion membrane had the ERM tightly adherent to the retinal surface, creating a Ziploc effect. The ERM must be lifted to identify the true surgical plane between the FVP and the retina. In the lower panel, macular thickening and elevation on the nasal side of the macula were noted in the preoperative OCT image. (Courtesy of Dr. Chung-May Yang)

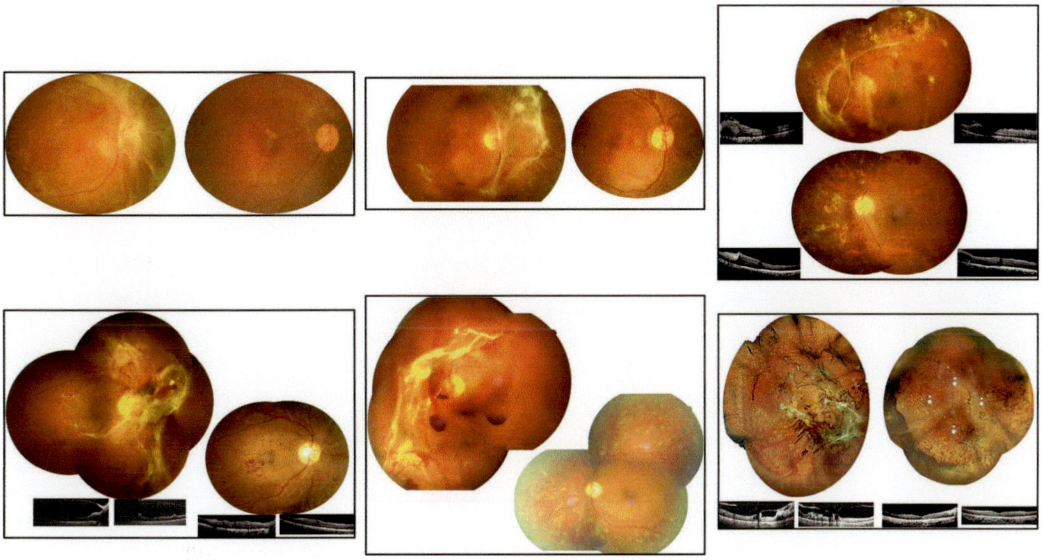

Fig. 1.6 Six sets of color photos/OCT images showing pre- and postoperative retinal changes in eyes in which the FVP was distributed mainly in the disc, nasal and arcade areas. The proliferation may be moderate or severe (grade 3 severity in the lower right panel). (Courtesy of Dr. Chung-May Yang)

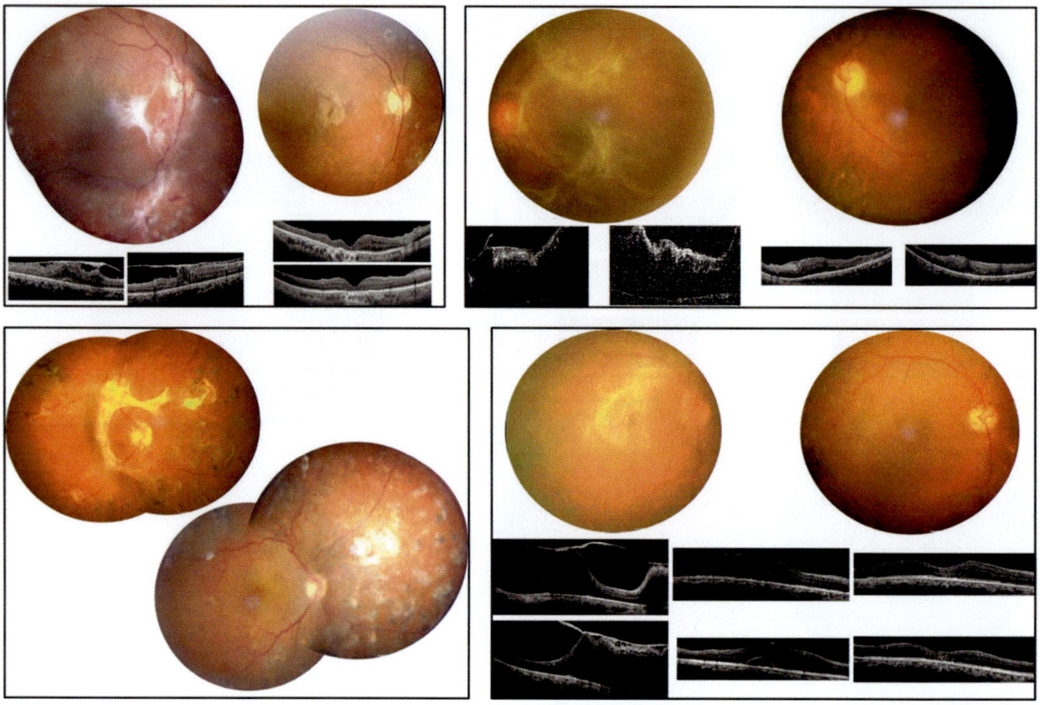

Fig. 1.7 Four sets of color photos/OCT images showing pre- and postoperative retinal changes in eyes with FVPs distributed mainly in the macular area. Condensed premacular tissue caused either macular schisis (upper left and lower right) or TRD (upper right). All four patients had predominantly fibrotic proliferation. (Courtesy of Dr. Chung-May Yang)

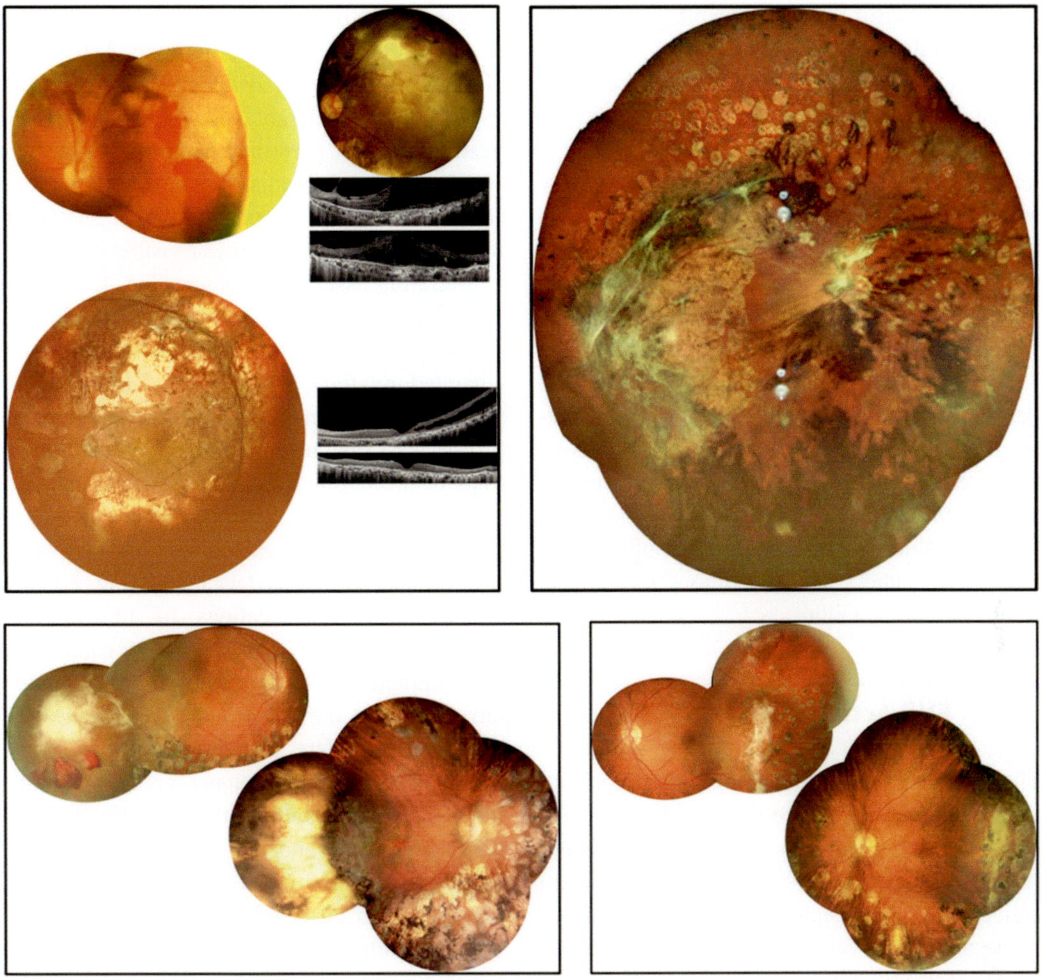

Fig. 1.8 Four sets of images showing retinal changes with the FVP mainly in the midperiphery outside the arcade. In the upper left panel, the FVP is on the temporal side (upper left composite color photo); after vitrectomy and SB on the temporal side, there was extensive temporal retinal schisis (right upper color photo and OCT images); after further operation to remove residual temporal-side proliferative tissue, the retina was reattached with residual retinoschisis (lower wide angle color photo and OCT). The upper right panel shows the attached retina with mainly the midperipheral active FVP and VH. The lower two panels show pre- and postoperative composite color photos of the two eyes of the same patient. After surgery, the FVP tissue on the temporal side of the left eye was isolated without removal (lower right composite color photo in the lower right panel). (Courtesy of Dr. Chung-May Yang)

1.4 Adhesion Severity

FVP tissues are integrated with the PH and connect with the retina at multiple sites through point adhesion or through broad adhesion, which consists of multiple point adhesions. Point adhesion most likely occurs on the disc, with PVD present elsewhere. Broad adhesion is usually present adjacent to the disc, nasal to the disc, or along the arcade, especially at the bending end of the TU or TL arcade. Thickened broad adhesions usually spare the macula, but condensed tissue may adhere to the foveal or parafoveal area. Two broad adhesion membranes may be connected to each other by a thin FVP membrane or a PH. They may form irregular full or incomplete circles around the arcade. Contraction of the broad adhesion membrane causes macular folding, schisis, or TRD. This is a major challenge for surgeons because of the difficulty of complete removal and the possibility of postoperative traction or bleeding.

When a broad adhesion membrane extends to the equator or beyond, instrument accessibility for its removal is compromised, and AP traction release becomes difficult because the PH is close to the retina. The edge of the broad adhesion membrane frequently has an ERM tightly adherent to the retinal surface, creating a Ziploc effect, making identification of the surgical plane between the FVP and the retina difficult (Fig. 1.5, upper right). The most severe FVP-induced adhesion pulled the peripapillary retina toward the central region, creating a funnel-shaped TRD with thick FVP tissue within the funnel and on the surface of the detached retina, forming a table top-like configuration—the so-called table top traction (TTT) configuration. Surgery to address such conditions most likely results in surgical failure.

1.5 FVP Activity

The FVP may be active, meaning that proliferation is an ongoing process; VR adhesion may become stronger with time, and the risk of VH or preretinal hemorrhage is high. NVs of different calibers may be visible within the FVP membrane, along with various amounts of VH/preretinal hemorrhage. Alternatively, the FVP may be mainly or predominantly fibrotic or inactive, meaning that fibrotic tissue predominates in proliferative tissue. In the latter condition, retinal vessel sheathing is frequently observed. The retina becomes thin and atrophic. Tissue traction, however, may persist. Unlike the avascular PVR membrane, the proliferative tissue contains leaking NVs, which is evident by FA examination. Because of adhesions to retinal vessels, bleeding may occur during the removal of such inactive tissue. In some cases, certain areas may exhibit an inactive pattern, while other areas exhibit an active FVP proliferation pattern.

Case examples of FVP of various severities, distributions, and activities are shown in Fig. 1.9.

For study or description convenience, the activity, severity, and location of FVP are classified or graded as follows [1, 2]:

Disease activity can be classified as active proliferation or fibrous proliferation. Active proliferation is defined as visible new vessels within the proliferative membranes with any degree of fresh vitreous or preretinal hemorrhage. Fibrous proliferation is defined as predominantly preretinal fibrosis with widespread vascular sheathing without active hemorrhages or visible NV in the proliferating tissue or elsewhere (Fig. 1.10).

The severity of FVP is assessed according to the preoperative and intraoperative findings and is separated into three grades. Grade 1 (mild): no or only point adhesions at ≤ 3 sites. Grade 2 (moderate): at least one but less than three broad adhesions or proliferative tissues at the disc, macula, and arcade. Grade 3 (severe): broad adhesion at ≥ 3 sites, proliferation extending to the periphery, or no posterior vitreous detachment (Fig. 1.11).

The distribution/locations of fibrovascular proliferation can be divided into four categories. (a) Complete arcade type: fibrous proliferation surrounds both the upper and lower arcade vessels. (b) Incomplete arcade type: fibrous proliferation surrounds only upper or lower arcade vessels. (c) Juxtapapillary type: proliferative tissue is present around the disc and nasal to the disc (Figs. 1.5 and 1.6). (d) Central type: proliferating tissue is observed mainly in the macular area. (e) Midperipheral type: proliferative tissue distributes mainly but not limited to the midperiphery (Fig. 1.8).

The macular area is defined as the area with a diameter of approximately 5.5 mm centered on the foveal depression. The central retinal depression of the macula, which is 1.5 mm in diameter, is named the foveal area. The parafoveal area is a ring 0.5 mm in width surrounding the fovea.

Various fundus changes may occur subsequent to the development of FVP: VH, preretinal hemorrhage, diffuse or irregular macular thickening, macular folds, macular traction schisis TRS, macular TRD, combined RRD and TRD (CTRRD), macular edema, lamellar macular hole (LMH), MH, and vitreopapillary traction (Figs. 1.12 and 1.13) Because of the severe consequences, progressive FVP has become an indication for surgery. We considered surgery for progressive FVP if the total area of the active

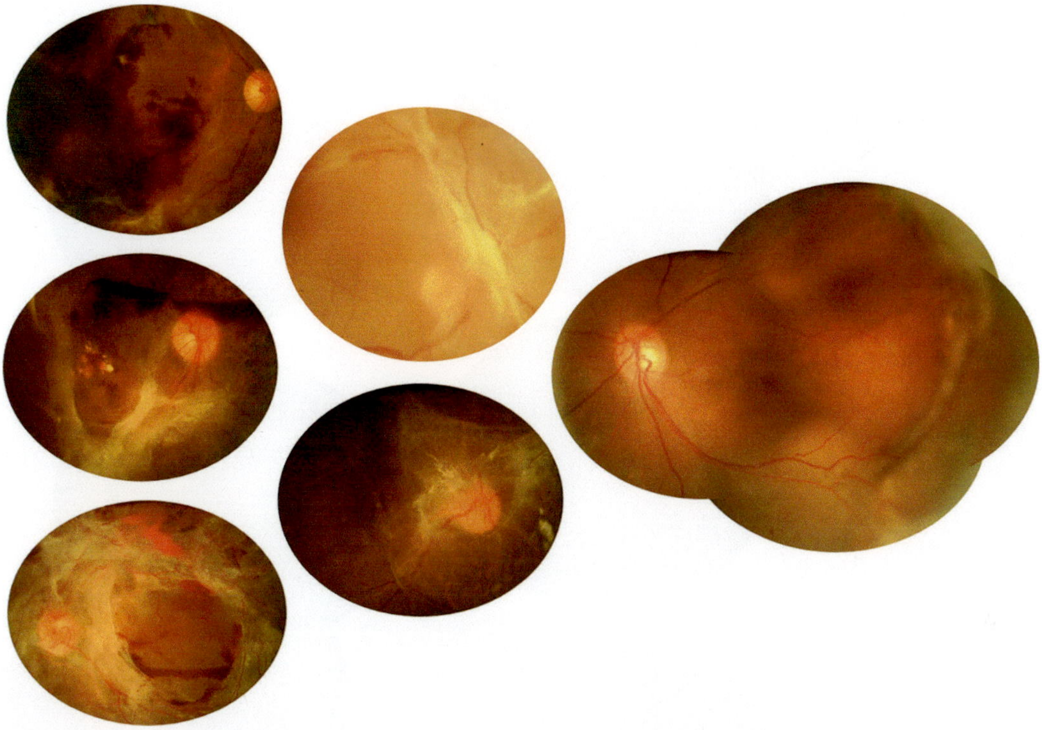

Fig. 1.9 Six examples of retinal changes in eyes with FVP of various severities, distributions, and activities. The three color photos in the left column show active FVPs of different severities. The two color photos in the middle column show mainly fibrotic proliferation. The FVP distribution is mainly along or surrounding the arcade in the 3 color photos in the left column; at the disc, nasal side, and arcade in the upper color photo in the middle column; in the disc area in the lower color photo in the middle column; and in the midperiphery in the right composite color photo. The lower left color photo shows the most severe proliferation, with the active FVP growing around the arcade for 360°. (Courtesy of Dr. Chung-May Yang)

FVP within the equator was equal to or greater than three disc areas, combined with the following features: (1) significant VH, causing BCVA to decrease to 0.1 or less; (2) significant macular structural changes, such as thickening, folding, irregular elevation, and LMH, causing BCVA to decrease to 0.2 or less; or FTMH, regardless of BCVA level.

The most important and frequent complication of untreated progressive FVP is TRD.

Thus, the TRD will be the focus of the following discussion.

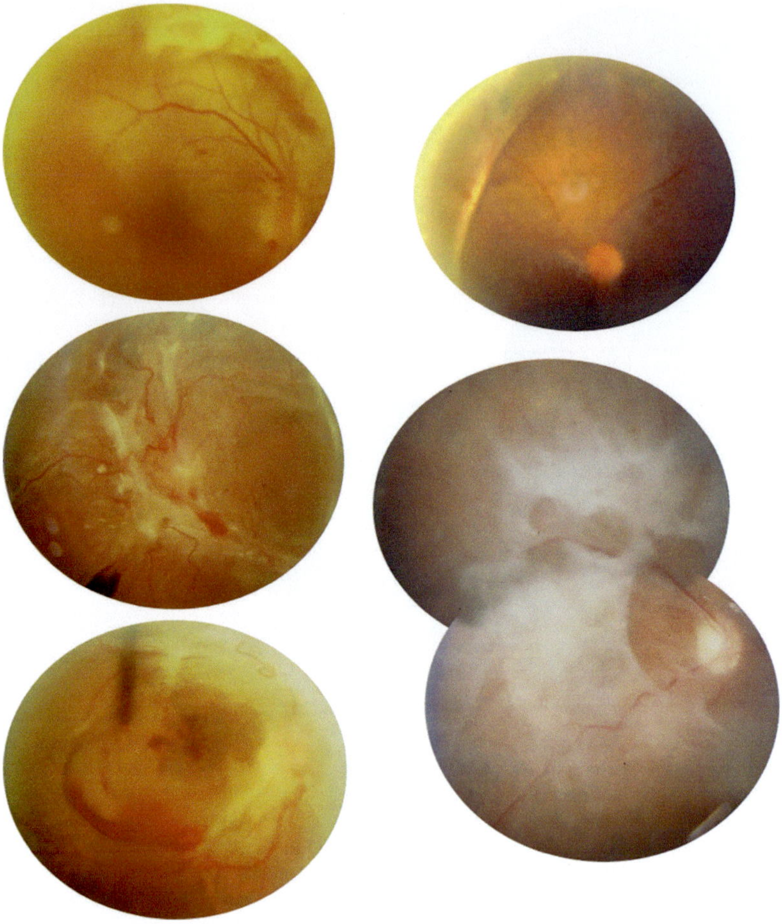

Fig. 1.10 Color photos of active FVPs (left column) and mainly fibrotic FVPs (right column). (Courtesy of Dr. Chung-May Yang)

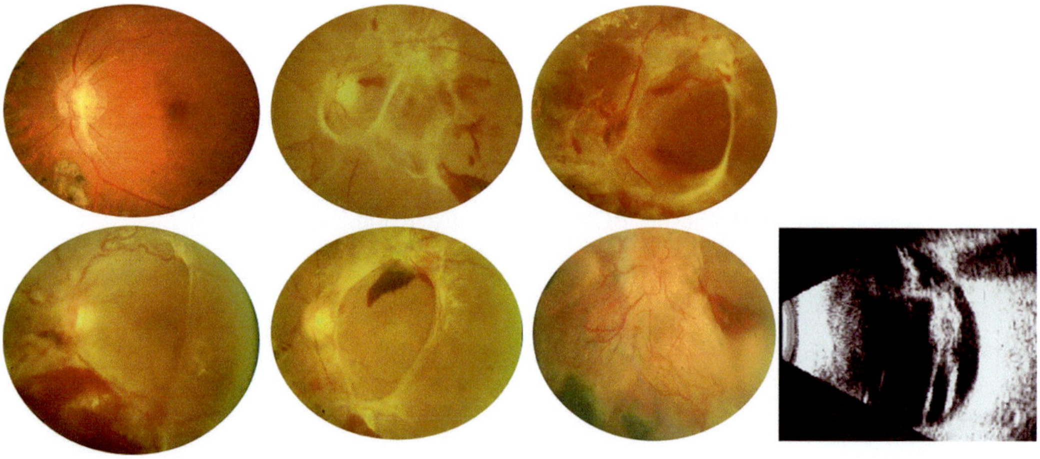

Fig. 1.11 Severity grading of FVP in PDR. Grade 1: no or focal adhesions at ≤ 3 sites (left side two color photos). Grade 2: at least 1 but less than three broad adhesions or proliferative tissues at the disc, macula, and arcade (center 2 images). Grade 3: broad adhesion at ≥3 sites, proliferation extending to the periphery, or no posterior vitreous detachment (right side two color photos). The right lower ultrasonography image corresponding to the right lower color image shows TRD with the table-top traction (TTT) configuration. (Courtesy of Dr. Chung-May Yang)

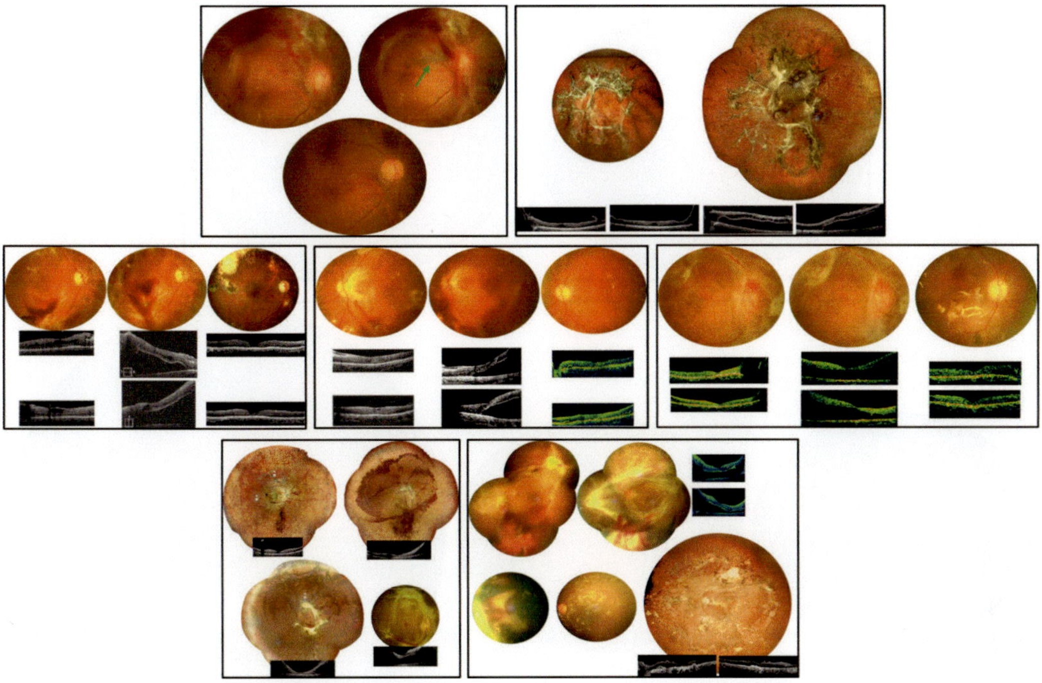

Fig. 1.12 Seven sets of color photos/OCT images showing the development or extension of the TRD from the FVP. The left upper panel shows the advancement of the TRD and the appearance of subretinal blood (green arrow). The right upper panel shows the development of TRD from severe fibrotic proliferation. All other patients had active FVP. The lower left panel shows only preoperative changes. (Courtesy of Dr. Yi-Ting Hsieh). The middle left and middle central images were obtained from the two eyes of the same patient. (Courtesy of Dr. Chung-May Yang)

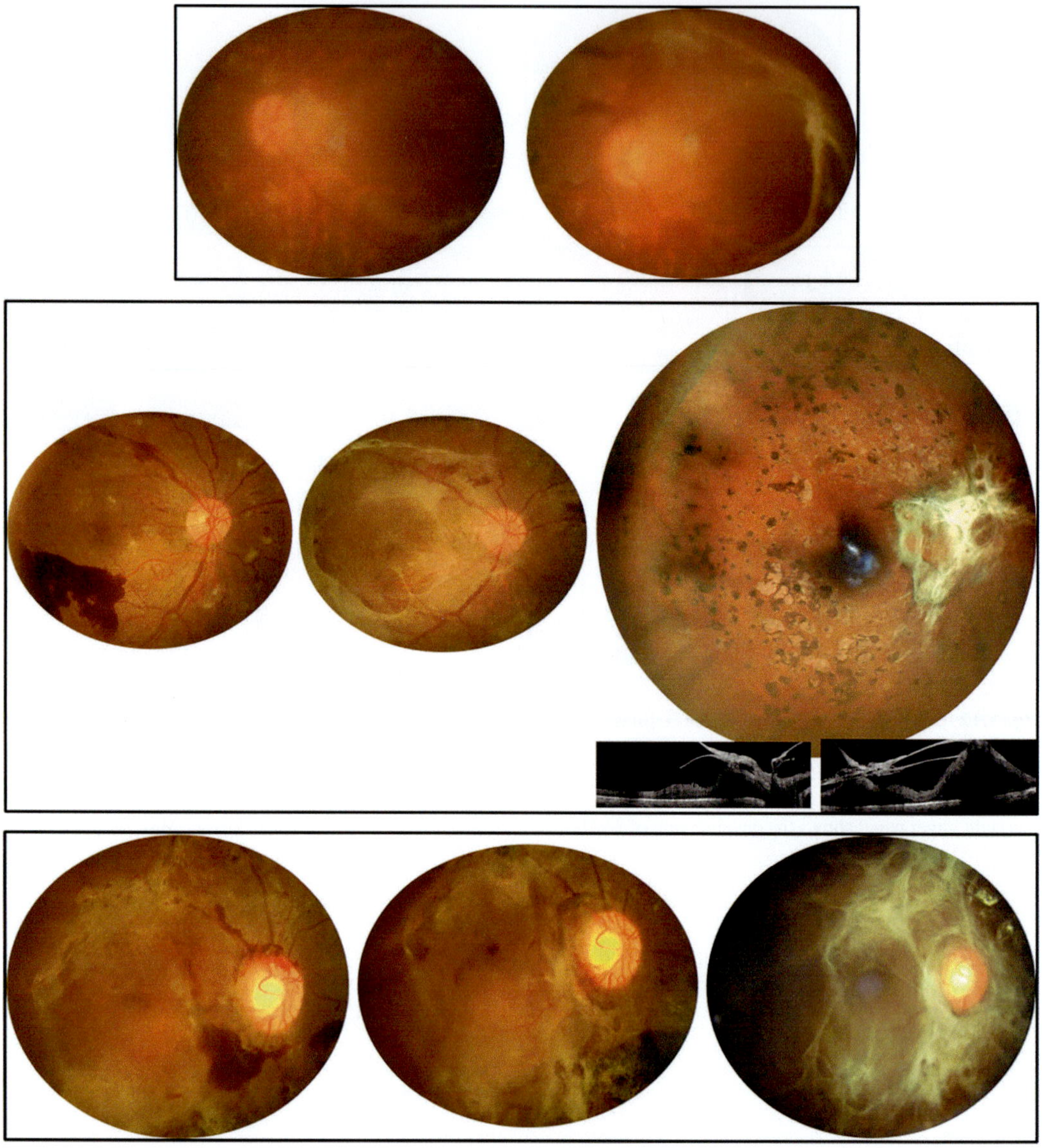

Fig. 1.13 Progression and evolution of FVP in three patients. The upper panel shows the advancement of FVP causing CTRRD at 7 months. The middle panel shows NV with preretinal hemorrhage that progressed to FVP within 4 months and then to TRD 7 years later (right side-wide angle color photo and OCTs). The lower panel shows the progression of FVP at 2 months and to extensive fibrosis at 2.5 years. (Courtesy of Dr. Chung-May Yang)

1.6 TRD: Development

TRD may have a rapid onset, causing decreased vision in a short time, or may persist for a long time in the extramacular area before gradually approaching the macula. The FVP may be active or predominantly fibrotic. Laser, cryo-, and anti-VEGF agents may cause vitreous contraction and subsequent TRD.

1.7 TRD: Traction Force

Tangential traction and AP traction are usually present to induce TRD, which most likely occurs in the context of broad adhesion with peripheral vitreous detachment. Broad adhesion without vitreous detachment usually causes localized shallow elevation, folding, or schisis only (please see Chap. 10 on TMS). A thickened vitreous schisis membrane may be the source of AP traction, even though the true PH remains pliable and is attached to the peripheral retina.

1.8 TRD: Clinical Pictures

The TRD may be localized within the arcade or extend to the periphery but never to the ora serrata. RD extending to the ora is caused by retinal break(s), and RD is usually a combination of rhegmatogenous and tractional RD. The degree and shape of retinal elevation varied: a small area of the TRD presented a concave shape, peaking at the site with the highest AP traction force within the FVP area; if the area of the TRD was large, the retinal surface became wavy and had a more convex shape resembling an RRD configuration.

TRD may be associated with subretinal fibrosis, depending on the duration of detachment. In RRD, subretinal fibrosis appears if RD persists for more than 3 months. In TRD, subretinal fibrosis may develop earlier because of the pro-proliferative environment in the vitreous cavity and within the subretinal space. In addition, subretinal blood may be present without visible retinal breaks, especially in eyes with a large TRD. However, whether microbreaks occur, vitreous or preretinal blood seeps through, or intraretinal blood spontaneously permeates into the subretinal space remains unknown. Please see Chap. 22 on subretinal blood.

The contraction of the FVP may increase vessel permeability, which in turn may create massive amounts of hard exudates (HEs), and this occurs most frequently at the junction of FVP-retina adhesions. In young patients with active FV, the strong traction is counterbalanced by the equally strong RPE pumping action, resulting in prominent folding with or without shallow detachment and HE (please see Chap. 24 on young PDR and Chap. 9 on massive HE).

The membrane above the macula is usually thin, in contrast to the thick membrane at the arcade. This is because of the effect of the premacular vitreous fluid pocket, which creates a thin membrane loosely adhering to the macula. In certain cases, vitreous condensation or plaque may adhere to the fovea or parafoveal area, generating macular/foveal traction; foveal tissue avulsion may occur during membrane peeling (please see Chap. 15 on MH during DV).

We considered surgery for TRD if there was an impending macula-off TRD or a macula-involved TRD, and we adopted a close follow-up strategy for eyes with an extramacular TRD, especially an extra-arcade TRD. The aims of surgery are to remove the opacified vitreous, release tangential and AP traction on the retina, reattach the retina, reinforce retinal ablation, and prevent further vitreous hemorrhage and ERM or FVP recurrence.

Many factors influence functional outcomes after successful operation of progressive FVP or TRD: (1) Duration of macular detachment; (2) Perfusion of the macula; (3) The severity of disc atrophy; (4) The severity of retinal atrophy; (5) Severe structural abnormalities, such as macular edema, macular pucker, macular scarring, macular atrophy, or macular holes; (6) History of submacular blood; (7) Duration of high intraocular pressure (IOP) or the presence of NVG.

1.9 Vitrectomy Procedures

The first step is the removal of opacified vitreous fluid for better visualization of vitreoretinal abnormalities. AP traction release is then carried out. A vitreous cutter was used to cut the connection between the FVP and the hyaloid membrane. The circumferential release of AP traction should be performed to the largest extent as safely as possible. This procedure serves two purposes: releasing AP traction and creating free edges to facilitate better membrane engagement at different angles during FVP removal. Surgical success is greatly enhanced if 360°AP traction release can be performed smoothly. Occasionally, scissors may be required to sever the PH too close to the retinal surface in the periphery. AP traction release starts from the mobile PH. PH engagement may become difficult when the PH is too close to the retina because of peripheral VR adhesion. In such cases, there is no need to attempt to complete the 360° AP traction release because a retinal break may be created. These connection sites can be treated later during FVP membrane-retina separation, working from the posterior retina to the periphery. If complete AP traction release fails, one may either leave the PH alone, if the tissue is redundant and causes no significant traction, add a segmental SB, or even perform limited or wide peripheral retinectomy to release traction.

When there is widespread VR attachment without PVD, it becomes impossible to approach the peripheral hyaloid membrane for AP traction release. In such cases, one should perform FVP membrane-retina separation in the posterior pole and work toward the periphery.

The third step is the removal of FVP. Commonly employed techniques for FVP removal include segmentation, delamination, en bloc dissection, and various bimanual approaches, all of which can be used in combination. Although it is safer to work from the posterior to the periphery, the so-called inside-out approach, with the help of a wide-angle viewing system and a micro-incision vitrectomy probe, a handy "outside-in" approach moving from the periphery toward the disc side has been more frequently applied.

Segmentation involves separating the FVP membrane into smaller isolated islands, and delamination involves separating the individual epicenter between the FVP membrane and the retina so that the FVP can be completely removed. Segmentation is possible because even widespread FVP membranes are composed of several broad adhesion areas connected by thickened nonadherent membranes or thin PHs. Therefore, there is always space available for instrument engagement within or between broad adhesion patches to perform segmentation. Segmentation can be performed with a cutter or scissors. Curved horizontal scissors with thinner blades can provide better access to the space between the retina and the membrane than vertical scissors (Fig. 1.14). Prominent proliferative vessels

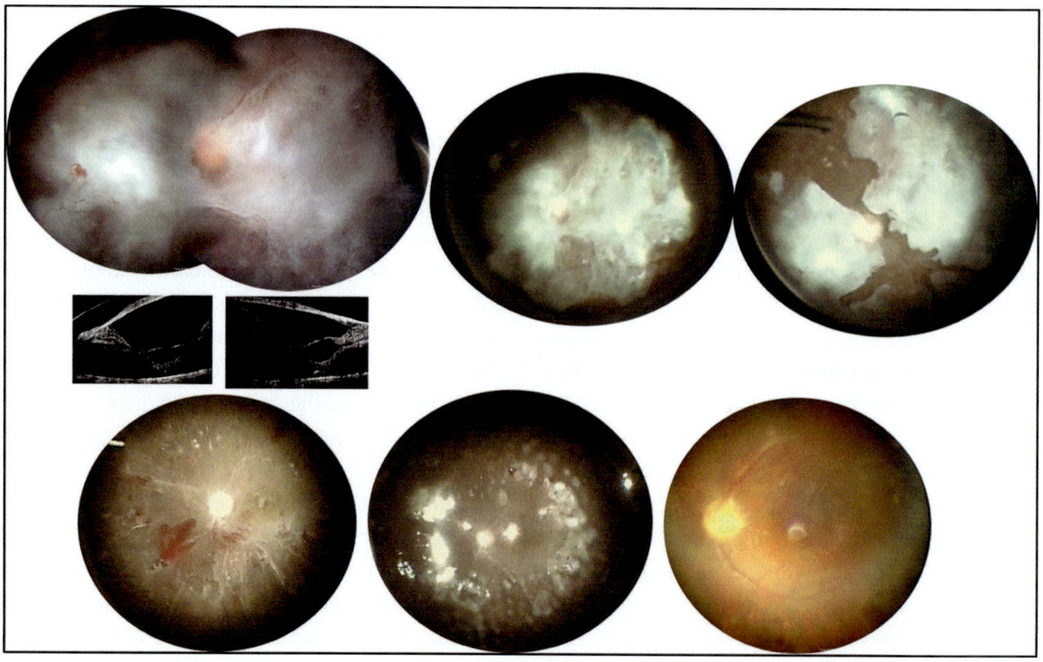

Fig. 1.14 One set of images showing pre-, intra-, and postoperative retinal changes in an eye with extensive preretinal fibrosis and TRD. Composite color images and OCT images before surgery are shown on the upper left; intraoperative video images are shown on the upper center, upper right, lower left, and lower center. The segmentation technique was used to facilitate membrane removal (upper right). After surgery, the retina was attached, and the FVP tissue was removed (lower right). (Courtesy of Dr. Chung-May Yang)

should be bypassed if possible to decrease bleeding during segmentation. Scissors have been advocated for performing delamination because of their ability to pass through the tiny space between the retina and the overlying FVP and to cut off the epicenter with precision. However, as smaller gauged instruments become more popular, scissors may be replaced by cutters to perform both segmentation and delamination. A great advantage of the new 27G system is the substantial reduction in the necessity of frequent instrument changes and bimanual manipulation, as the 27G beveled-tip vitrector can combine the functions of forceps, scissors, picks, and dissectors in one instrument. Several techniques, such as lift and shave, blunt dissection, and back-shave manipulations, may successfully manage very adherent abnormal tissues without inadvertent damage to the underlying retina [3, 4]. LED-illuminated instruments may provide adequate endoillumination of 27G systems [5, 6]. A reduction in the cutter speed to 5000–7500 cpm may facilitate the efficient removal of very rigid membranes while reasonably maintaining minimal tissue movement underneath [4]. Despite these advantages, current 27-gauge instruments are prone to bend during peripheral dissection. A larger gauge vitrector may be required for very thick membranes or for peripheral dissection. Alternatively, mixing gauges can facilitate dissection in such cases. A 23/25-gauge instrument through valved cannulas is applied to treat peripheral lesions, while a 27-gauge probe can be introduced for posterior lesions [7].

Identification of the true surgical plane is of utmost importance for membrane removal. FVP growth along the inner vitreous schisis membrane may create a false surgical plane, while ERM growing from the edge of the FVP tissue may obliterate the surgical plane. Only after lifting the outer vitreous schisis membrane or ERM can the true surgical plane be exposed. One way to find the surgical plane is through peeling of the thin ERM on the macular area. Lifting the membrane and extending the separation to the arcade makes the surgical plane and epicenter more easily visible. Although lifting the FVP tissue from the optic disc is an easy way to find the true surgical plane, this manipulation sometimes causes excessive bleeding from the torn disc vessels, thus compromising the surgical view, or even creates a retinal tear on a thin and detached retina adhering to the FVP membrane. It is better to remove the FVP tissue around the disc, if possible, to reduce these complications.

When an iatrogenic break is created, adjacent traction should be released as thoroughly as possible, ensuring that there is no connection to other FVP areas; otherwise, bullous RD may develop during further membrane dissection. Furthermore, postoperative recurrent RD may occur.

Broad membranes with complex adhesions may be trimmed to several smaller isolated FVP islands and left in place under conditions of no traction on the macular area and no connection with the peripheral hyaloid, even if the individual islands contain multiple adhesions. This approach is a better surgical choice than the attempt to remove all the membrane, which results in breaks or bleeding, causing more complications. One should bear in mind that the unremoved isolated FVP islands may become the source of postoperative late recurrent vitreous hemorrhage. On the other hand, widespread fibrotic membranes around the arcade and/or connected to the vitreous base through thin and semitransparent membranes are difficult to remove entirely without causing iatrogenic breaks. In such cases, conservative treatment involves removal of the premacular membrane and vertical incisions at one or multiple sites around the arcade fibrosis circle to relax the circumferential traction. This manipulation may effectively enhance the recovery of macular structures without causing significant complications [8].

With the preferential use of MIVS, especially the 27G instrument, many complicated cases can be successfully treated with unimanual techniques. However, a bimanual technique using chandelier light for illumination is still needed for the dissection of large and highly adherent FVPs or for severe combined RD where the FVP membrane adheres to the floating retina, making unimanual dissection difficult and dangerous. In such cases, forceps are used to stabilize and grasp the membrane to expose the epicenter for quicker and safer dissection via either a cutter or scissors.

Some important surgical anatomy related to the surgery is shown in Fig. 1.15.

Other specific manipulations include retinectomy and subretinal band removal. They are briefly described in the following chapter.

Bleeding should be checked promptly and vigorously to avoid compromising the surgical plane. To reduce the possibility of excessive bleeding during surgery, patients should discontinue the use of anticoagulants or aspirin for 10 days or more before surgery. Many patients are receiving regular hemodialysis (H/D), which may require anticoagulants to prevent obstruction of the shunt; patients should consult with physicians in the H/D service to taper off the use of anticoagulants. Patients with liver cirrhosis are in the easy bleeding group because of inadequate production of coagulation factors. The use of anti-VEGF therapy shortly before surgery in patients with active FVP prompted new vessel constriction and reduced the severity of intraoperative bleeding.

Hemostasis may be achieved by temporal elevation of the intraocular pressure, mechanical compression of the bleeding point using a cutter tip or a soft-tipped cannula, simultaneous suction and endodiathermy with a tissue manipulator (combining illumination, aspiration or infusion, and diathermy functions), an extrusion needle with coaxial diathermy function, endophotocoagulation, or a combination of the above techniques. Air, thrombin, viscoelastic substances, perfluorocarbon liquids, and silicone oil have been used for hemostasis. Prompt elevation of IOP is feasible with newly developed vitrectomy machines or can be achieved by simply raising the infusion bottle for at least 1 min. No cutting or suction should be performed during this time to maintain a high IOP. Afterwards, the IOP should be slowly lowered to check for

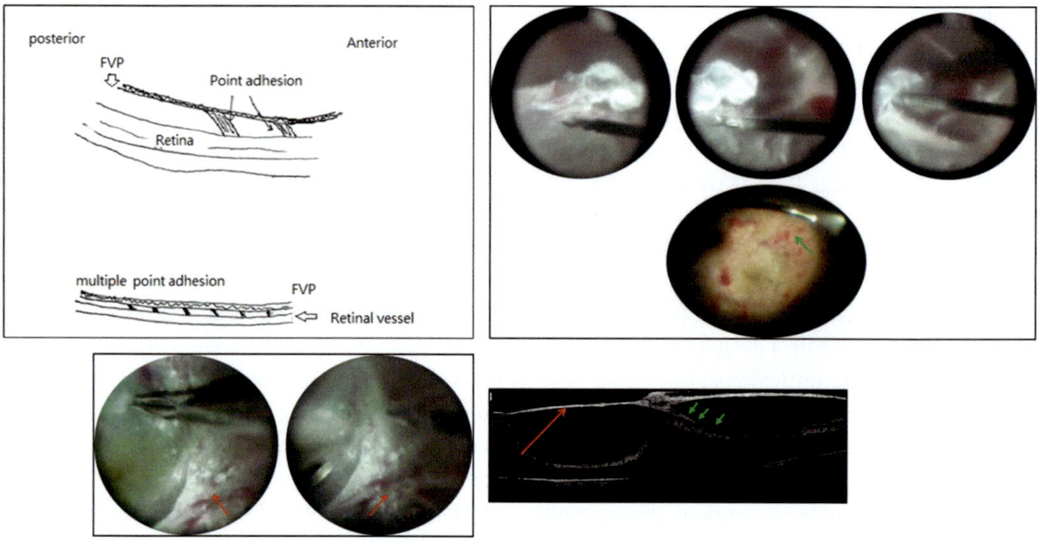

Fig. 1.15 Three sets of images and one set of drawings showing some of the important surgical anatomies of the DV. In the upper left panel, the simplified drawing shows multiple adhesion points along a vessel. Note that there are gaps between the adhesions; also note the more anteriorly located adhesion base on the retina and the more posteriorly located adhesion tip on the FVP membrane. This oblique orientation makes inside-out scissor dissection more efficient than outside-in dissection. The upper right panel shows how the tip of a scissor blade can be inserted between the adhesion gaps to break the adhesions according to sequential intraoperative video images. The lower left intraoperative video images show the compact adhesion points (red arrows) at the bending end of the temporal upper or lower arcade after removal of the FVP membrane. This adhesion pattern indicates that more time and effort may be needed for FVP dissection in this area. The lower right panel shows the thick FVP-related membrane (long red arrow) and the ERM removed from the adhesion, which is the true surgical plane (short green arrows). (Courtesy of Dr. Chung-May Yang)

further bleeding. The procedure can be repeated a few times, with gradual prolongation of high IOP duration, but the duration of IOP elevation should never exceed 3 min. Although a few studies have shown that prolonged IOP increase does not cause significant visual harm, high IOP in a circulation-compromised eye may cause optic nerve or retinal damage. Mechanical compression can be promptly achieved by using the tip of the vitreous cutter or other instruments, such as a soft-tip extrusion needle. Commercially available soft-tip instruments, especially those designed for intraoperative hemostasis, can also be used. The IOP should be kept high during this manipulation. Endodiathermy or an endolaser can be used to stop further bleeding. A multifunction instrument with simultaneous suction and diathermy is appropriate for this purpose, as blood aspiration clearly exposes the bleeder for direct instrument tip contact. Care is taken not to damage the surrounding retina. This can be achieved by slightly tilting the instrument tip and using the side of the tip to engage the bleeder. Excessive diathermy should be avoided because it may cause further bleeding or tissue necrosis and iatrogenic breakage during or after surgery. In doubt, the treated area should be surrounded by one or two cycles of mild laser irradiation. Elevated large NVs can be treated before tissue dissection to minimize bleeding. Bleeding from small NVs may be left untreated, as further separation of the tissue from the retina may cause spontaneous cessation of bleeding. Green light endophotocoagulation can also achieve proper hemostasis, as hemoglobin may absorb laser energy. It is less likely to damage retinal tissue as diathermy would. If possible, blood should be removed before it becomes sticky clots. When the above techniques fail to stop the bleeding and the surgical field becomes compromised, air or other vitreous substitutes, such as Healon or perfluorocarbon liquids, may be used. The hemostatic effects come from mechanical compression or restriction of blood spreading; the concentration of coagulation factors may also play a role. Thrombin and hemocoagulase (a hemocoagulating enzyme isolated from snake venom) have been used for treating intractable bleeding, but postoperative inflammation is a major concern. Sticky clots may form with their use.

After the bleeding has been controlled, sheets of blood clots may be removed first by careful suction at the thinner margin of the clot to obtain partial detachment of the clot edge from the retina and then by working toward the thicker center part. The part of the clot freeing from the retina can be removed with a vitreous cutter using minor suction. A large sheet connecting several bleeding sources can be segmented into several smaller parts by suction and cutting; blood clots surrounding the bleeding sites are then trimmed to small islands. Excessive pulling and trimming of blood clots may result in recurrent bleeding.

In TRD, whether the subretinal fluid (SRF) should be drained through iatrogenic breaks is debated. We did not drain the SRF if the detachment area was localized but routinely drained the SRF in the TRD extending beyond the arcades. First, I did not find iatrogenic breaks for SRF drainage or lasers around the break would increase traction or the rate of detachment; furthermore, this practice may allow earlier macular reattachment and possibly a more rapid clearance of excessive growth factors within the SRF. Even so, sometimes a prolonged period is required for complete reattachment. Laser photocoagulation around retinal breaks and PRP (or supplementary PRP) up to the ora serrata is then performed, followed by appropriate tamponade. Please see Chap. 6 for the choice of tamponade agent. Various presentations of the TRD and surgical results are shown in Figs. 1.16, 1.17, 1.18, and 1.19.

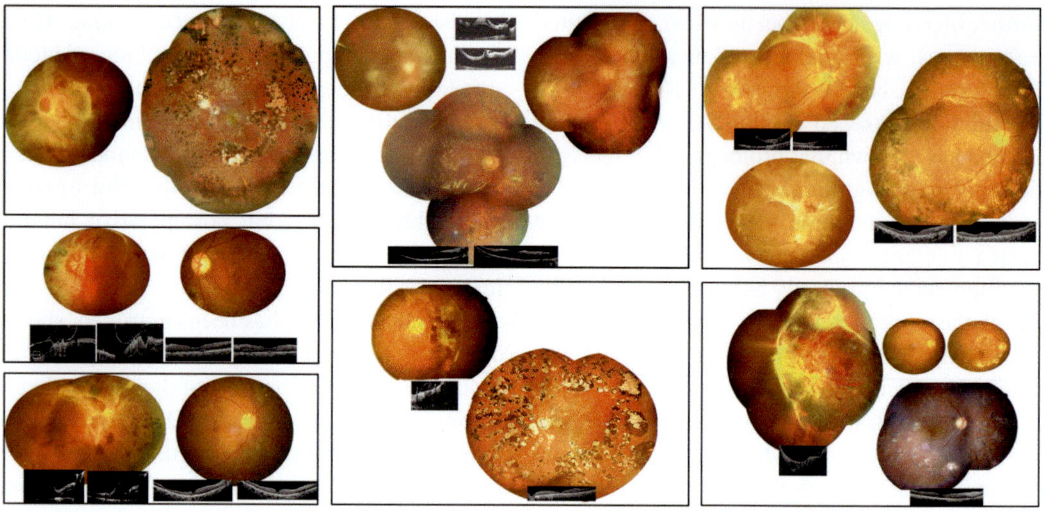

Fig. 1.16 Seven sets of pre- and postoperative color photos/OCT images of retinal changes in eyes with moderately active FVP and TRD. An intraoperative video image is shown on the lower left side of the upper right panel. Note the delay in SRF reabsorption shown in the 6-month postoperative images (right) in the left middle panel. (Courtesy of Dr. Chung-May Yang)

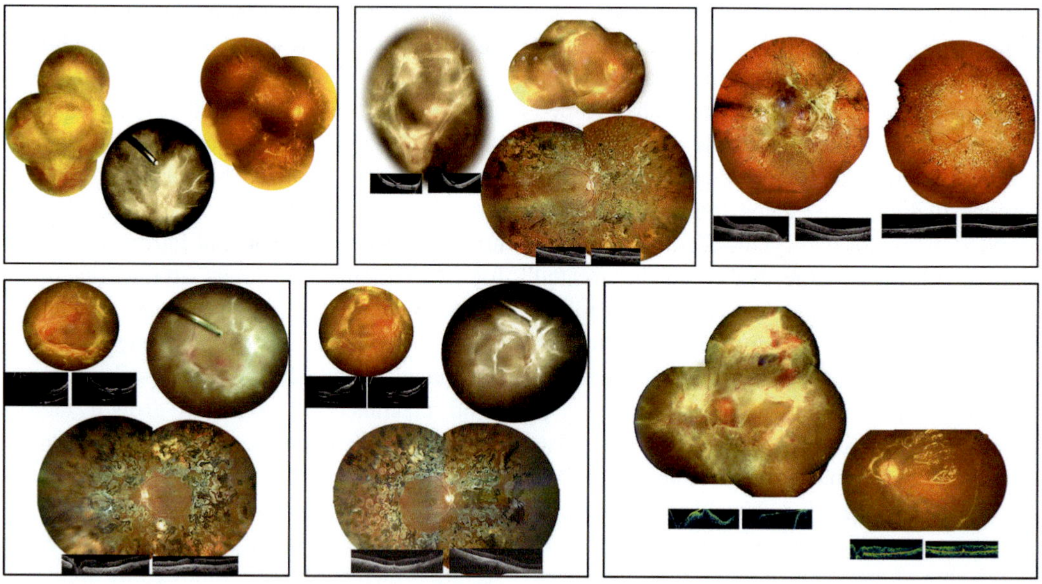

Fig. 1.17 Six sets of pre- and postoperative color photos/OCT images of retinal changes in eyes with severe active FVP and TRD. Intraoperative video images are shown in four panels: upper left panel, upper center panel, and lower left and lower center panels. (Courtesy of Dr. Chung-May Yang)

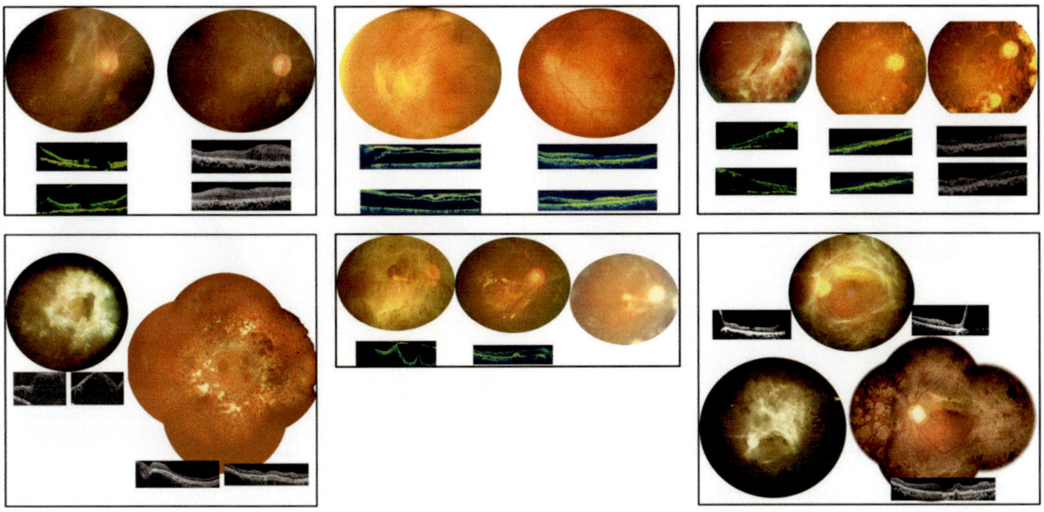

Fig. 1.18 Six sets of pre- and postoperative color photos and OCT images showing retinal changes in eyes with different severities and distributions of FVP. Eyes with severe proliferation are shown in the center panel and the two lower panels. (Courtesy of Dr. Chung-May Yang)

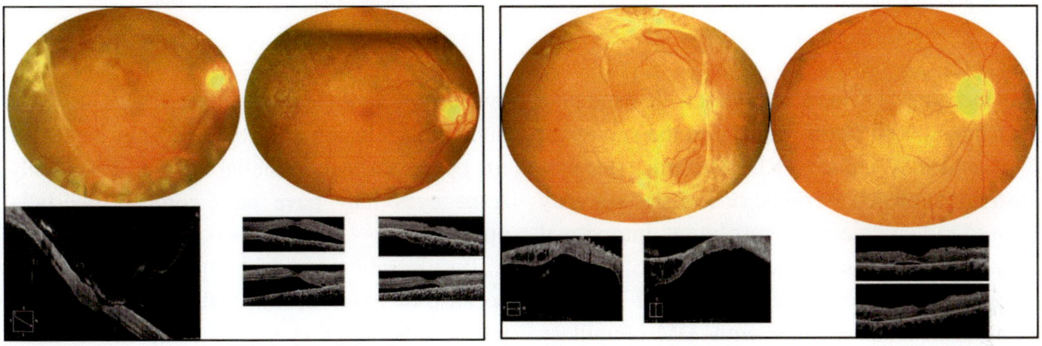

Fig. 1.19 Two examples of pre- and postoperative images showing delayed SRF reabsorption in eyes with TRD. In the left panel, OCT images on the right were taken 8 months and 12 months after surgery. In the right panel, residual SRF was noted 6 months after surgery (right OCT images). (Courtesy of Dr. Chung-May Yang)

1.10 Postoperative Complications

Major postoperative complications include intraocular inflammation, accompanied by fibrin formation in the anterior chamber and in the vitreous cavity; high IOP; persistent corneal epithelial defects; early and later recurrent vitreous hemorrhage; anterior hyaloidal FVP (AHFVP); recurrent RD; macular structural changes, such as LMH, MH, macular pucker; and NVG.

Prolonged operation time or surgery involving complicated FVP, excessive PRP, or cryotherapy may cause excessive postoperative inflammation. Combined cataract operation and vitrectomy also exacerbate postoperative inflammation. This reaction may induce postoperative intravitreal fibrin, AC fibrin formation, choroidal thickening, lower exudative RD, and macular exudative RD. Transient lower RD is not uncommon, with SRF reabsorbed within 1–2 weeks. Macular exudative RD occurs less often but may cause a marked decrease in VA before fluid reabsorption (Figs. 1.20 and 1.21). Intravitreal fibrin or transvitreal fibrinoid reactions usually appear on the first or second day after surgery, forming strands, bands, nets, or veins within the vitreous cavity. Although spontaneous resolution is the rule, it

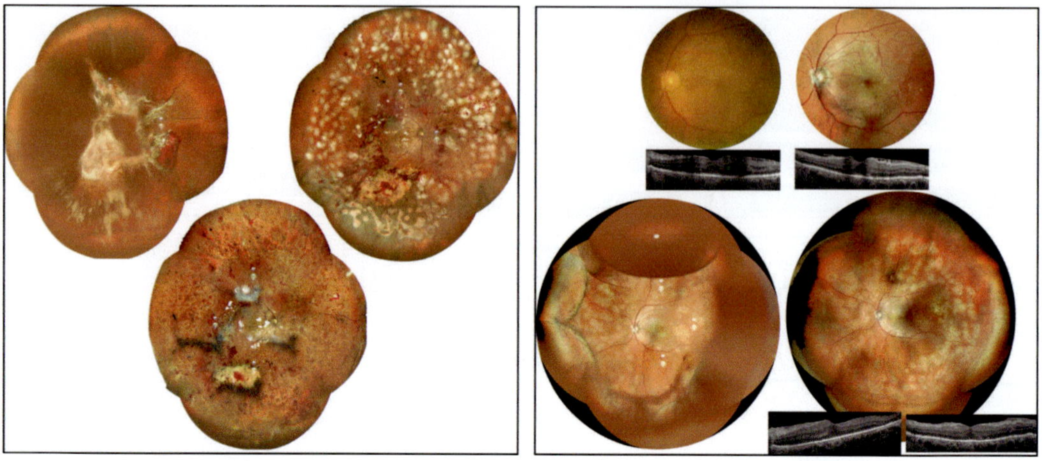

Fig. 1.20 Two sets of images showing postoperative exudative RD (left panel) and CD (right panel). In the left panel, severe FVP with VH was noted (upper left wide angle color photo). Immediately after vitrectomy, intraoperative PRP, and SO infusion, lower exudative RD developed, as shown by the green color in the lower field in the wide angle color photo (upper right). Two weeks later, the RD subsided (lower wide angle color photo). In the left panel, preoperative color images and OCT images show macular thickening and ERM (upper); after vitrectomy with ERM/ILM peeling and mild scattered PRP, peripheral CD at 360° developed (lower left); 2 weeks later, the CD subsided, and the macular condition improved (lower right). (Courtesy of Dr. Chung-May Yang)

may become severe, associated with exudative detachment with fibrin material in the subretinal fluid, and may induce TRD. Systemic steroids, posterior subtenon steroids, or IVI steroids may be used to facilitate fibrin resolution. Intravitreal TPA may, on rare occasions, be needed (Fig. 1.21). Systemic steroids should be used with caution in patients with DM. Pupillary blocks from ciliary body effusion, ciliary body anterior rotation, anterior chamber fibrin, or posterior synechiae should be carefully examined and treated depending on the underlying causes. Notably, when one has simultaneous cataract surgery and DV complicated by moderate or severe FVP that requires prolonged gas or SO tamponade or a prolonged facedown position, the AC reaction may be more severe (please see Chap. 6), and posterior synechia refractory to laser iridotomy is prone to occur, causing pupillary block and increased IOP. In such cases, surgical peripheral iridectomy during surgery may be important.

Corneal epithelial defects may be prolonged. Corneal specialists should be consulted early. Autoserum or insulin may shorten the time for reepithelialization. The use of preservative-free eye drops, therapeutic contact lenses, or even punctum occlusion or lid suturing may be needed for better corneal epithelial healing. Eventually, some eyes may have faint corneal superficial opacity.

Postoperative transient high IOP is common because of inflammation and choroidal thickening. In a SO-filled eye, the incompressive nature of the SO aggravates the choroidal thickening effect on IOP. It is of utmost importance to reduce IOP as soon as possible because the optic nerve is vulnerable to IOP increases in eyes with PDR. AC tapping should be performed if the IOP increases to 35 mmHg or more. Hyphema or VH-induced ghost cell glaucoma (usually occurring 3 weeks or more after surgery) are other causes of high IOP.

AHFVP (Fig. 1.22), RI, and NVG are severe postoperative complications. They are characterized by excessive angiogenic factors. They are briefly discussed in Chap. 26 on post-DV glaucoma.

Other complications, such as fibrosis, ERM, and recurrent RD, will be discussed in other chapters.

Causes of surgical failure include iatrogenic breaks with incomplete traction release, either

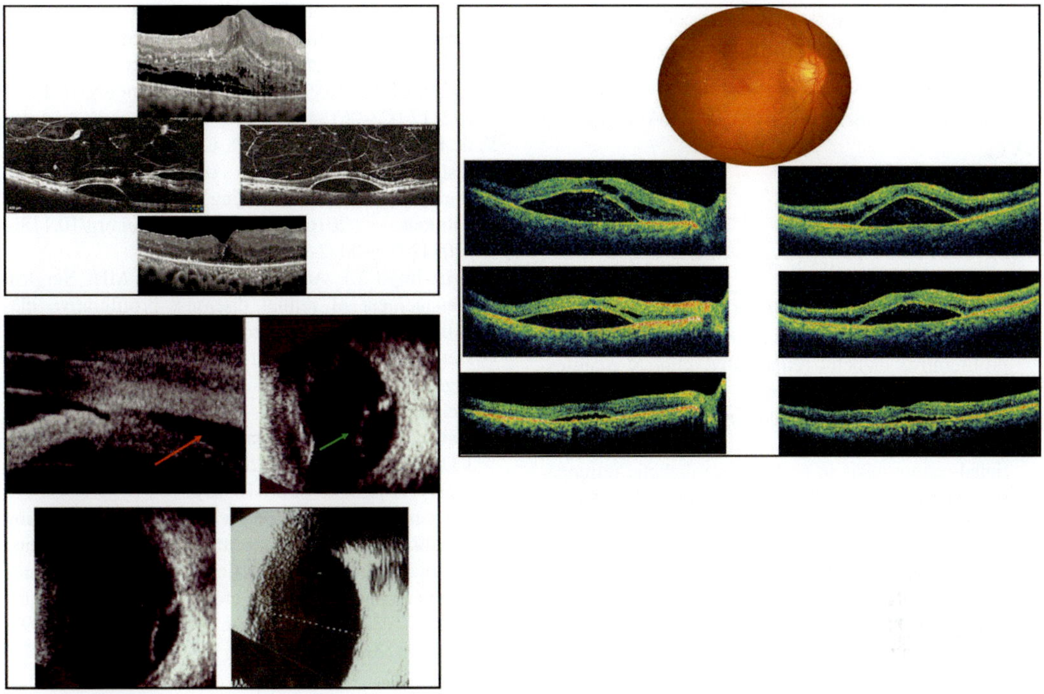

Fig. 1.21 Three sets of images showing postoperative transvitreal and subretinal fibrin reactions (upper left panel) and macular exudative RD (all three panels). All three patients had FVPs with VH but without TRD before surgery. In the upper left panel, postoperative macular RD with fibrin-like material was noted (upper OCT image); transvitreal fibrin material and membrane were also noted (middle 2 OCT images). After the IVI of 50 μg of TPA, 4 mg of suprachoroidal TPA on postoperative day 6, followed by vitreous lavage and IVI of 25 μg of TPA on day 9, the vitreous became clear, and the retina was reattached on day 14 (lower OCT image) (courtesy of Dr. San-Ni Chen). In the lower left panel, ultrasound biomicroscopy on postoperative day 1 revealed ciliary detachment (upper left; red arrow points to the ciliary detachment). Marked macular detachment was detected on day 5 by US (upper right). It persisted on day 7 (lower left) and resolved on day 11 (lower right). In the right panel, fundus examination on post-DV day 30 revealed 3 DD macular detachments (upper color photo). Sequential OCT performed at 6 M, 7 M, and 8 M after surgery revealed improvement but persistent macular detachment (3 rows of OCT images). Note the possible presence of subretinal fibrin material in the subretinal fluid on post-DV 6 M and 7 M. (Courtesy of Dr. Chung-May Yang)

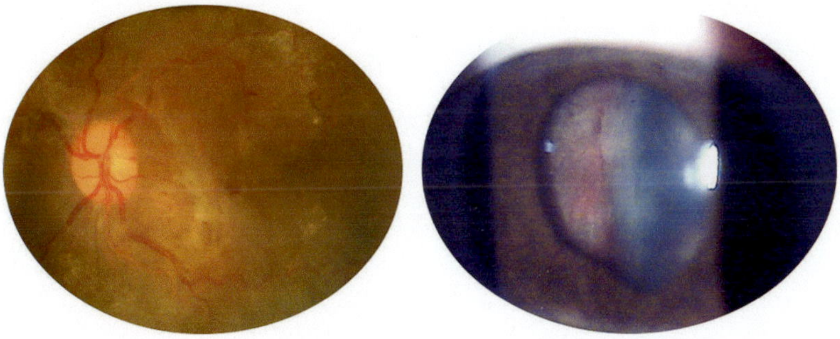

Fig. 1.22 An example of AHFVP in a young woman. A preoperative fundus color photo is shown on the left; prominent AHFVP, seen with a slit lamp biomicroscope, developed 6 weeks after surgery (left). (Courtesy of Dr. Chung-May Yang)

because the FVP is too severe or because massive bleeding occurs, preventing further surgery; missed breaks; SO infusion before traction release; and persistent high IOP, AHFVP, or NVG.

References

1. Yang CM, Su PY, Yeh PT, Chen MS. Combined rhegmatogenous and traction retinal detachment in proliferative diabetic retinopathy: clinical manifestations and surgical outcome. Can J Ophthalmol. 2008;43(2):192–8. https://doi.org/10.3129/i08-007.
2. Su CC, Yang CH, Yeh PT, Yang CM. Macular tractional retinoschisis in proliferative diabetic retinopathy: clinical characteristics and surgical outcome. Ophthalmologica. 2014;231(1):23–30. https://doi.org/10.1159/000355078.
3. Berrocal MH. All-probe vitrectomy dissection techniques for diabetic tractional retinal detachments: lift and shave. Retina. 2018;38 Suppl 1:S2–4. https://doi.org/10.1097/IAE.0000000000001884.
4. Chen SN, Chen SJ, Wu TT, Wu WC, Yang CH, Yang CM. Refining vitrectomy for proliferative diabetic retinopathy. Graefes Arch Clin Exp Ophthalmol. 2023;261(12):3659–70. https://doi.org/10.1007/s00417-023-06134-w.
5. de Oliveira PR, Berger AR, Chow DR. Vitreoretinal instruments: vitrectomy cutters, endoillumination and wide-angle viewing systems. Int J Retina Vitreous. 2016;2:28. https://doi.org/10.1186/s40942-016-0052-9.
6. Cruz-Inigo YJ, Acaba LA, Berrocal MH. Surgical management of retinal diseases: proliferative diabetic retinopathy and traction retinal detachment. Dev Ophthalmol. 2014;54:196–203. https://doi.org/10.1159/000360467.
7. Oellers P, Mahmoud TH. Surgery for proliferative diabetic retinopathy: new tips and tricks. J Ophthalmic Vis Res. 2016;11(1):93–9. https://doi.org/10.4103/2008-322X.180697.
8. Berrocal MH, Acaba-Berrocal L. Minimal, relaxing membranectomies for the management of opacified hyaloid with diabetic tractional retinal detachments in monocular patients: a novel surgical technique. Retina. 2022;43(12):2144–7. https://doi.org/10.1097/IAE.0000000000003524.

Special Consideration in Diabetic Vitrectomy

2

Abstract

In this chapter, the bimanual technique, retinectomy, and removal of subretinal fibrosis will be briefly discussed as supplements to the surgical techniques discussed in the previous chapter.

2.1 Bimanual Techniques

In complex situations involving broad adhesion, especially when membranes are extremely adherent, bimanual dissection is employed to facilitate the removal of fibrovascular proliferation (FVP) [1, 2]. This technique is also likely to be required in eyes with preexisting retinal breaks with severe proliferation or iatrogenic breaks created at or close to a prominent FVP tissue in the early stage of surgery, as the bullous and mobile features of retinal detachment that develop or exacerbate during surgery may hamper safe, unimanual proliferative tissue dissection.

Bimanual dissection is possible with the use of an instrument that has the dual functions of stabilizing or lifting the membrane and illuminating the membrane. Such an instrument has the limitations of low light intensity, and the instrument can create shadows. Alternatively, the technique can be achieved with the placement of a fixed extra light source. The latter has gained popularity as the light intensity has improved. Several types of chandelier light designs are available for performing bimanual surgery. Which to choose depends on the surgeon's preference, instrument familiarity, or availability.

The decision to use bimanual dissection should be made before surgery. The severity and extent of broad adhesion and mobility of the retina are the main considerations for choosing to use an extra illuminating system. The common place for inserting the illuminator is in the nasal lower quadrant. However, it may be adjusted to other places. The area of the most complex adhesions may guide the choice of location to set up the illuminator. Twin-headed illuminators placed at different sites may provide a brighter view and less shadowing by the FVP tissue or the instrument.

Sclerotomy using the trocar cannula system should be directed perpendicular to the scleral surface to avoid light scattering from the crystalline lens or intraocular lens (IOL). Bimanual dissection usually proceeds with forceps or other gentle suction devices to lift and stabilize the FVP membrane and scissors or cutters in the other hand (usually the dominant hand (Fig. 2.1). However, instrument exchange between the two hands may be necessary to facilitate engagement of the FVP-retina adhesion point. Cutter and scissors may be used alternately. Bimanual dissection usually alternates with unimanual dissection. The common practice is to perform unimanual dissection first, which changes to the

C.-M. Yang, *Surgery for Complications of Diabetic Retinopathy*,
https://doi.org/10.1007/978-981-96-2848-3_2

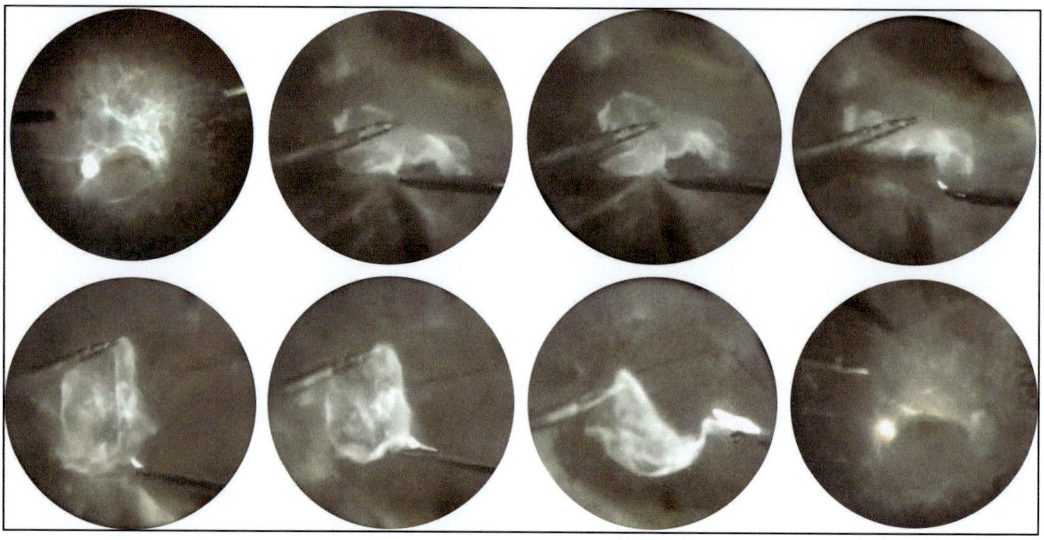

Fig. 2.1 One set of intraoperative images showing the most commonly used bimanual manipulation. Overview images at the beginning and at the end of the surgery are shown in the upper left and lower right, respectively. In this particular patient, a widespread broad FVP membrane was noted in the temporal upper quadrant of the left eye. The bimanual technique with scissors and forceps was used to engage and separate each adhesion point between the retina and the FVP membrane (three right-sided images and two lower-left images). After all the adhesions were released, the FVP membrane was detached from the retina (lower second right). (Courtesy of Dr. Chung-May Yang)

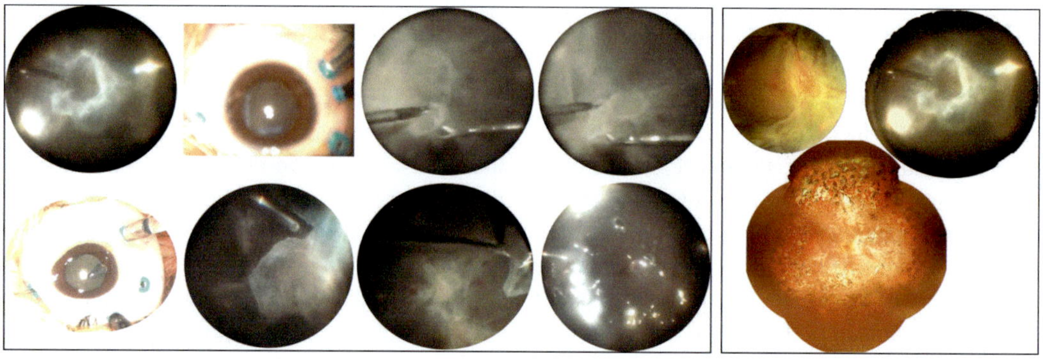

Fig. 2.2 Two sets of images of the same patient. The left panel shows the intraoperative video images of the bimanual maneuver with different positions of the Chandelier illuminator for better visualization of tissue dissection. The right panel shows pre-, intra-, and postoperative color photos of this patient. In the left panel, overview images at the beginning and at the end of the surgery are shown in the upper left and lower right, respectively. The sclerotomy for the chandelier illuminator (black tip) was positioned on the temporal side. Bimanual dissection with forceps and scissors is shown on the two upper right images. The Chandelier illuminator was repositioned at the temporal upper quadrant for a brighter view of the nasal lower large FVP membrane (lower left). Cutter segmentation (lower second left) and bimanual dissection of the nasal lower FVP membrane continued (lower second right) under wide-angle viewing. In the right panel, pre- and intraoperative images show extensive FVP around the arcade and widespread FVP in the nasal and nasal lower regions (upper 2 images). Postoperative wide angle color photo shows the attached retina with minimal residual FVP tissue. (Courtesy of Dr. Chung-May Yang)

bimanual technique when dissection becomes difficult. The two techniques may shift back and forth depending on which maneuver provides an easier way to achieve membrane removal. Steady instrument handling may be facilitated by resting the wrists on an adequately adjusted armrest.

Examples of various bimanual techniques for treating proliferative diabetic retinopathy (PDR) with severe FVP are shown in Figs. 2.2, 2.3, and 2.4.

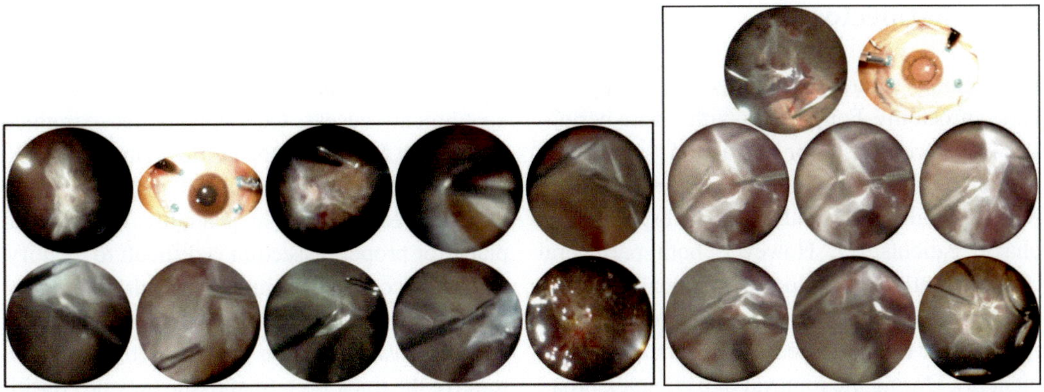

Fig. 2.3 Two sets of intraoperative video images showing bimanual maneuvering in both eyes of the same patient. The left panel shows the right eye, and the right panel shows the left eye. Please see Fig. 1.1, Chap. 1 for the pre- and postoperative retinal changes in this patient. Overview images at the beginning and at the end of the surgery are shown in the upper left and lower right panels, respectively. For sclerotomy, the chandelier illuminator (black tip) was positioned in the nasal lower quadrant for both eyes. In the left panel, AP traction release was performed first (upper center), followed by cutter segmentation (upper second right); bimanual dissection with forceps and scissors followed (upper right and lower left); further bimanual cutter segmentation was performed (lower second left). The scissors were changed to the nondominant left hand for better accessibility of the retina-FVP membrane adhesion points (lower center and lower second right). In the right panel, bimanual manipulation with scissors in the nondominant left hand for dissection of FVP tissue nasal to the arcade is shown in the middle row. Images of lower tissue dissection are shown in the lower left and lower center. (Courtesy of Dr. Chung-May Yang)

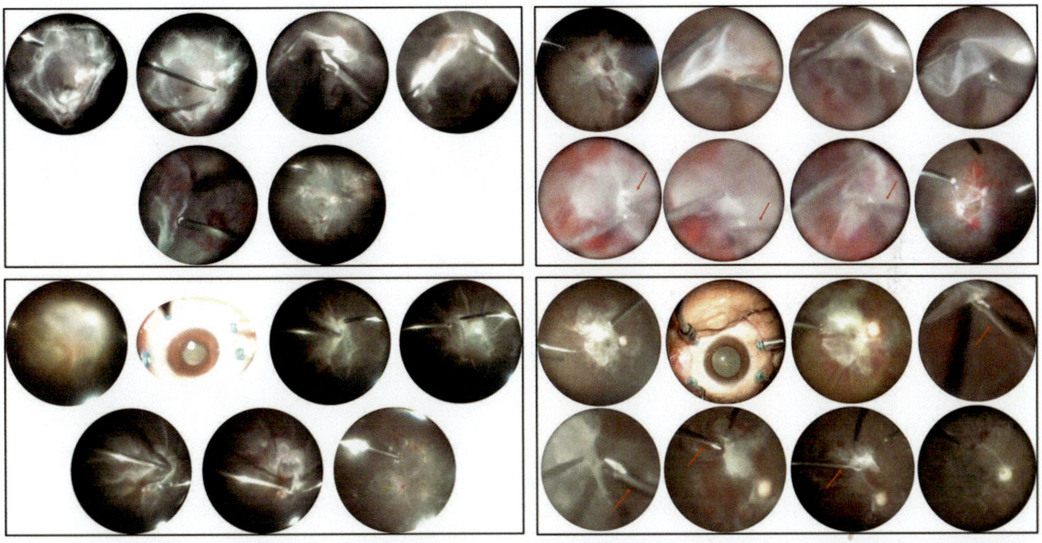

Fig. 2.4 Four sets of images showing various manipulation techniques for bimanual dissection of the FVP membrane. In each panel, overview images at the beginning and at the end of the surgery are shown in the upper left and lower right, respectively. In the upper left panel, severe proliferation was noted, and tissue segmentation was performed first (upper second left), followed by bimanual dissection with scissors and forceps (upper second right and upper right). The scissors were then changed to cutters for further dissection (lower left). Please see the upper middle panel of Fig. 1.17 in Chap. 1 for the pre- and postoperative retinal changes in this patient. In the lower left panel, bimanual manipulation was achieved with a cutter and forceps (2 upper right images, lower left and center images). In the upper right panel, an overview image shows a widespread broad FVP membrane in both the upper and lower retina (upper left). Bimanual inside-out dissection was performed to remove the lower FVP membrane (three upper images), while an outside-in approach was adopted to remove the upper FVP membrane (lower row except the lower right images). Red arrows point to the scissors. Gentle tissue lifting with forceps and precise adhesion separation with scissors are important. In the lower right panel, after cutter segmentation (upper second right), bimanual techniques under a high-magnification lens were performed (upper right and lower left). More peripheral dissection was performed under a wide angle lens (2 center images in the lower row). Good stereopsis was compromised for adequate visualization. (Courtesy of Dr. Chung-May Yang)

2.2 Retinectomy

Retinectomy is rarely performed in primary diabetic vitrectomy. For patients with severe peripheral anterior-posterior traction with a rhegmatogenous etiology, an adjuvant scleral buckle should be considered first, especially in phakic patients [2]. However, both peripheral circumferential retinectomy and localized mid-peripheral retinectomy may sometimes be required for traction release and retinal reattachment [3]. During the removal of a complex broad adhesion membrane with multiple epicenters, multiple breaks are likely to occur, and a local or limited retinectomy is thus preferred. In some cases, the FVP may extend all the way to the far periphery, and scleral buckling may be insufficient to relieve traction and/or reproliferation. Therefore, circumferential retinectomy to remove FVP-induced traction becomes necessary for anatomical success. Occasionally, an extrathick membrane formed by the cortical vitreous mixed with a thick blood clot and FVP may be encountered, especially in young adults. The surgical plane for proper dissection is difficult to identify, and it becomes extremely difficult to remove such tissue without damaging the underlying retina. To ensure traction release, retinectomy to remove the thick preretinal tissue may be considered. Silicone oil (SO) infusion is usually needed after these procedures.

Examples of pre- and postoperative retinal changes in eyes undergone retinectomy are shown in Fig. 2.5.

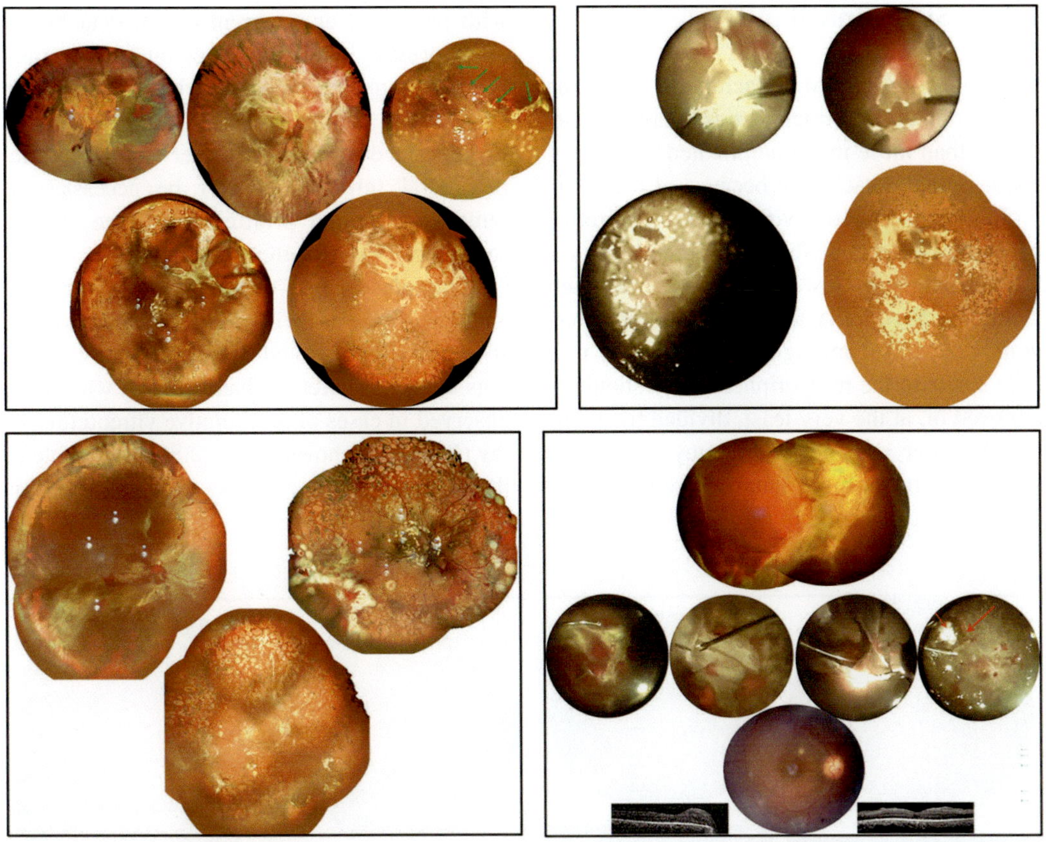

Fig. 2.5 Four sets of images showing pre- and postoperative retinal changes after vitrectomy combined with various types of retinectomy. In the upper 2 panels, 2 patients underwent focal midperipheral retinectomy to release retinal traction. In the lower two panels, peripheral retinectomy was performed in 2 patients to release anterior traction. SO was used in all patients after primary surgery, and the retina remained attached after SO removal in all four patients. In the upper left panel, the FVP membrane mixed with a thick blood clot prevented adequate tissue dissection. A large midperipheral retinectomy was performed (green arrows in the upper right wide angle color photo). After surgery with SO infusion, the retinectomy bed developed fibrotic bands and membranes (lower left and right), but the retina was attached after SO removal (lower right). Please see Fig. 2.9 for intraoperative video images of this patient. In the upper right panel, a smaller retinectomy was performed to release a highly adherent and easily bleeding FVP membrane. Intraoperative postretinectomy and postlaser video images are shown on the lower left. The retina was attached after SO removal (lower right). In the lower left panel, the temporal lower peripheral FVP extending to the vitreous base was noted before surgery (upper left wide angle color photo). A wide angle color photo on the first postoperative day is shown on the upper right. The retina was attached after SO removal (lower wide angle photo). In the lower right panel, the patient had PDR and endophthalmitis. After extensive medical treatment, the patient's left eye had no light perception. In the right eye, the patient developed active FVP with VH and retinal detachment (upper composite color photo). Intraoperatively, a granuloma-like scar in the temporal upper far periphery was noted. Bimanual vitrectomy with peripheral retinectomy bypassing the granuloma scar was performed (intraoperative video images in the middle row). The red arrows point to the retinectomy edge, and the white color indicates a granuloma-like scar. After surgery and subsequent SO removal, the retina remained attached (lower color photo and OCT images). (Courtesy of Dr. Chung-May Yang)

2.3 Subretinal Bands

In PDR with retinal detachment, subretinal fibrosis and subretinal bands may develop sooner than those in uncomplicated rhegmatogenous retinal detachment because of the strong proliferative microenvironment. Subretinal bands located outside the posterior pole may be left undisturbed. However, if retinal reattachment or a smooth macular contour is interfered with by a band spanning the macula or by multiple bands in the midperiphery, they should be removed or, at the very least, divided by microforceps after creating retinotomy at suitable sites. Sometimes more than one retinotomy is needed for proper traction release [3]. In eyes with persistent or recurrent retinal detachment after primary diabetic vitrectomy, subretinal proliferation and bands may be prominent. In such cases, retinal inversion to expose the undersurface of the retina after circumferential peripheral retinectomy may be necessary to remove subretinal proliferative tissue (please see Chap. 19—Recurrent RD).

Examples of pre- and postoperative retinal changes in eyes with subretinal bands are shown in Figs. 2.6 and 2.7. The pathology findings of these subretinal bands, along with those observed in cases of proliferative vitreoretinopathy (PVR), are shown in Fig. 2.8. An example of the three surgical techniques used in one eye is shown in Fig. 2.9.

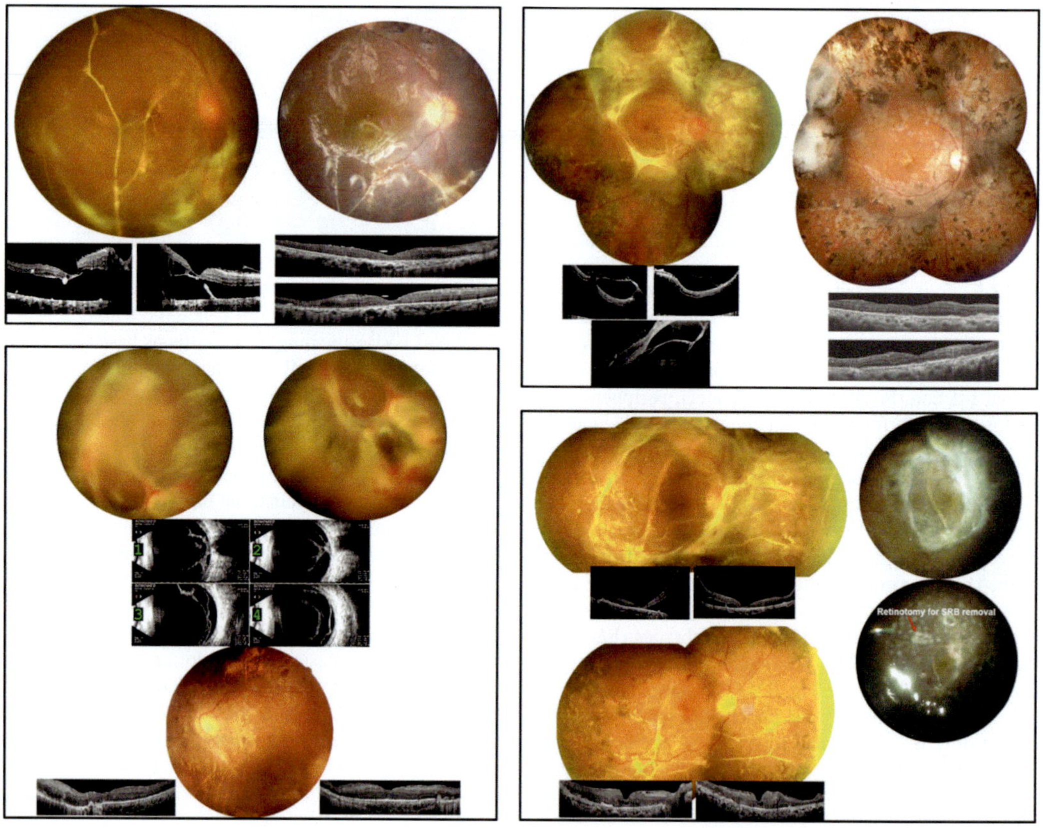

Fig. 2.6 Four sets of images showing pre- and postoperative retinal changes in eyes with PDR, RD, and subretinal bands. All subretinal bands were partially or completely removed. Note that the subretinal bands running across the subretinal space may attach to the retina at one end and to the RPE at the other end (preoperative OCT images on the left side of the upper left panel). Postoperative color photos and/or OCT images are shown on the right side or in the lower row of the panels. All patients had reattached retinas after surgery. The SO was not removed in the patient in the upper left panel. (Courtesy of Dr. Chung-May Yang)

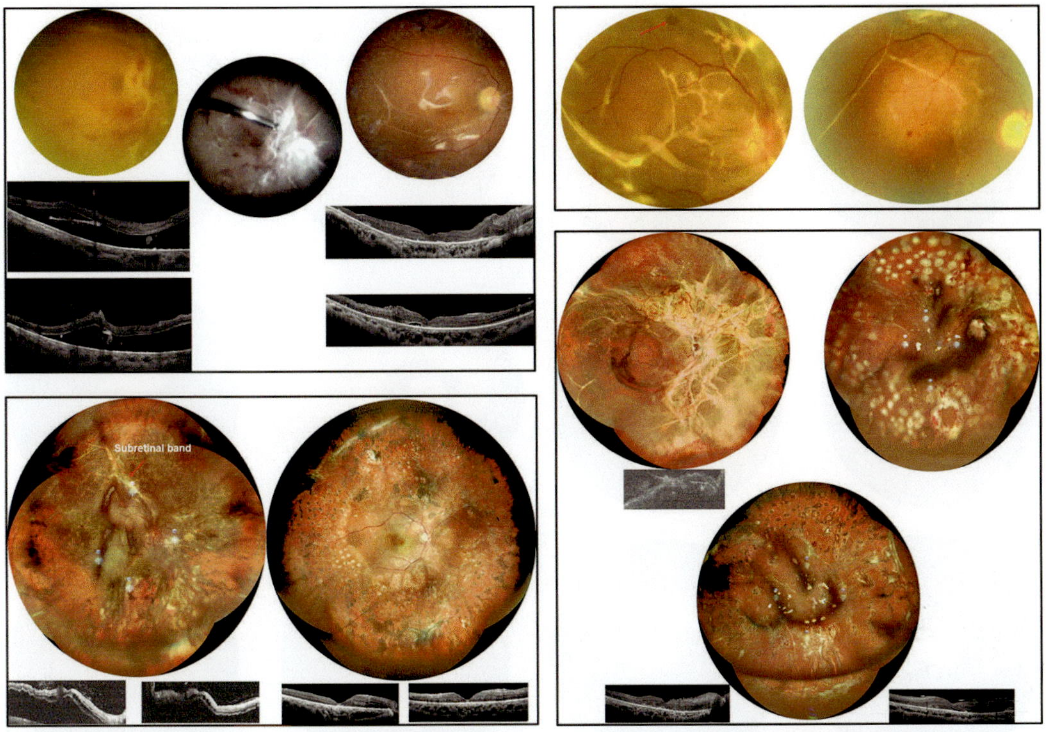

Fig. 2.7 Another four sets of images showing pre- and postoperative retinal changes in eyes with PDR, RD, and subretinal bands. All subretinal bands were partially or completely removed. Postoperative color photos and/or OCT images are shown on the right side or in the lower row of the panels. All patients had reattached retinas after surgery. The SO was not removed in the patients in the upper left or lower right panels. (Courtesy of Dr. Chung-May Yang)

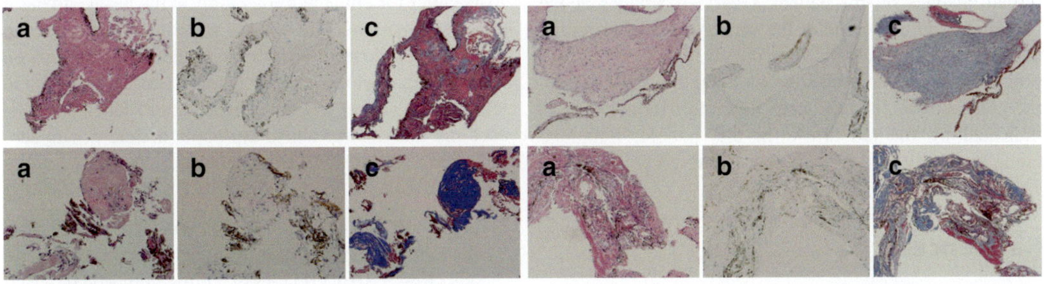

Fig. 2.8 Histopathological specimens of subretinal proliferation membranes or bands in PDR (left 2 images) and PVR (right 2 images) patients. Special staining methods were used for all the samples. (**a**) Represents H&E staining; (**b**) represents CD34 staining (mainly for vascular endothelial cells); (**c**) represents Masson's trichrome staining (mainly for epithelial cells and muscles). All specimens were CD34 negative, indicating that there were no vascular components in these specimens. The subretinal band in PDR is mainly composed of epithelial cells and myofibrotic tissue, while the subretinal bands in PVR are mainly composed of fibrotic tissue (blue staining via Masson's trichrome stain) with glial cells or RPE cell-derived epithelial cells. Thus, both subretinal bands in PDR and PVR are avascular tissues. The components in the PDR and PVR bands might be different. (Courtesy of Dr. Po-Ting Yeh)

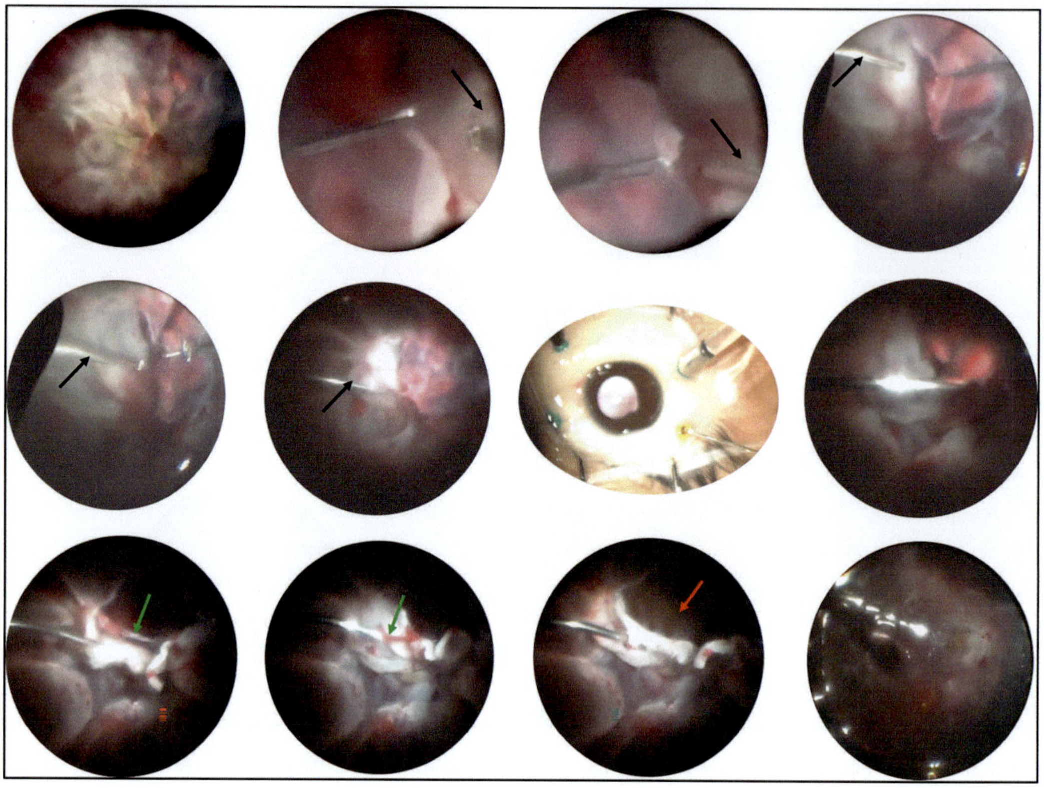

Fig. 2.9 One set of images showing bimanual manipulation, subretinal band removal, and retinectomy. Please see Fig. 2.5, upper left panel for the pre- and postoperative retinal changes of this patient. Overview images at the beginning and at the end of the surgery are shown in the upper left and lower right, respectively. The black arrows point to the vitrector, the subretinal band is indicated by the green arrows, and the bare RPE after retinectomy is indicated by the red arrow. In this patient, bimanual manipulations with a 25G cutter and forceps are shown in the three images in the upper row and the middle left image. When a very thick membrane was encountered (middle second left), the 25G cutter was replaced by the 23-G cutter for efficient retinectomy at the nasal and nasal upper mid-periphery to release traction (middle second right and middle right). The subretinal band was removed with forceps after the subretinal space was exposed by the retinectomy (lower left and lower second left). The retinectomy margin was above the upper arcade (lower second right). (Courtesy of Dr. Chung-May Yang)

References

1. Shroff CM, Gupta C, Shroff D, Atri N, Gupta P, Dutta R. Bimanual microincision vitreous surgery for severe proliferative diabetic retinopathy: outcome in more than 300 eyes. Retina. 2018;38(Suppl 1): S134–S45. https://doi.org/10.1097/IAE.0000000000002093.
2. Oellers P, Mahmoud TH. Surgery for proliferative diabetic retinopathy: new tips and tricks. J Ophthalmic Vis Res. 2016;11(1):93–9. https://doi.org/10.4103/2008-322X.180697.
3. Chen SN, Chen SJ, Wu TT, Wu WC, Yang CH, Yang CM. Refining vitrectomy for proliferative diabetic retinopathy. Graefes Arch Clin Exp Ophthalmol. 2023;261(12):3659–70. https://doi.org/10.1007/s00417-023-06134-w.

3 Treatment of Persistent Vitreous Hemorrhage in Proliferative Diabetic Retinopathy

Abstract

Vitreous hemorrhage (VH), including preretinal hemorrhage, is a major aspect of proliferative diabetic retinopathy (PDR) and an important cause of vision loss (Michels, Retina 1:1–17, 1981). The presence and growth of NV are the most important risk factors for VH. Conventional treatment methods include indirect laser panretinal photocoagulation (PRP) if the VH is not too dense or panretinal cryotherapy intended to enhance blood reabsorption and inhibit neovascularization (Avery et al., Ophthalmology 113:1695 e1–e15, 2006; Mason et al., Ophthalmol 142:685–688, 2006; Spaide and Fisher, Retina 26:275–278, 2006). However, PRP is usually inadequate in the presence of VH, and panretinal cryotherapy may have other limitations, such as causing significant intraocular inflammation or inducing traction retinal detachment (TRD) (Mosier et al., Am J Ophthalmol 100:440–444, 1985; Benedett et al., Ophthalmology 94:612–619, 1987). Recently, antivascular endothelium growth factor (anti-VEGF) has been shown to be effective in reducing the severity of recurrent vitreous hemorrhage (Spaide and Fisher, Retina 26:275–278, 2006). Ultimately, vitrectomy may be needed for persistent vitreous hemorrhage. The optimal timing of vitrectomy for persistent/nonclearing VH has been debated. The Diabetic Retinopathy Vitrectomy Study (DRVS) showed a benefit of early surgery (1–6 months after the onset of VH) for patients with type 1 DM and severe VH (Group TDRVSR, Arch Ophthalmol 103:1644–1652, 1985; Group TDRVSR, Arch Ophthalmol 108:958–64, 1990). However, advances in VR surgery have led many to advocate earlier surgery for all patients. The proper presurgical management, surgical timing, and surgical features will be discussed in this chapter.

3.1 Case Report

A 58-year-old woman with fairly controlled HT and DM for more than 10 years. One year prior, the patient had complete panretinal photocoagulation (PRP) in both eyes. She visited our clinic complaining of sudden onset blurred vision in the right eye 3 days before her visit without improvement. On examination, best-corrected visaul acuity (BCVA) was counting fingers at 100 cm in the right eye and 0.8 in the left eye. Intraocular pressure (IOP) was normal in both eyes. There was no rubeosis iridis (RI) in either eye. Mild cataracts were noted bilaterally. Fundus examinations revealed diffuse VH in the right eye, with optic disc and retinal vessels undiscernible. A clear fundus with a PRP scar was observed in the left eye. US revealed dense VH without vitreoretinal adhesion. Three weeks after

C.-M. Yang, *Surgery for Complications of Diabetic Retinopathy*,
https://doi.org/10.1007/978-981-96-2848-3_3

the visit, the patient's condition did not improve. Under peribulbar anesthesia, intravitreal Avastin (1.25 mg/0.05 mL) was given along with peripheral anterior retinal cryotherapy (ARC; 4 quadrants; 3 spots in each quadrant). VH decreased significantly 2 weeks after the treatment. The optic disc and posterior vessels became visible. Supplementary PRP was administered. VH gradually subsided, and BCVA improved to 0.7. Optical coherence tomography (OCT) did not show macular edema. The fundus showed lower peripheral residual VH.

3.2 Persistent VH in PDR

VH is the most common complication of PDR. It usually causes a sudden decrease in vision. Some patients were first diagnosed with PDR only after VH in one eye was detected. In many patients, VH is the first signifying the development of PDR from BDR. Some patients developed VH after or during PRP treatment sessions. Although short-term, single episodes of VH may occur, PDR-affected eyes most often experience repeated bleeding, either after the previous hemorrhage has been largely reabsorbed or during the reabsorption process of the earlier hemorrhage, thus disturbingly prolonging the visual impairment time. VH in patients with a history of diabetic retinopathy almost always results from retinal neovascularization (NV), even if clinical examination fails to reveal the presence of NV. Hemorrhage may rarely be caused by peripheral retinal vessel avulsion and/or tear during the PVD process. Blood located in the preretinal space or within the vitreous cavity may contain significant amounts of various growth factors or cytokines, which, along with factors released from the ischemic retina, serve as further stimuli for fibrovascular proliferation, especially in young adults, forming a self-catalyzing process [2]. The development of NV under an opacified vitreous allows for recurrent bleeding from the initial bleeding site and fresh bleeding from different sites of neovascularization. Rebleeding may occur either spontaneously or through vitreoretinal traction. The severity grading system was the same as that used for the vitreous opacity grading system: grade 0: mild VH with clear fundus view; grade 1: faint opacity with visible retinal vessels and disc detail; grade 2: moderate opacity with clear disc detail but without visible retinal vessels; grade 3: marked opacity with invisible retinal vessels and hazy disc details; and grade 4: no fundus view (Fig. 3.1).

Before any treatment is initiated, systemic risk factors should be sought for and reversed as best as possible. There are many systemic factors that

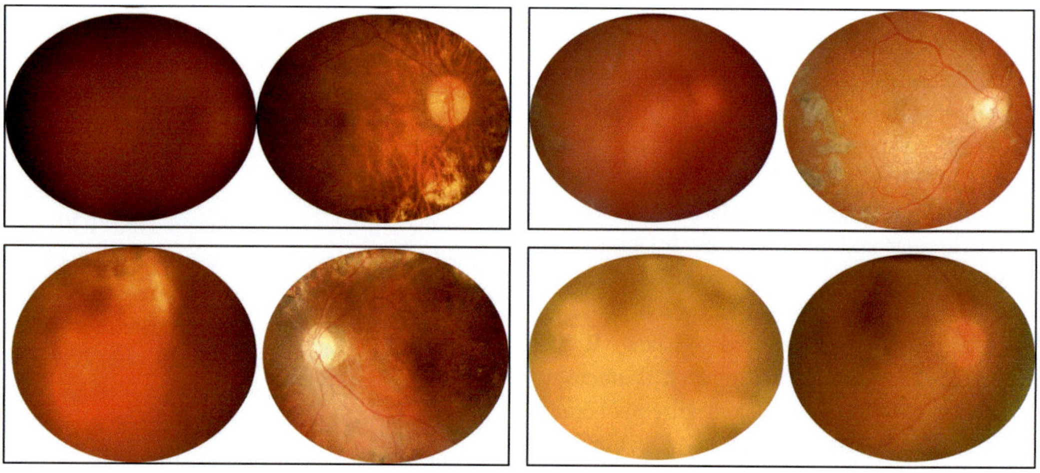

Fig. 3.1 Four sets of color photos showing pre- and postoperative fundus changes of various severities of VH. VH decreased from dense (upper left) to moderate (upper right and lower left). Chronic moderate VH is shown in the lower right panel. (Courtesy of Dr. Chung-May Yang)

may increase the possibility of recurrent VH, such as the intake of aspirin, anticoagulant therapy, and certain herbal drugs aimed at "enhancing" general health, circulation, or energy [3, 4]. Patients receiving hemodialysis for renal failure are prone to recurrent VH, partly because of the use of heparin during the procedure to prevent blood clotting. Poorly controlled hypertension and habitual smoking may disrupt vascular integrity and aggravate retinal ischemia [5]. For treatment, prompt PRP should be performed, if possible, to areas unobstructed by VH, followed by further laser to the exposed area during reabsorption of VH. Supplementary or fill-in PRP should be performed when active FVP can be detected. Care should be taken not to use high-power or high-density laser spots adjacent to the fibrotic or active NV to reduce vitreous contraction and further bleeding. Recently, antivascular endothelium growth factor (anti-VEGF) agents, either alone or in combination with PRP, have been advocated for the treatment of persistent VH [1, 6]. Anti-VEGF agents can promptly reduce the activity of NVs, thus preventing further bleeding during the reabsorption process, and this, in turn, may reduce the duration of vitreous opacity. It may also decrease preexisting macular edema or macular edema induced by PRP.

When a fresh hemorrhage is too dense to allow good fundus visualization or adequate laser treatment, US should be performed to assess the vitreoretinal interface condition. If no evidence of vitreoretinal broad adhesion or multiple point adhesions exists, either intravitreal anti-VEGF, peripheral ARC, or a combination of both may be used to accelerate the reabsorption of VH and prevent recurrent VH [6, 7]. The rationale behind the use of ARC is that, on the one hand, this modality may partially replace PRP to inhibit angiogenesis, and on the other hand, it may introduce inflammatory cells into the vitreous cavity to carry away blood cells. The combination of both treatments inhibits NV through the combined action of cryotherapy and anti-VEGF therapy while taking advantage of anti-VEGF therapy to reduce the likelihood of NV formation or macular edema secondary to cryotherapy-induced inflammation. ARC is performed under peribulbar anesthesia. A total of two to three spots with a 4-s duration for each spot are applied in each quadrant. After partial or complete clearance of the vitreous blood, PRP should be promptly performed. If no visual improvement or vitreous clearance can be detected 3–4 weeks after intravitreal anti-VEGF therapy with or without peripheral ARC and US shows no prominent vitreoretinal adhesion, repeated IVI of anti-VEGF agent may be performed. In one of our studies regarding persistent VH, we evaluated the efficacy of IVI bevacizumab with PRP in the treatment of PDR with VH. An IVI injection of 1.25 mg of bevacizumab was given to 40 patients with PDR and persistent VH, followed by PRP when visualization of the peripheral fundus could be obtained. A second injection was administered 4–6 weeks after the first injection if no signs of a decrease in VH were noted. Vitrectomy was performed if VH lasted more than 12 weeks. The times for vitreous clear-up in the posterior fundus (VCUT) and the rate of vitrectomy were compared with those in a historical control group (40 eyes in 40 patients) who were treated with conventional methods. Thirty-one eyes received one injection, and nine eyes (22.5%) received two injections. The VCUTs in the study and control groups were 11.9 ± 9.5 weeks and 18.1 ± 12.7 weeks ($p = 0.02$), respectively. The percentages of patients who required vitrectomy were 10% in the study group and 45% in the control group. This study suggested that one or two intravitreal injections of 1.25 mg of bevacizumab with PRP are associated with a more rapid regression of VH and may reduce the need for vitrectomy [6]. In another study, we further evaluated the efficacy of IVI bevacizumab injection (IVB) combined with ARC in the treatment of PDR with VH [7]. In the study group, transconjunctival ARC (a total of 12 spots) followed by IVB (1.25 mg) was administered in the same manner; in the control group, only IVB was given. PRP was performed during follow-up when possible. Repeated IVB was performed in both groups if VH persisted for more than 4 weeks following the initial treatment. Vitrectomy was performed if VH showed no improvement for 12–16 weeks. The vitreous clear-up time (VCUT) at the posterior pole and the rate of vitrectomy were compared between the two groups. Our study showed that although combined treatment with ARC and IVB might not decrease the eventual vitrectomy rate, it was associated with more rapid clearing of VH in eyes with PDR than IVB alone.

The presence of vitreoretinal broad adhesion or multiple point adhesions is a contraindication for using cryotherapy or anti-VEGF to speed up VH reabsorption because severe TRD or even combined RD may develop secondary to vitreous contraction (Fig. 3.2).

For a discussion on premacular hemorrhage, please see Chap. 4.

If the above methods fail to improve vision within 3–4 months, vitrectomy may be performed as the last resort to improve vision and prevent further deterioration of retinal function. Vitrectomy should be performed earlier if there is suspected RD, if patients have type 1 DM with HT, or if the RI develops during FU. Early surgery may be considered if the eye with VH is the only functioning eye (Fig. 3.3).

In eyes with diffuse VH, VR adhesions are usually not severe, most often at the disc or at one or two other sites, so blood can easily access the vitreous cavity. Preoperative US is valuable for providing a general assessment of VR interface conditions. Vitrectomy starts where the vitreous is mobile. Poor mobility indicates VR adhesion underneath. Bleeding or tear may occur if the cutter suction is too strong. Old blood has a yellow color. Yellow sand-like precipitates from blood degradation products may be observed on the retinal surface. When mixed with fresh blood, the vitreous may have a multilayered membrane with a branching pattern on the surface, resembling retinal vessels (Figs. 3.4 and 3.5) Subhyaloid hemorrhages may settle on the retina, forming a thick layer of blood (Fig. 3.6). It may take time to

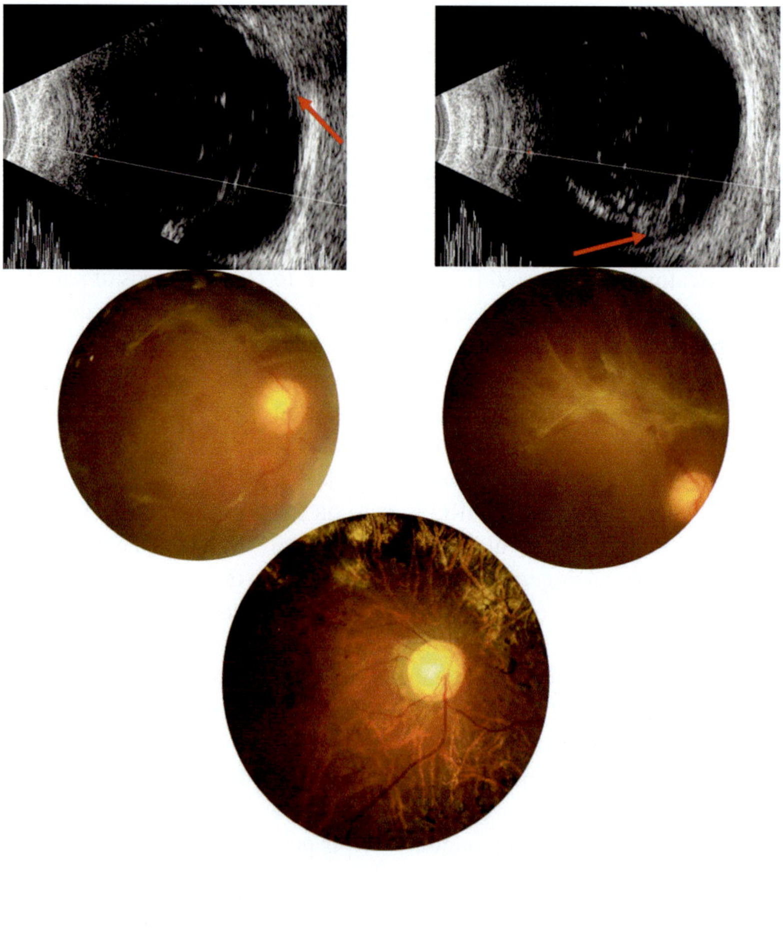

Fig. 3.2 This 46-year-old man had VH in the right eye and broad VR adhesion (upper row). Red arrows point to the sites of broad adhesion. CTRRD developed after ARC and IVI Avastin injection (middle row). The retina eventually reattached after surgery (lower color photo). BCVA improved from ND 50 cm to 0.1. (Courtesy of Dr. Chung-May Yang)

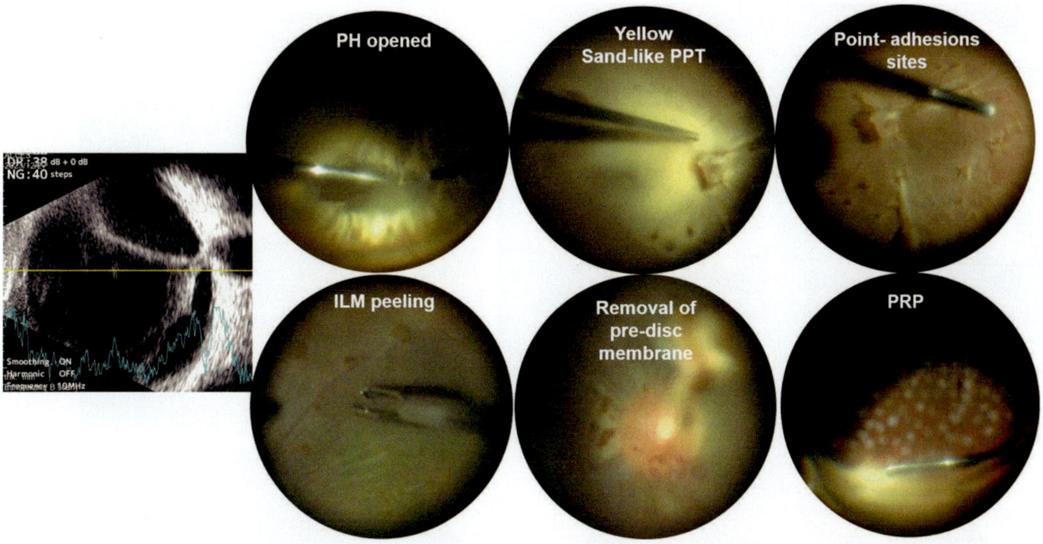

Fig. 3.3 One image set showing a case example of PDR with long-standing nonclearing vitreous hemorrhage. Preoperative ultrasonography revealed a thick vitreous membrane with vitreopapillary adhesion. The configuration resembles retinal detachment, but the presence of echogenic materials in the submembrane space instead of an echo-free space indicates that the membrane is not the retina (left ultrasonography image). Intraoperative video-captured images (right side 6 images) show yellow-colored vitreous opacity, yellow sand-like precipitates, point adhesion sites, and vitreopapillary adhesion. ILM peeling and PRP were performed in this patient. (Courtesy of Dr. Chung-May Yang)

remove it by putting the instrument into the subhyaloid space. Blood within the space between the retina and the adherent posterior hyaloid may present as a multilayered slab with a mixed dark red color or a dark green or brown color. It may become accessible only after breaking the overlying transparent posterior hyaloid. After preretinal blood removal, there may be a brownish pigmented thin or rug-like thick vitreous membrane formed by the posterior hyaloid fragment or epiretinal membrane mixed with blood degradation substance (Fig. 3.7). Care should be taken during removal because of multiple-point adhesions to the retina. FVP of various severities may be present after blood removal, and the surgeon should judge whether complete removal of the FVP is necessary (Fig. 3.8). One may occasionally encounter an extrathick membrane formed by the cortical vitreous mixed with a thick blood clot, especially in young adults. A larger gauged cutter may be required for its removal. The removal of FVP and such thick tissue is discussed in Chap. 2.

After removal of the opacified vitreous and the FVP, internal limiting membrane (ILM) removal in the macular area is necessary to remove the epimacular membrane and prevent recurrence of epiretinal fibrosis [8–10]. Adding supplementary PRP to the untreated area up to the ora is important for preventing postoperative NV. During vitrectomy, oral breakage or dialysis may occur because the vitreous may become less stretchable when it is mixed with blood. It is necessary to check the retinal periphery using indentation (Fig. 3.9).

The author routinely injects anti-VEGF at the end of surgery to prevent early NV formation and rebleeding [11].

If there is no further bleeding, gradual vitreous clear-up is expected. Haziness may persist for some time because the residual blood in the vitreous base may disperse into the vitreous cavity, and blood clots created during surgery may disseminate into the vitreous cavity after lysis. US should be performed during FU to ensure that there is no RD. A sudden decrease in IOP suggested RD. If an RI appears, underlying abnormalities should be identified. Post-DV recurrent bleeding is discussed in Chap. 18.

Case examples of VH with no or mild VR adhesion or with broad adhesions are shown in Figs. 3.10 and 3.11.

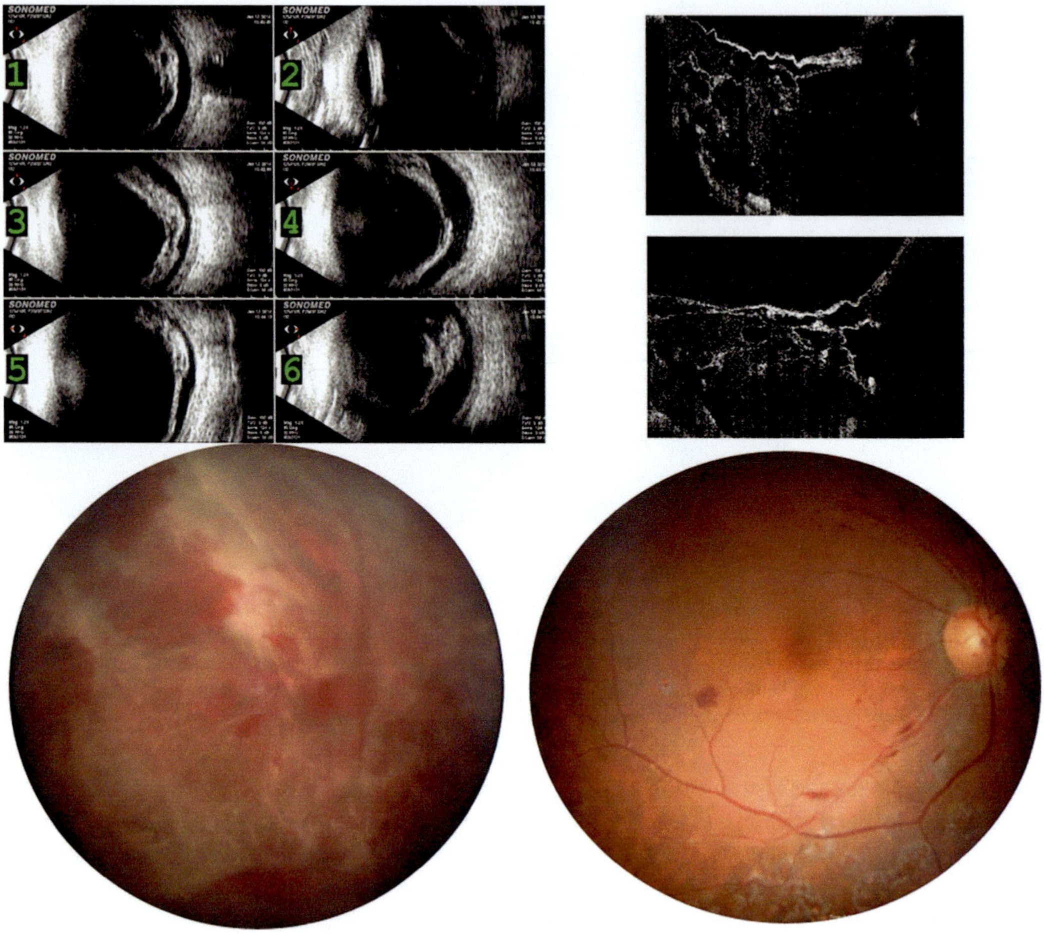

Fig. 3.4 This 71-year-old woman had right eye VH condensing into a multilayered thickened membrane (US images: upper left; OCT images: upper right; color photo: lower left). After surgery, the fundus became clear. BCVA improved from hand motion to 0.1. (Courtesy of Dr. Chung-May Yang)

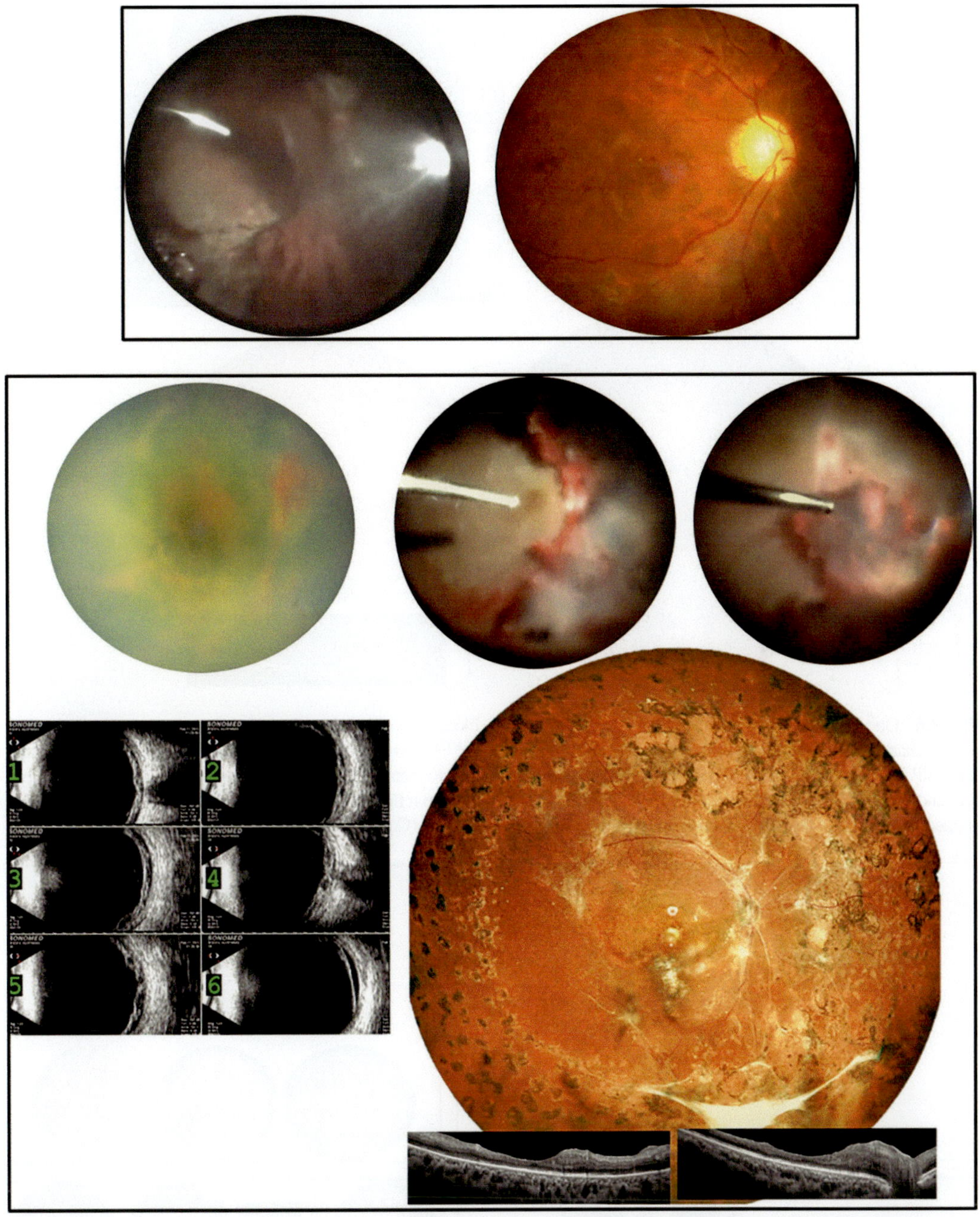

Fig. 3.5 Two examples of active PDR with a thick vitreous membrane mixed with blood are shown. The pre- and postoperative fundus images of a 34-year-old man are shown in the upper panels. BCVA improved from counting fingers 20 cm to 0.4. The lower set was a 28-year-old woman with type 2 DM. US images, pre- and intraoperative color images, and postoperative wide angle color images and OCT images are shown. The vitreous was green or red before surgery (left upper color photo). The patient underwent vitrectomy with SO injection followed by SO removal 5 years later. The BCVA improved from hand motion 100 cm to 0.1 cm. (Courtesy of Dr. Chung-May Yang)

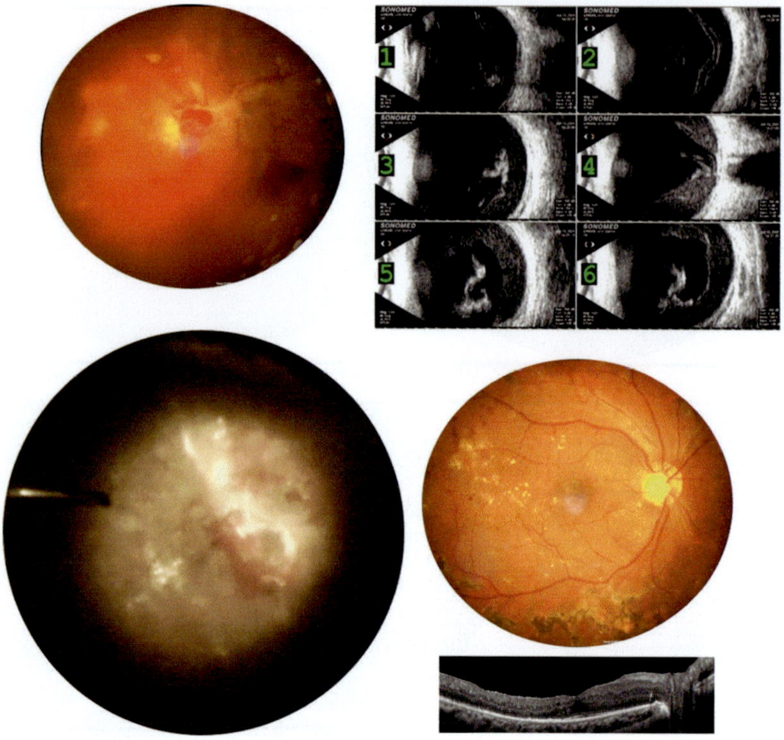

Fig. 3.6 One set of images showing pre-, intra-, and postoperative changes in a patient with PDR with VH, subhyaloid H, and FVP. Preoperative color photo and US images showing the VH and subhyaloid H, along with some FVP around the disc (upper). The extent of the FVP was more clearly observed after blood removal. Subhyaloid blood was compartmentalized by the FVP tissue, thus taking time to remove (lower left intraoperative video image). After surgery, the medium became clear, and the retina was attached (lower right color photo and OCT image). (Courtesy of Dr. Chung-May Yang)

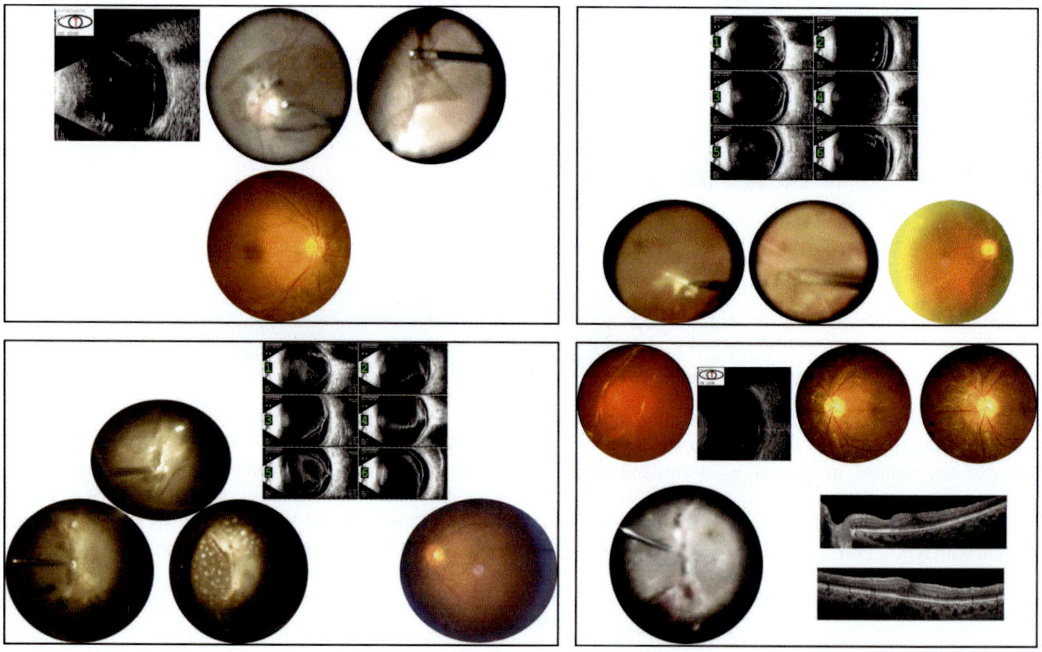

Fig. 3.7 Four sets of photos (US images; intraoperative and postoperative color images in the upper two and lower left sets; US images; pre-, intra-, and postoperative color images; OCT images in the lower right set) showing a thin pigmented membrane (upper two panels) and a rug-like thick pigmented membrane (lower two panels). (Courtesy of Dr. Chung-May Yang)

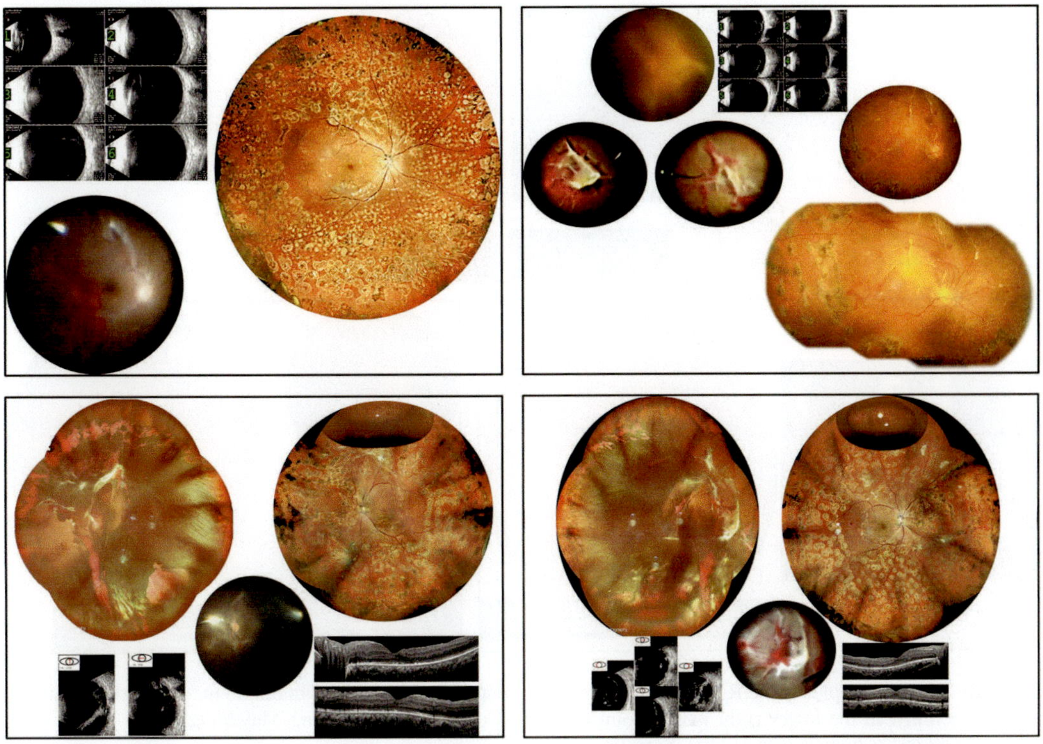

Fig. 3.8 Four sets of images (US images; intra- and postoperative color photos in the upper two panels; US images; pre-, intra-, and postoperative color photos; OCT images in the lower two panels) showing VH with various severities of the FVP. In the upper left panel, an upper arcade FVP band is visible (lower left intraoperative video image). In the upper right panel, a broad adhesion FVP with prominent folds is shown (upper left 2 intraoperative video images). Thick vitreous membranes mixed with blood (US images) and more severe FVP, mainly on the nasal side (center intraoperative video images), are noted in the lower two sets. The lower two sets are from the two eyes of a 36-year-old woman with type 2 DM. Please see Chap. 25 for more details on DV in both eyes. (Courtesy of Dr. Chung-May Yang)

Fig. 3.9 This 58-year-old woman had dense VH in the left eye (right). During surgery, supplementary PRP up to the ora was performed (left). BCVA improved from 0.01 to 0.3. (Courtesy of Dr. Chung-May Yang)

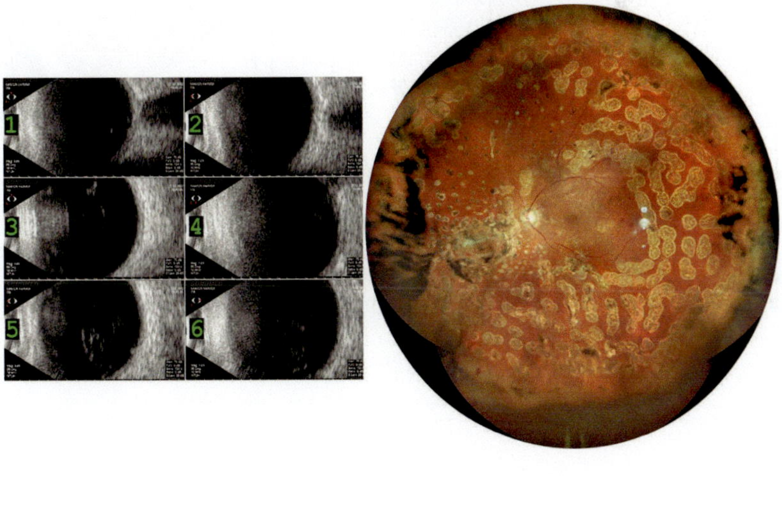

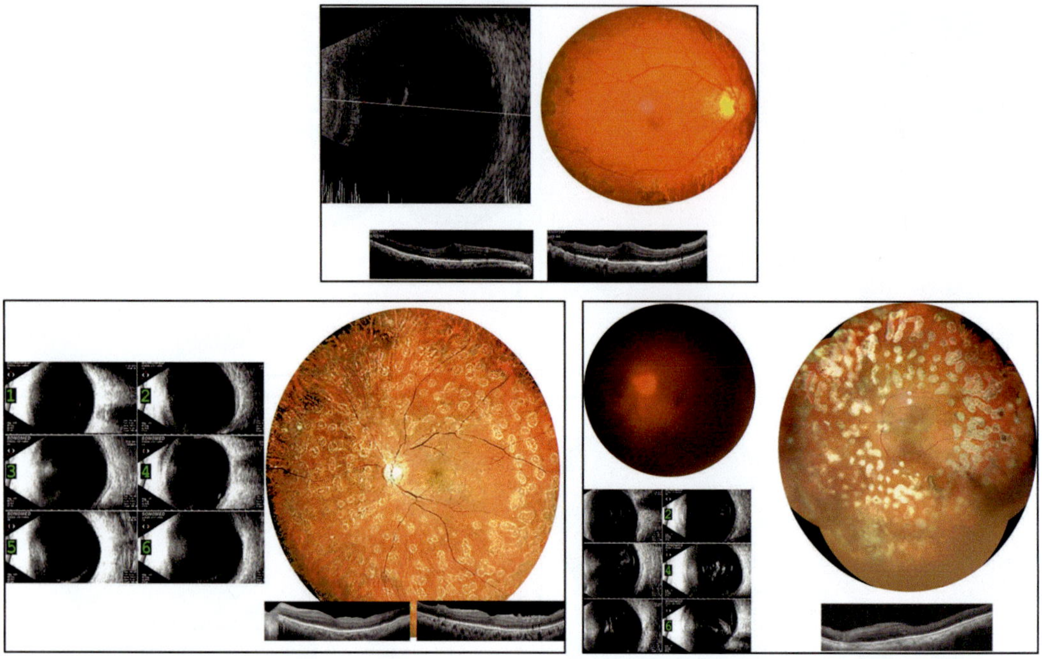

Fig. 3.10 Three examples of PDR with VH before and after vitrectomy. In the lower right panel, point adhesion is noted in US images (lower left). Significant VA improvement was obtained in all three patients. (Courtesy of Dr. Chung-May Yang)

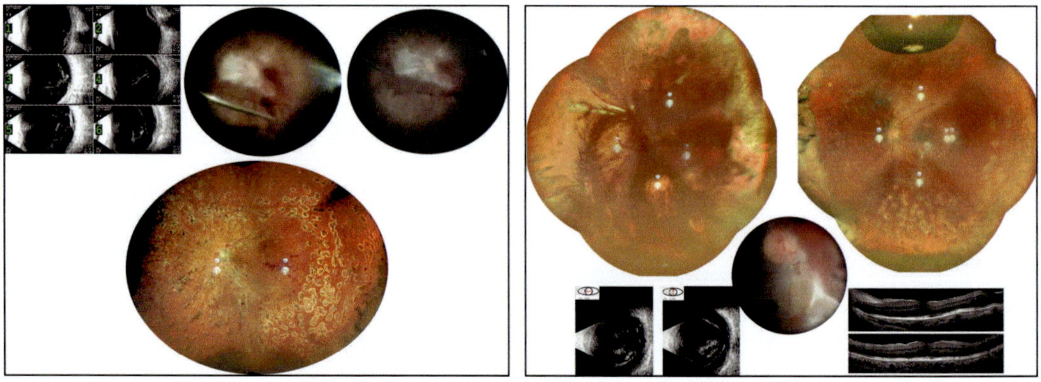

Fig. 3.11 Two examples of VH with FVP are shown. FVP membranes are more clearly visible in the intraoperative video images (upper right 2 images in the upper left panel; lower center image in the right panel). VA improved significantly after surgery. Broad adhesion can be observed in the US images in the two panels. (Courtesy of Dr. Chung-May Yang)

References

1. Spaide RF, Fisher YL. Intravitreal bevacizumab (Avastin) treatment of proliferative diabetic retinopathy complicated by vitreous hemorrhage. Retina. 2006;26(3):275–8. https://doi.org/10.1097/00006982-200603000-00004.
2. Chen E, Park CH. Use of intravitreal bevacizumab as a preoperative adjunct for tractional retinal detachment repair in severe proliferative diabetic retinopathy. Retina. 2006;26(6):699–700. https://doi.org/10.1097/01.iae.0000225351.87205.69.
3. Chung KF, Dent G, McCusker M, Guinot P, Page CP, Barnes PJ. Effect of a ginkgolide mixture (BN 52063) in antagonizing skin and platelet responses to platelet activating factor in man. Lancet. 1987;1(8527):248–51. https://doi.org/10.1016/s0140-6736(87)90066-3.
4. Rosenblatt M, Mindel J. Spontaneous hyphema associated with ingestion of Ginkgo biloba extract. N Engl J Med. 1997;336(15):1108. https://doi.org/10.1056/NEJM199704103361518.
5. Jeganathan VS, Sabanayagam C, Tai ES, Lee J, Sun C, Kawasaki R, et al. Effect of blood pressure on the retinal vasculature in a multiethnic Asian population. Hypertens Res. 2009;32(11):975–82. https://doi.org/10.1038/hr.2009.130.
6. Huang YH, Yeh PT, Chen MS, Yang CH, Yang CM. Intravitreal bevacizumab and panretinal photocoagulation for proliferative diabetic retinopathy associated with vitreous hemorrhage. Retina. 2009;29(8):1134–40. https://doi.org/10.1097/IAE.0b013e3181b094b7.
7. Hsieh MC, Yeh PT, Yang CM, Yang CH. Anterior retinal cryotherapy and intravitreal injection of bevacizumab in the treatment of nonclearing vitreous hemorrhage in proliferative diabetic retinopathy. J Ocul Pharmacol Ther. 2014;30(4):353–8. https://doi.org/10.1089/jop.2013.0104.
8. Chang PY, Yang CM, Yang CH, Chen MS, Wang JY. Pars plana vitrectomy for diabetic fibrovascular proliferation with and without internal limiting membrane peeling. Eye (Lond). 2009;23(4):960–5. https://doi.org/10.1038/eye.2008.334.
9. Michalewska Z, Bednarski M, Michalewski J, Jerzy N. The role of ILM peeling in vitreous surgery for proliferative diabetic retinopathy complications. Ophthalmic Surg Lasers Imaging Retina. 2013;44(3):238–42. https://doi.org/10.3928/23258160-20130503-05.
10. Rush RB, Del Valle Penella A, Reinauer RM, Rush SW, Bastar PG. Internal limiting membrane peeling during vitrectomy for diabetic vitreous hemorrhage: a randomized clinical trial. Retina. 2021;41(5):1118–26. https://doi.org/10.1097/IAE.0000000000002976.
11. Cheema RA, Mushtaq J, Al-Khars W, Al-Askar E, Cheema MA. Role of intravitreal bevacizumab (Avastin) injected at the end of diabetic vitrectomy in preventing postoperative recurrent vitreous hemorrhage. Retina. 2010;30(10):1646–50. https://doi.org/10.1097/IAE.0b013e3181d6def0.

4 Premacular Hemorrhage

Abstract

Premacular hemorrhage (PMH) is defined as blood located between the posterior hyaloid and the retina or between the internal limiting membrane and the neurosensory retina (Mennel, Br J Ophthalmol 91:850–852, 2007; Michels, Retina 1:1–17, 1981). It may exist in both spaces. Diseases commonly associated with premacular hemorrhage include but are not limited to arterial macroaneurysms, branch retinal vein occlusion (BRVO), Terson syndrome, child abuse, ocular trauma, and Valsalva maculopathy (Russell and Hageman, Retina 12:346–50, 1992). Proliferative diabetic retinopathy (PDR) is another entity that may be complicated by premacular hemorrhage (Michels, Retina 1:1–17, 1981). As neovessels (NVs) usually grow along the posterior hyaloid, PMHs are almost always distributed between the posterior hyaloid (PH) and the retina. Because this complication may greatly disturb central vision for a long period of time and may be an important stimulant of fibrovascular proliferation, intervention is usually indicated. Treatment methods ranging from tissue plasminogen activator (TPA) injection to YAG laser membranotomy to vitrectomy have been suggested (Chung, Ophthalmic Surg Lasers 32:7–12, 2001; Raymond, Ophthalmology 102:406–11, 1995; O'Hanley and Canny, Ophthalmology 92:507–11, 1985); however, the best treatment method has not been established. The clinical features and treatment methods used are discussed in this chapter.

4.1 Case Report

This is a 20-year-old woman with type 1 DM. Both eyes were treated with panretinal photocoagulation (PRP) for PDR. She complained of sudden onset of blurred vision in the right eye. Her BCVA decreased from 0.3 to 0.05 in the right eye. Fundus examinations revealed premacular hemorrhage and minor vitreous hemorrhage in the right eye. There was no significant fibrovascular prolifertaion (FVP). IVI Avastin (1.25 mg/0.05 mL) and C3F8 (0.3 mL) were administered 2 weeks later when the patient's condition did not improve. The patient assumed a face-facing position for 2 days. Postoperative vitreous blood collection prevented adequate fundus examination. Three weeks later, the fundus became clear, and mild FVP was observed on the disc. In the following year, two IVIs of Avastin and supplementary PRP were given to treat FVP. IVI Avastin and PRP were also given to the left eye. Her BCVA improved to 0.5 in both eyes, and the conditions stabilized for 15 years (Fig. 4.1).

C.-M. Yang, *Surgery for Complications of Diabetic Retinopathy*,
https://doi.org/10.1007/978-981-96-2848-3_4

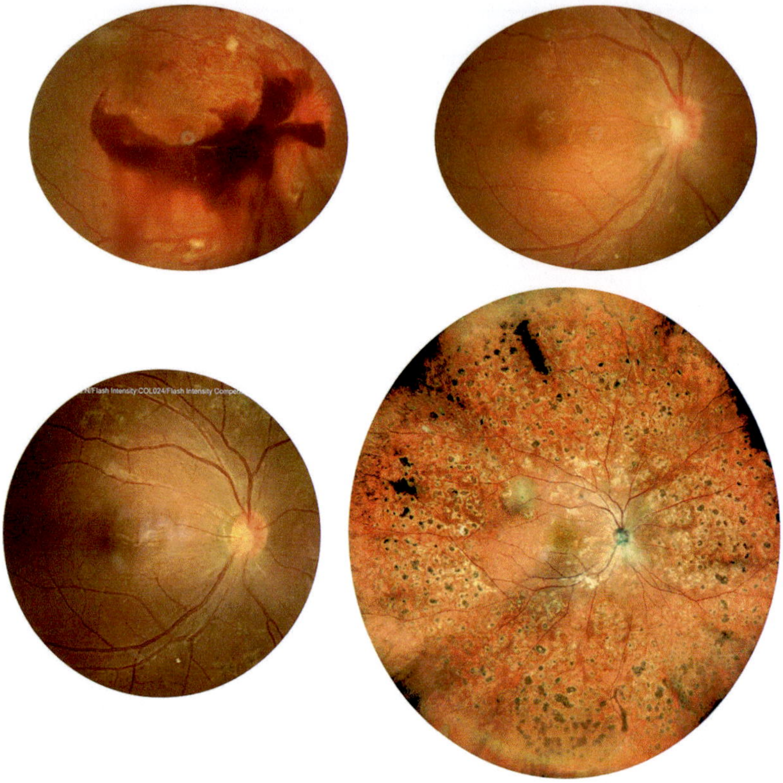

Fig. 4.1 Premacular hemorrhage in the right eye of a young woman with PDR (upper left color photo). The hemorrhage subsided after IVI of Avastin and gas; minor FVP was noted adjacent to the disc (upper left). After further PRP and anti-VEGF treatment, the retina became quiet for more than 10 years (lower 2 color photos). (Courtesy of Dr. Chung-May Yang)

4.2 Premacular Hemorrhage in DR

In PDR, PMH may be part of a more complex change associated with significant FVP or the major lesion in the fundus. Diabetic PMH occurs when blood from preretinal neovascular tissue is entrapped between the retina and the posterior hyaloid in the macular area. It may occur spontaneously or secondary to traction from a localized posterior vitreous detachment (PVD). Diabetic PMHs may have various presentations or associated abnormalities.

The fundus may not have visible NV or may show active NV or FVP adjacent to or remote from the PMH patches. A wide area of preretinal hemorrhage accompanied by significant FVP tissue may present as an FVP island surrounded by red blood, obscuring the underlying retina (Fig. 4.2). Preretinal hemorrhage may take a boat-shaped configuration when the space between the PH and the retina is substantial or may have irregular contours and various sizes at different locations when the space is tight with only a focal area PVD. It may have a bright red, dark red, or even black color. The thicker the blood is, the darker the color. Sometimes, two layers of blood with different colors may coexist. This is because vitreous splitting creates different compartments. An irregular light reflex may exist from the PMH surface membrane. Prominent HE may be observed. The fellow eye may have a similar presentation or may have other PDR changes.

PMH may undergo different evolutionary processes. It may resolve spontaneously or break into the vitreous cavity, causing VH, or turn to yellow-colored fibrin, then gradually reabsorb or have a prolonged presence; it may be reabsorbed but, at the same time, prompt the formation of premacular fibrosis at the original PMH area or nearby, inducing macular traction (Fig. 4.3). In PDR, the possibility of VA being affected by the PMH is high because of the disease itself, and from the subsequent changes, it should be treated.

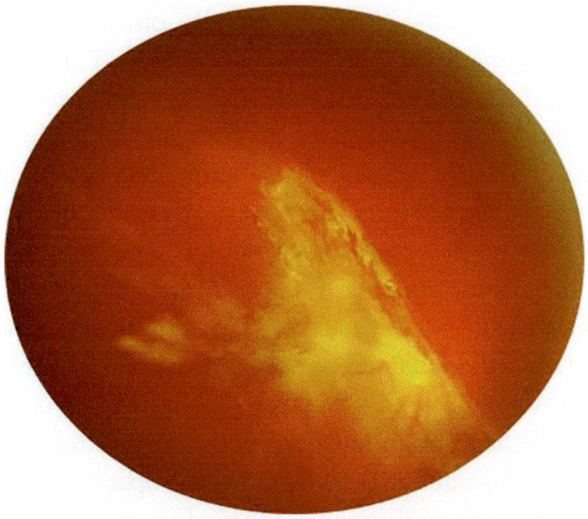

Fig. 4.2 Clinical image of preretinal hemorrhage around the FVP island. The blood under the posterior hyaloid connects with the FVP tissue, allowing the proliferative tissue to stand out. (Courtesy of Dr. Chung-May Yang)

As the presence of PMH indicates an active proliferative stage, PRP or supplementary PRP should be applied first before breakthrough VH occurs. Treatment strategies aimed at the PMH include the use of a YAG laser to disrupt the overlying hyaloid membrane for blood drainage and reabsorption; vitrectomy to remove the PH and blood; the use of intravitreal gas or IVI gas plus tissue plasminogen activator (TPA) to displace the blood away from the macular area or into the vitreous cavity [1]; and the use of IVI gas and anti-VEGF to displace the blood and render neovascularization less active, thus decreasing the likelihood of recurrent hemorrhage [2].

We reported the effect of intravitreal injection of TPA and gas for the treatment of diabetic premacular hemorrhage in five eyes of five consecutive

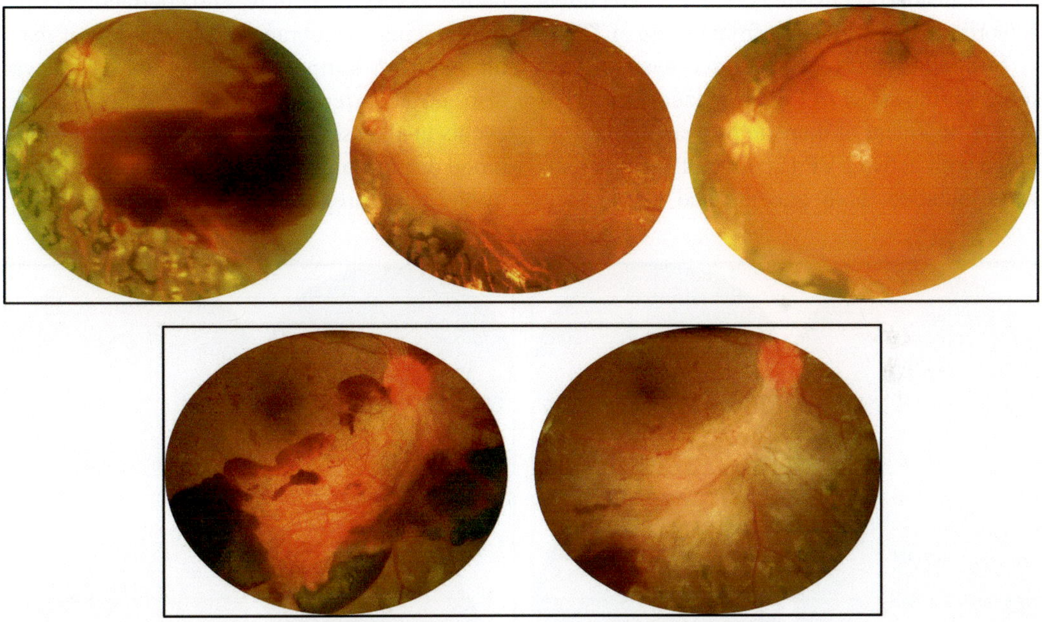

Fig. 4.3 Two patients experienced disease progression after the reabsorption of preretinal hemorrhage without treatment. In the upper panel, a dense preretinal fibrotic sheet was noted (center), and surgery was performed (right). In the lower panel, active NVs were transferred to the FVP membrane in the lower arcade (right). (Courtesy of Dr. Chung-May Yang)

patients [1]. Gas was used to displace the blood, while TPA was used to make the blood more mobile for a better gas effect. All five eyes had fresh diabetic premacular hemorrhage and previous PRP. An intravitreal injection of 50 mg of TPA and 0.3 mL of sulfur hexafluoride were performed. After the procedure, patients maintained a prone position for 3 days and were followed for an average of 7 months (range 6–8 months). All treated eyes exhibited clearing of the premacular hemorrhage with improved visual acuity. Three eyes with no visible fibrovascular proliferation required 3 weeks to resorb the blood, and two eyes with active fibrovascular proliferation needed 2 months for the intravitreal hemorrhage to resorb. This small series showed that intravitreal injection of TPA and gas may be an effective way to treat fresh diabetic premacular hemorrhage. Although the results seemed satisfactory, the major concern is the possibility of recurrent hemorrhage and the toxicity from the use of TPA.

In another study, we reported a small case series on the effect of IVI bevacizumab and gas for the treatment of diabetic premacular hemorrhage with active FVP [2]. Overall, six patients were included. Four patients had hemorrhage confined to the macular area only, one had hemorrhage around the disc and scattered in the parafoveal area, and one had minor vitreous hemorrhage in addition to premacular hemorrhage. After treatment, patients maintained a face-down position for 3 days. The time interval between the premacular hemorrhage and the intravitreal injection ranged from 1 to 6 weeks (average: 3 ± 1.5 weeks). This duration seems shorter than that of our previous technique using TPA and gas. All six eyes had complete hemorrhage absorption and a reduction in fibrovascular proliferation. Transient vitreous opacification from the breakthrough of the blood was observed in all eyes. An average of 3.8 ± 1.8 weeks (range, 1–6 weeks) was required for the clearing of premacular hemorrhage. Visual acuity improved in all six eyes after the removal of the premacular hemorrhage. There was no contraction of the fibrovascular membrane or progression of macular traction during the follow-up. There was also no recurrent bleeding or other adverse events in all cases (Fig. 4.4). One mechanism of blood displacement may be the creation of PVD by the intravitreal expansible gas. However, in

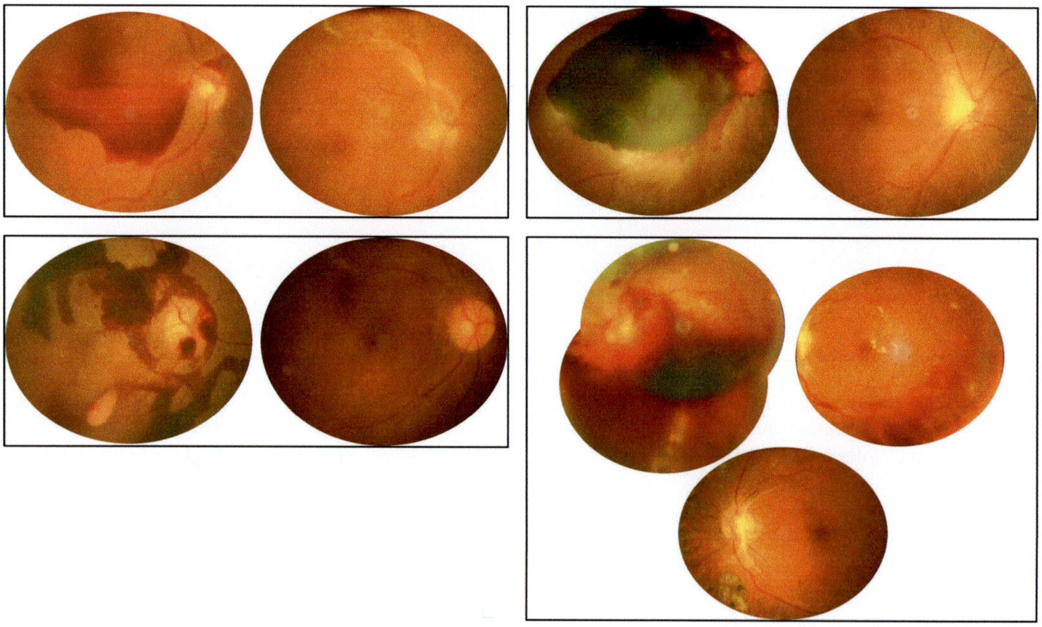

Fig. 4.4 Four patients with premacular hemorrhage were treated with IVI of Avastin and gas. All patients had minor FVP after blood reabsorption, but the macula was not affected, and no further operation was performed. In the lower right panel, pretreatment changes are shown in the upper left composite color image. The posttreatment changes are shown in the upper right and lower color photos. (Courtesy of Dr. Chung-May Yang)

our case series, we did not observe separation of the hyaloid from the underlying retina in the macular area after blood reabsorption. Adherent fibrovascular proliferation might have prevented gross PVD. Alternatively, the blood may first be displaced into the peripheral preretinal area where posterior vitreous hyaloids are more loosely attached to the retina or a partial PVD has already occurred. From there, the blood escapes into the vitreous cavity. The main purpose of anti-VEGF agents is to inhibit NY and further bleeding. VEGF may play a definite role in platelet aggregation and fibrin formation [3]. Anti-VEGF therapy may enhance fibrinolysis under pathological conditions. It is possible that bevacizumab may play a role in making the preretinal blood more mobile for displacement. In proliferative diabetic retinopathy, because the blood is primarily located between the retina and the posterior hyaloid, it may be more susceptible to the possible effect of bevacizumab. While bevacizumab may have potential benefits in treating this disease, further comparative studies may be needed to determine whether gas alone can achieve similar results. Complete laser pretreatment may not be mandatory with these combined injection techniques since bevacizumab may rapidly inhibit further proliferation. However, as the effect is only transient and peripheral vitreous clearance may be prolonged, retinal photocoagulation, at least in the peripheral retina before treatment, is recommended. Complete PRP after the vitreous becomes clear remains necessary to prevent disease progression on a long-term basis. We suggest that this procedure be used in patients with mild rather than severe fibrovascular proliferation to reduce the incidence of contraction of the fibrovascular membrane and progression of macular traction, which may be caused by intravitreal injection of bevacizumab. Although not observed in our case series, a peripheral retinal tear caused by pneumatic displacement is a potential complication. However, the overall complication rate caused by intravitreal gas should remain much lower than that of other vitreoretinal procedures, such as pars plana vitrectomy.

After treatment, long-term follow-up is necessary because reproliferation may develop. Timely anti-VEGF therapy and supplementary PRP may still be needed.

In those cases where the PMH is only a part of a more complicated structural abnormality, surgery is still the better option (Fig. 4.5).

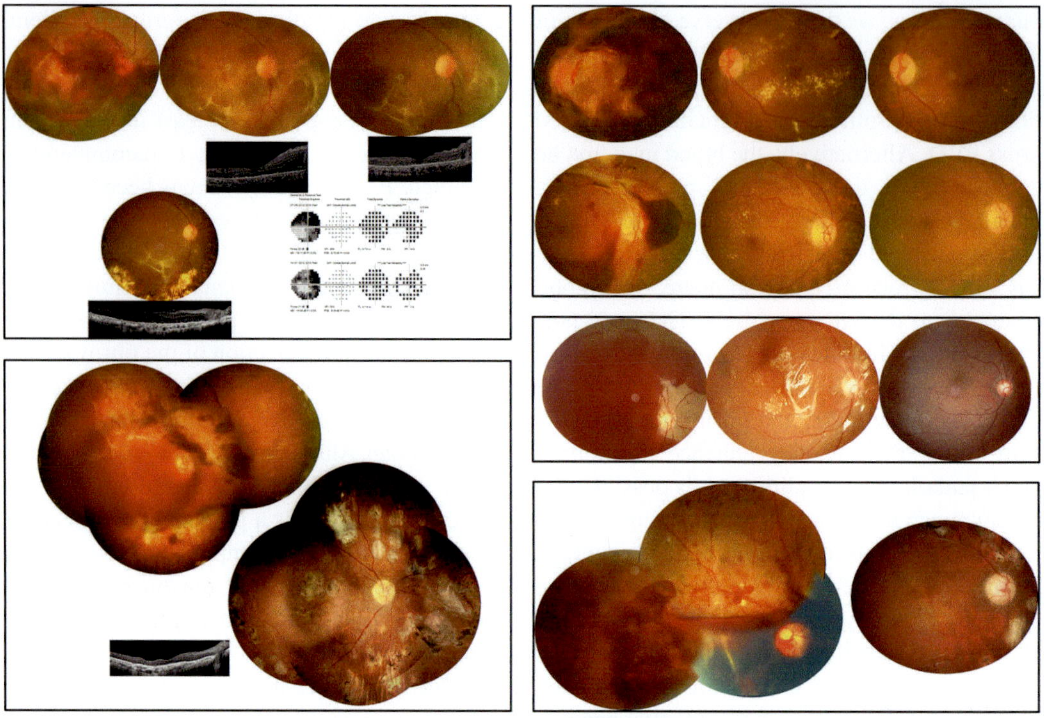

Fig. 4.5 Five examples of premacular hemorrhage associated with FVP treated with vitrectomy. In the upper left panel, the patient initially had widespread preretinal hemorrhage and VH (upper left composite). The patient elected to receive FU instead of surgery. One year later, the hemorrhage subsided, but fibrotic tissue nasal to the disc caused disc traction and nasal macular thickening (upper center and right color photos and OCT images). After surgery, the disc color improved, and the retina was attached. The subretinal bands in the lower macula suggested previous TRD (lower left). Compared with the preoperative findings, the VF improved (lower right). Please see Chap. 14 for the details of vitreopapillary traction. In the upper right panel, both eyes from the same patient had preretinal hemorrhage and FVP (upper and lower left color photos). After surgery, hard exudates gradually reabsorbed, and the retina became clear in both eyes (center and right color photos in the two rows). The other three panels show three cases of wide areas of preretinal hemorrhage and FVP (left-side color photos in each panel). After surgery, the retina became quiet. In the middle panel on the right side, SO infusion was used (center color photo), followed by cataract surgery and SO removal (right color photo). (Courtesy of Dr. Chung-May Yang)

References

1. Yang CM, Chen MS. Tissue plasminogen activator and gas for diabetic premacular hemorrhage. Am J Ophthalmol. 2000;129(3):393–4. https://doi.org/10.1016/s0002-9394(99)00393-1.
2. Shih CW, Yang CM, Chen MS, Wang TJ. Intravitreal injection of bevacizumab and gas for diabetic premacular hemorrhage with active fibrovascular proliferation. Graefes Arch Clin Exp Ophthalmol. 2008;246(11):1547–51. https://doi.org/10.1007/s00417-008-0902-8.
3. Verheul HM, Jorna AS, Hoekman K, Broxterman HJ, Gebbink MF, Pinedo HM. Vascular endothelial growth factor-stimulated endothelial cells promote adhesion and activation of platelets. Blood. 2000;96(13):4216–21.

5 Combined Tractional and Rhegmatogenous Retinal Detachment in Proliferative Diabetic Retinopathy

Abstract

Combined tractional and rhegmatogenous retinal detachment (combined RD, CTRRD) is a serious complication of proliferative diabetic retinopathy (PDR). The detached retina has a rhegmatogenous detachment-like convex configuration, usually extending to the ora serrata, and is associated with fibrovascular tissue of varying severity (Thompson et al., Arch Ophthalmol 105:503–572, 1987; Rice et al., Am J Ophthalmol 95:34–44, 1983). Retinal breaks are likely to appear when tractional force acts on the thin retina in PDR patients and are usually situated adjacent to the proliferative tissue or at previous laser scars. Thick proliferative membranes, retinal folds, or vitreous opacity may obstruct the detection of retinal breaks. Although it occurs less frequently than pure tractional retinal detachment (TRD), this complication warrants prompt vitreous surgery. There are few studies on the clinical manifestations and surgical results of this complication as a distinct entity (Yang et al., Can J Ophthalmol 43:192–198, 2008; Hsu et al., J Ophthalmol 2014:917375, 2014; Cruz-Inigo and Berrocal, Int J Retina Vitreous 3:38, 2017). As the use of anti-vascular endothelial growth factor (VEGF) agents became more common, either alone or in combination with other agents, in treating PDR complications, clinical features and surgical success rates were likely altered because anti-VEGF agents may induce fibrous contractions, possibly causing more TRD or combined RD. The clinical presentations, risk factors, treatment methods, and outcomes are discussed in this chapter.

5.1 Case Report

Patient 1: A 55-year-old man with DM who was under OHA control (recent HbA1c: 5.8%). He had a history of bilateral panretinal photocoagulation (PRP) after PDR diagnosis and was followed up at our clinic with a stable extramacular TRD in the right eye. Rapid onset of progressive RD with inferior macular involvement was noted during one OPD visit. On examination, best-corrected visual acuity (BCVA) was 0.5 in the right eye and 1.0 in the left eye. Fundus examination revealed the FVP over the superior and inferior arcades and the inferior RD extending to the ora. A diagnosis of combined RD was made, and vitrectomy was performed. During surgery, one round hole was noted adjacent to and partly covered by fibrovascular proliferation (FVP) tissue in the lower arcade. After surgery, the retina was reattached (Fig. 5.1).

Patient 2: A 38-year-old man with DM and dyslipidemia. He had been treated with insulin and OHA, and his ophthalmic history was sig-

C.-M. Yang, *Surgery for Complications of Diabetic Retinopathy*,
https://doi.org/10.1007/978-981-96-2848-3_5

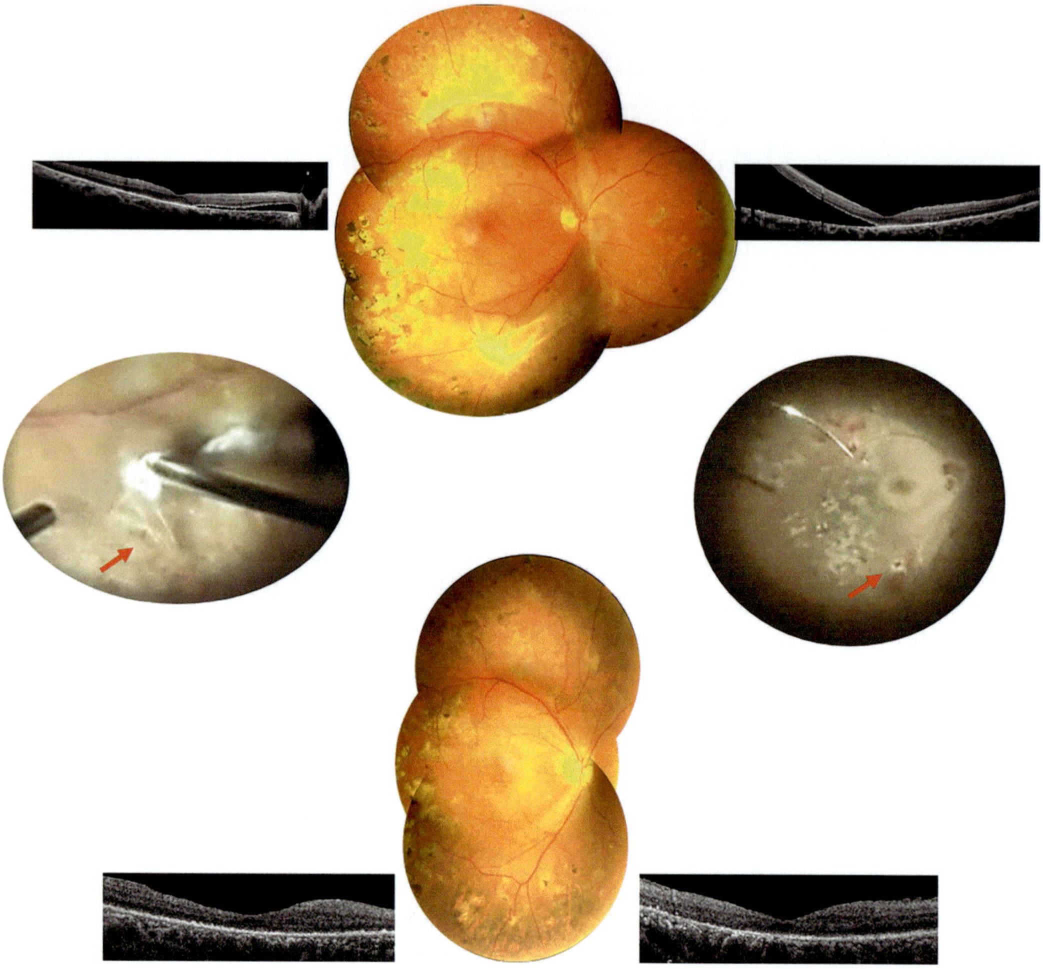

Fig. 5.1 Preoperative (top color composite color photo and OCT images), intraoperative (middle 2 video images), and postoperative (bottom composite color photo and OCT images) retinal changes in the right eye in Patient 1. The red arrow points to the break. (Courtesy of Dr. Chung-May Yang)

nificant for PDR with diabetic macular edema in both eyes. PRP and IVI of anti-VEGF were performed several times in both eyes. During follow-up at another hospital, a black shadow in the right eye developed. The patient came to our outpatient clinic for further treatment. On examination, BCVA was 0.1 in the right eye and 0.5 in the left eye. Fundus examinations revealed FVP in the peripapillary area and along the arcade, subtotal RD sparing the superior periphery, and VH sparing the lower vitreous cavity in the right eye. The left eye also had FVP around the arcade, with a mild lower VH. During right eye surgery, one round hole was noted at the edge of a lattice degeneration in the temporal upper periphery; a subretinal band in the upper midperiphery was noted and removed. After surgery with silicone oil (SO), the retina was reattached. Subsequent phacoemulsification with posterior chamber intraocular lens (PCIOL) and SO removal were performed. Her BCVA improved to 0.6 approximately 13 months after the primary surgery. The operation in the left eye was uneventful (Fig. 5.2).

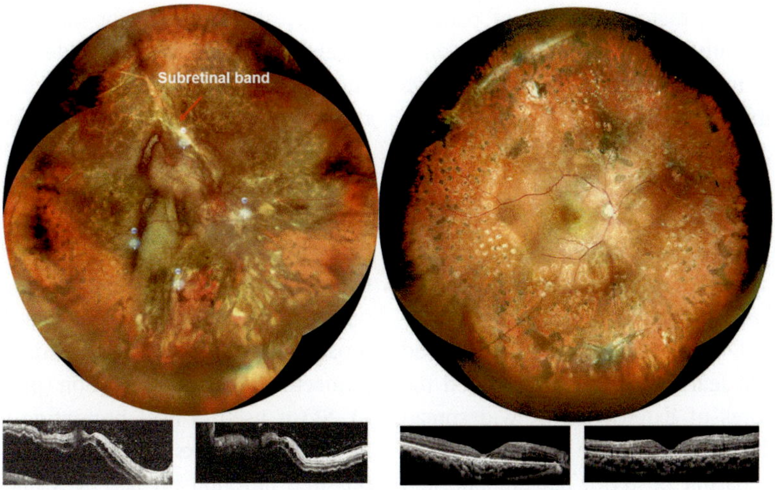

Fig. 5.2 Preoperative (left wide angle color photo and OCT images) and postoperative (right wide angle photo and OCT images) manifestations of CTRRD in the right eye of Patient 2. The superior FVP, subtotal RD (greenish area), and lower VH were noted before surgery (left). A prominent subretinal band can be seen in the upper part (red arrow). After surgery, the retina reattached (right). (Courtesy of Dr. Chung-May Yang)

5.2 Combined RD in PDR

CTRRD is a rare but serious complication of PDR. A literature review revealed that 7–35% of patients who underwent PPV for complications of diabetic retinopathy had CTRRD [1, 3, 4, 5]. The disease is characterized by the existence of retinal break(s) associated with FVP of various severities. The break(s) are mostly slit-like, round, or oval. They may be hidden within the retinal folds or covered by adjacent FVP tissue. Alternatively, peripheral lattice degeneration or previous laser scarring may be the source of break(s), as in Patient 2. The macular hole may sometimes be the only break in such cases. Only approximately half of the patients experienced break(s) before surgery. The detachment has a convex configuration and usually reaches the ora serrata in at least some area, but the extent of the detachment may be limited by PRP scars. As the use of anti-VEGF agents, either alone or in combination with other agents, becomes more common for treating PDR complications, combined RD may occur more frequently [6, 7]. Although anti-VEGF agents may induce the regression of active neovascularization and prevent the development of neovascular glaucoma (NVG), they may also induce fibrous contractions. Our study revealed that the percentage of recent (within 3 months of the development of combined RD) PRP and/or IVI anti-VEGFs in patients with CTRRD was greater than 10% [3]. Although definite statistical support is lacking, this result suggests that one should perform PRP or IVI of anti-VEGF agents with caution, as these procedures may predispose eyes to increased traction or even CTRRD.

The severity of FVP varies. The FVP severity may be mild (several point adhesions or one or two band-like VR attachments), moderate (one to two broad attachments), or severe (three or more broad attachments with at least one extending to the equator or beyond). Please see Chap. 1 for details on the severity grading. Retinal detachment may be localized (fewer than 2 quadrants), subtotal detachment (at least 2 but fewer than 4 quadrants), or total detachment. Retinal atrophy, defined as diffuse retinal thinning with attenuation of more than 1 quadrant of retinal vessels with or without secondary optic nerve atrophy, is observed in approximately 10–20% of patients [2]. The proliferative features may be predominantly fibrotic, in which most of the proliferative tissue appears avascular, and predominantly active fibrovascular, in which a large part of the proliferative tissue contains visible vessels. We recently reported that the active and fibrotic ratio in CTRRD was 1.38, indicating more active FVP cases [3]. Except for a few patients who presented with a picture similar to that of pure rhegmatogenous RD with condensed strands and adjacent visible tears, most patients shared the common features of extensive RD, widespread and tightly adherent plaque-like preretinal proliferative tissue, partial posterior detachment, and retinal folds. In rare instances, the majority of FVPs are distributed in different areas from the break and detachment areas.

There may be a few possible pathways for the development of combined RD: first, active FVP with TRD undergoes further traction to induce break formation, as in Patient 1; second, the fibrotic tissue and the vitreous exert traction on the atrophic retina in a chronic PDR with or without TRD, causing break formation; third, vitreous anterior–posterior-oriented traction on the adherent FVP tissue induces flap tear formation; fourth, traction induced by PRP or anti-VEGF on the attached or detached retina causes the formation of breaks. Lattice degeneration with break(s) rarely causes RD in the presence of FVP elsewhere.

The highlights of surgical tips are as follows. Patients with active FVP but not fibrotic proliferation are treated with IVI anti-VEGF (1.25 mg of Avastin in our hospital) within 3 days before surgery; anterior-posterior vitreoretinal traction is released as much as possible first; scissors or cutter segmentation and delamination are used to remove thick fibrotic plaques; thin and pliable, nontaut peripheral hyaloid still adherent to the retina may be left unpeeled for fear of creating breaks; a bimanual technique is employed by using forceps in one hand and cutters or scissors in the other hand under chandelier light in patients with severe FVP or large breaks; severe and broad adhesion may be treated with localized retinectomy to release traction (please see Chap. 2). SO is used in eyes presenting with multiple large retinal breaks (preexisting or iatrogenic) or possible unfound breaks, eyes undergoing retinotomy or retinectomy, or those with residual vitreoretinal traction; an encircling buckle between the ora serrata and the equator should be placed in more severe cases where residual peripheral traction remains. IVI anti-VEGF can be used at the end of surgery.

The level of surgical difficulty depends on the severity of FVP, the degree of avascular proliferative changes, and the extent of mobility of the detached retina. With modern instruments and techniques, the reattachment rate is greater than 90%, although many patients require SO infusion [2, 3]. The final BCVA depends mainly on the preoperative BCVA, extent of RD, extent of intraoperative retinectomy, and extent of silicone oil use, all of which might be interrelated.

Case examples of CTRRDs with various presentations are shown in Figs. 5.3, 5.4, 5.5, 5.6, 5.7, and 5.8. For MH-induced CTRRD, please see Chap. 12 for details.

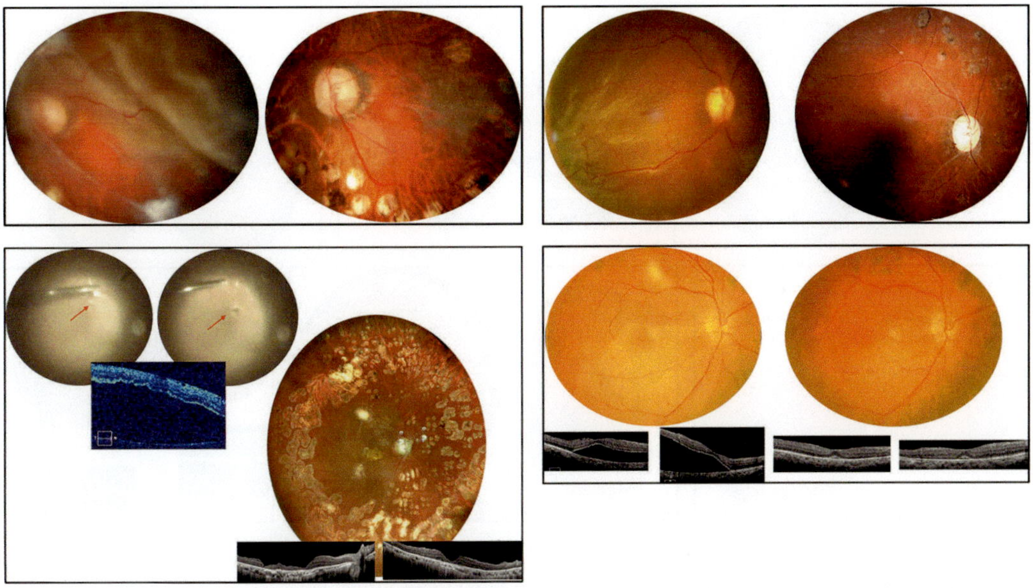

Fig. 5.3 Four sets of CTRRD associated with mild FVP. In each set, preoperative or intraoperative (left) and postoperative (right) images are shown. In the lower left panel, the red arrows point to the break which was found intraoperatively adjacent to an FVP patch (two intraoperative video images on the upper left). (Courtesy of Dr. Chung-May Yang)

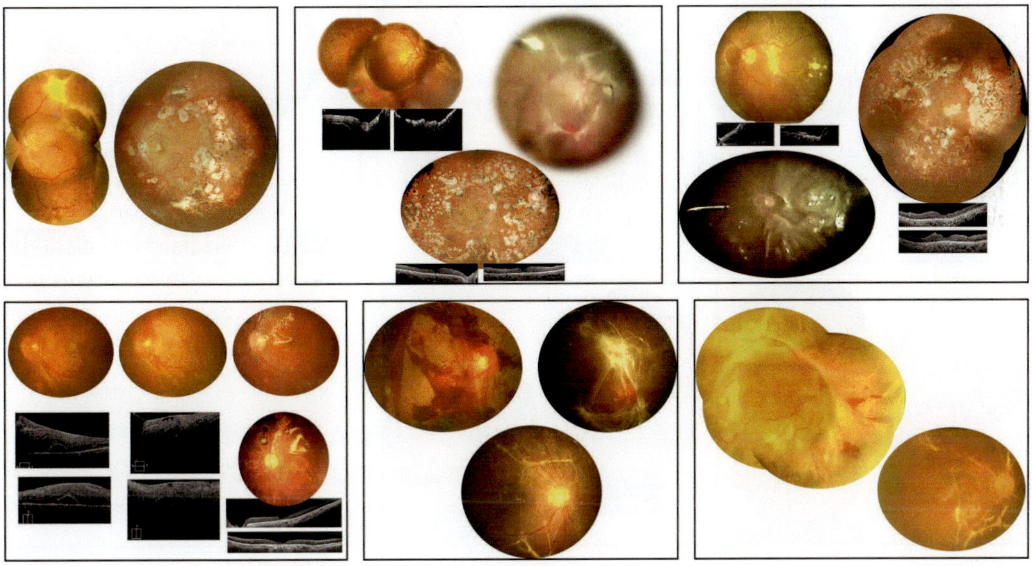

Fig. 5.4 Six sets of CTRRDs associated with moderate FVP. In the upper three panels, pre- and postoperative images are shown; the upper middle and right sets also show intraop wide-angle video images. In the lower left and lower middle panels, the progression of active FVP to CTRRD is shown; postop images are shown in the lower right (lower left panel) and lower center (lower middle panel) panels. In the lower right panel, vessel sheathing and subretinal bands are noted after surgery (lower right). (Courtesy of Dr. Chung-May Yang)

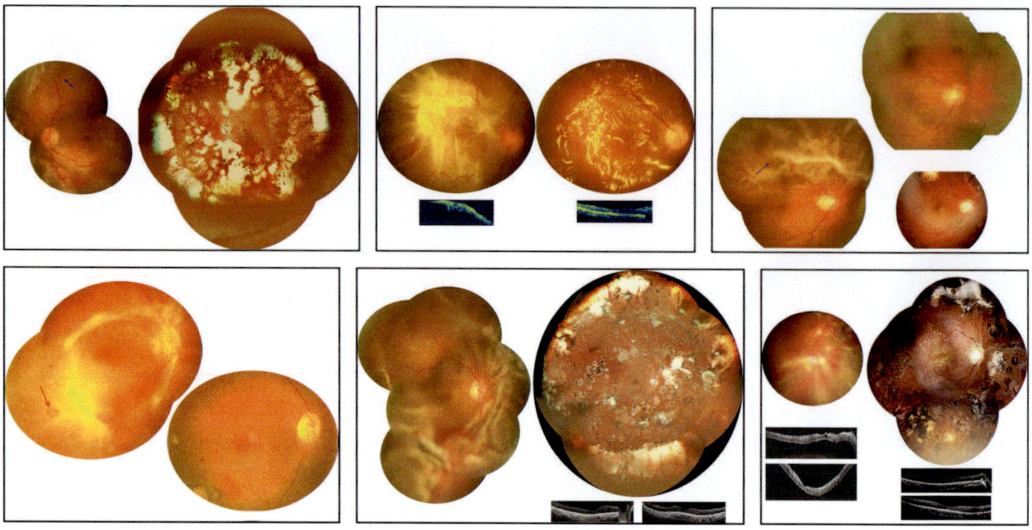

Fig. 5.5 Six sets of combined RD were associated with moderate FVP. In each panel, preop (left) and postop (right) images are shown. The blue arrow (upper left and upper right panel) and red arrow (lower left panel) point to the retinal break. (Courtesy of Dr. Chung-May Yang)

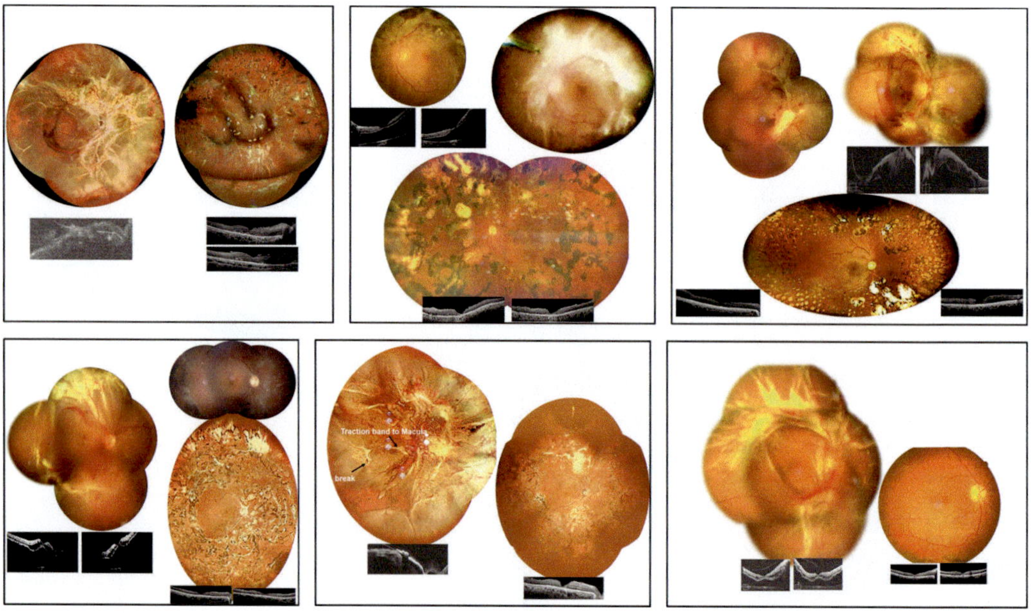

Fig. 5.6 Six sets of combined RD associated with severe FVP. In each panel, preop and postop images are shown. The images in the upper left panel are also shown in Fig. 2.7, Chap. 2. In the upper middle panel, an intraop wide-angle video image is shown (upper right). In the upper right panel, the preoperative progression of retinal changes is shown (upper left and upper right). In the lower center panel, within the wide angle color photo on the left side, the upper black arrow points to a traction band, and the lower black arrow points to the break. (Courtesy of Dr. Chung-May Yang)

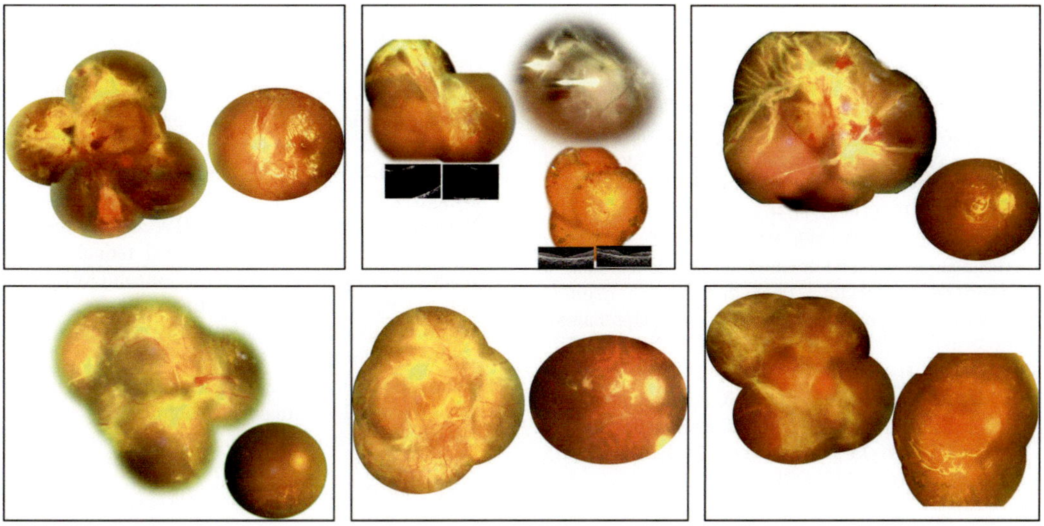

Fig. 5.7 Six additional sets of combined RD associated with severe FVP. In each panel, preoperative (left) and postoperative (right) images are shown. In the upper center panel, an intraoperative composite video image is also shown in the upper right. (Courtesy of Dr. Chung-May Yang)

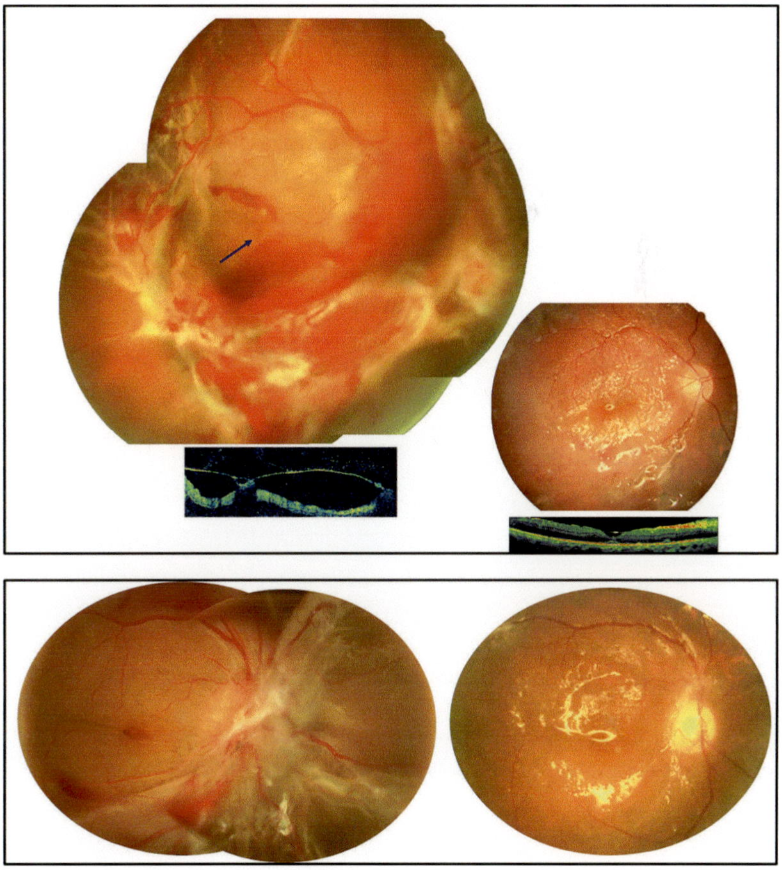

Fig. 5.8 Two sets of CTRRDs with MH. In each panel, preoperative (left) and postoperative (right) images are shown. In the upper panel, the blue arrow points to the MH. Please see Chap. 12 MH in DR for details. (Courtesy of Dr. Chung-May Yang)

References

1. Thompson JT, de Bustros S, Michels RG, Rice TA. Results and prognostic factors in vitrectomy for diabetic traction-rhegmatogenous retinal detachment. Arch Ophthalmol. 1987;105(4):503–7. https://doi.org/10.1001/archopht.1987.01060040073036.
2. Yang CM, Su PY, Yeh PT, Chen MS. Combined rhegmatogenous and traction retinal detachment in proliferative diabetic retinopathy: clinical manifestations and surgical outcome. Can J Ophthalmol. 2008;43(2):192–8. https://doi.org/10.3129/i08-007.
3. Hsu YJ, Hsieh YT, Yeh PT, Huang JY, Yang CM. Combined Tractional and Rhegmatogenous retinal detachment in proliferative diabetic retinopathy in the anti-VEGF era. J Ophthalmol. 2014;2014:917375. https://doi.org/10.1155/2014/917375.
4. Yang CM. Surgical treatment for diabetic retinopathy: 5-year experience. J Formos Med Assoc. 1998;97(7):477–84.
5. Aaberg TM, Abrams GW. Changing indications and techniques for vitrectomy in management of complications of diabetic retinopathy. Ophthalmology. 1987;94(7):775–9. https://doi.org/10.1016/s0161-6420(87)33528-6.
6. Arevalo JF, Maia M, Flynn HW Jr, Saravia M, Avery RL, Wu L, et al. Tractional retinal detachment following intravitreal bevacizumab (Avastin) in patients with severe proliferative diabetic retinopathy. Br J Ophthalmol. 2008;92(2):213–6. https://doi.org/10.1136/bjo.2007.127142.
7. Jonas JB, Schmidbauer M, Rensch F. Progression of tractional retinal detachment following intravitreal bevacizumab. Acta Ophthalmol. 2009;87(5):571–2. https://doi.org/10.1111/j.1755-3768.2008.01225.x.

6 Silicone Oil Use in Primary Diabetic Vitrectomy

Abstract

Despite advances in vitreoretinal surgery for the treatment of severe proliferative diabetic retinopathy (PDR), serious postoperative complications, such as recurrent retinal detachment (RD), neovascular glaucoma (NVG), and hypotony with subsequent phthisis bulbi, may lead to many cases that are unsalvageable (Shen and Yang, Eur J Ophthalmol 17:954–960, 2007; Chen et al., Graefes Arch Clin Exp Ophthalmol, 2023; Eliott et al., Retina. Philadelphia, PA: Elsevier Mosby 2438–2442, 2006). Although some of the complications may be reversed by the use of long-term silicone oil (SO) tamponade, SO itself may cause adverse effects, such as severe preretinal proliferation, high intraocular pressure (IOP), and emulsification, requiring eventual SO removal (Shen and Yang, Eur J Ophthalmol 17:954–960, 2007; Tsui et al., Eye (Lond) 34:2307–2314, 2020). The use of SO in DVs has been a controversial issue. The indications and time of its removal have not reached a general consensus among retinal surgeons. Early removal may avoid possible oil-related complications (Shen and Yang, Eur J Ophthalmol 17:954–960, 2007; Tsui et al., Eye (Lond) 34:2307–2314, 2020; Yeo et al., Ophthalmology 94:1109–1113, 1987, Scott et al., Am J Ophthalmol 130:745–750, 2000); however, premature SO removal may increase the possibility of recurrent vitreous hemorrhage (VH), recurrent RD, and phthisis bulbi (Shen and Yang, Eur J Ophthalmol 17:954–960, 2007; Tsui et al., Eye (Lond). 34:2307–2314, 2020; McCuen and Rinkoff, Arch Ophthalmol 107:677–682, 1989; Heimann et al., Graefes Arch Clin Exp Ophthalmol 227:152–156, 1989). Furthermore, the removal of SO may increase the risk of sudden visual loss in rare cases. In this chapter, we discuss the indications and complications of SO tamponade and removal, as well as the proper duration of SO removal.

6.1 Case Report

This 33-year-old man had a history of DM and hypertension for 10 years and was under oral medication control. He underwent vitrectomy for PDR in his left eye for complications of PDR at another hospital. He complained of blurred vision in the right eye for 4 months. On examination, best-corrected visual acuity (BCVA) was 0.02 in the right eye, and NLP in the left eye. Severe band keratopathy was noted in the left eye. Fundus examinations of the right eye revealed severe active fibrovascular proliferation (FVP) around the disc, nasal to the disc and in the lower arcade, extending to the midperiphery, and VH. Macular detachment with a prominent horizontal macular

C.-M. Yang, *Surgery for Complications of Diabetic Retinopathy*,
https://doi.org/10.1007/978-981-96-2848-3_6

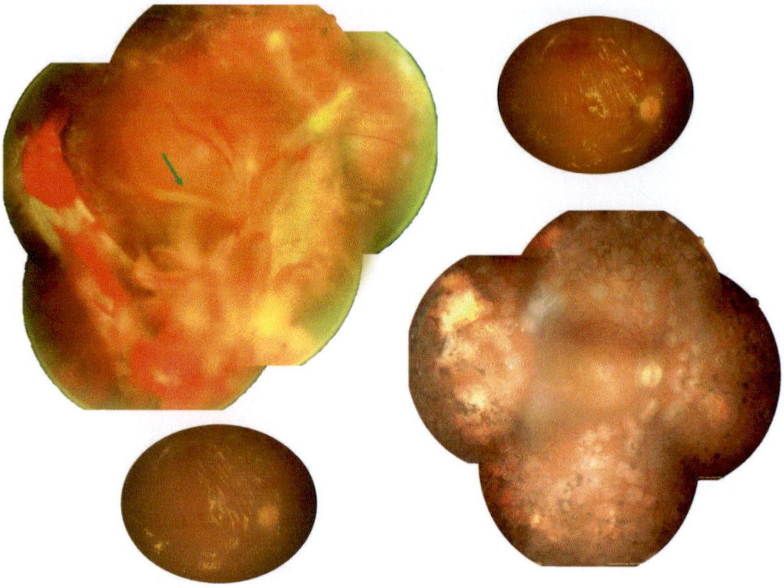

Fig. 6.1 Preoperative composite color photograph showing the FVP, VH, and TRD; the green arrow points to the prominent macular fold (upper left composite color photo). Thin and scattered preretinal blood under SO was noted in the early preoperative period (upper right color photo). The blood gradually disappeared (lower left color photo). After cataract surgery and SO removal, the retina remained attached (lower right composite color photo). (Courtesy of Dr. Chung-May Yang)

fold was also noted. He underwent vitrectomy, FVP tissue removal, PRP, SB for 360 degrees, and IVI of Avastin. Several iatrogenic breaks in different quadrants were made during surgery. SO infusion was performed. The retina reattached after surgery. Thin and scattered hemorrhagic patches, which gradually reabsorbed, were noted in the first week after surgery. He underwent cataract surgery and SO removal 2 years later. Her BCVA improved to 0.3 (Fig. 6.1).

6.2 Silicone Oil Use in Primary Diabetic Vitrectomy

In the surgical treatment of complicated PDR, SO may be used for long-term tamponade [1, 2, 3, 5–7]. In addition to early visual rehabilitation, the use of SO in PDR has the advantages of maintaining retinal attachment, lowering the rate and severity of recurrent bleeding, and reducing the possibility of RI [1, 2, 3, 4, 6–9]. However, SO may also be associated with adverse effects, including retinal ischemia, glaucoma, corneal edema, cataract formation, and peri-SO reproliferation [1, 3, 10–13]. In principle, the use of SO should be as conservative as possible.

The indications for SO injection are (1) severe proliferation in four quadrants with fibrovascular tissue extending beyond the equator in more than two quadrants and (2) the presence of residual traction or multiple breaks in different quadrants with suspected missed breaks after membrane dissection. (3) Large retinectomy was performed [1, 2, 3, 6, 7, 14]. Under these conditions, without long-term tamponade, the possibility of redetachment is high. Although SO removal on a later day is the general practice, some patients require permanent SO tamponade. The reasons for retaining SO include the following: the retina is judged not suitable for SO removal for fear of redetachment or hypotony; prominent RI with or without NVG is present; the visual potential is light perception or less; the duration of SO tamponade is too short; and finally, the patients opt not to undergo further surgery.

Intravitreal SO may affect the eye in several ways. Preretinal blood under SO is a common occurrence after surgery, resulting from retained blood at the end of the surgery or from postoperative recurrent bleeding. Because blood and the factors contained within it have been shown to be potent stimuli for cellular proliferation and SO may sequester these proliferation-stimulating factors in the space between the retina and the oil, preretinal blood may become an important source for peri-silicone oil proliferation, which is a major cause of surgical failure. On the other

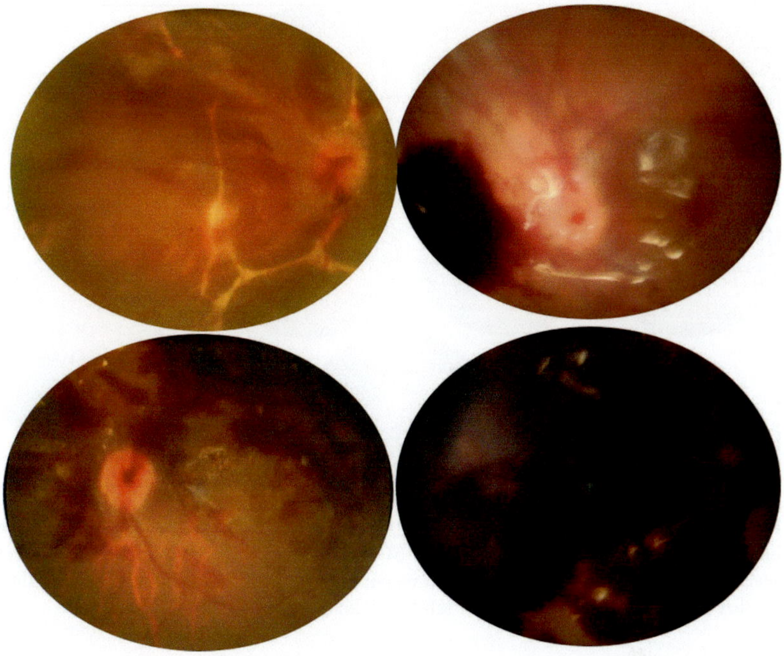

Fig. 6.2 Different severities of preretinal blood under SO. Thin and scattered patterns (upper left); thick and localized patterns (upper right); thick and scattered patterns (lower left); thick and confluent pattern (lower right). (Courtesy of Dr. Chung-May Yang)

hand, the mechanical effect and the compartmentalization of various factors, including anticoagulant factors, provided by SO may limit the frequency or severity of recurrent hemorrhage. Approximately 20% of patients with or without anti-vascular endothelial growth factor (VEGF) pretreatment had detectable recurrent hemorrhage under SO [6]. Maximal blood distributed in thin and scattered patterns (Grade 1), thick and localized patterns (Grade 2), or thick and scattered patterns (Grade 3) developed within 1 week after surgery and was largely reabsorbed within a month with improved postoperative vision. Thick and confluent blood extending to the midperiphery (Grade 4) resulted in severe fibrosis and detachment (Fig. 6.2) [7].

In most cases, reabsorption of the blood under the SO will not cause significant complications; however, in certain cases, a thick blood clot may evolve into a thick contractile fibrotic plaque. Visual function may be affected if the macula is involved. In rare instances, repeated hemorrhage under SO may occur and rapidly transform to fluffy, sticky, fibrin-like material. If SO is not removed promptly, RDs will soon develop, resulting in surgical failure (Figs. 6.3, 6.4, 6.5, and 6.6).

The amount of blood clots during surgery may directly influence the severity of preretinal blood after surgery. Apart from the judicious use of anticoagulants before surgery and careful intraoperative manipulations, presurgical anti-VEGF therapy has been advocated and shown to decrease intraoperative bleeding in patients with active NV [2, 6, 7, 14–16]. The effect of bevacizumab may be particularly beneficial in the treatment of severe active FVP, which is usually present in eyes with SO tamponade. Massive bleeding during surgery before the proper release of traction and peri-silicone oil proliferation after surgery are major causes of surgical failure [1, 6, 7, 17, 18]. Reproliferation is likely to occur in the presence of significant preretinal bleeding. Therefore, it is crucial to reduce intraoperative and postoperative preretinal hemorrhage during complicated diabetic vitrectomy with SO infusion. Our study showed that in eyes with severe active FVP, i.e., broad vitreous attachment around the disc and vascular arcade and extending to the periphery in at least 2 quadrants (≥grade 5 according to Eliott's grading system) [19], bevacizumab may significantly reduce the severity of intraoperative and postoperative bleeding (Fig. 6.3). Our observation revealed

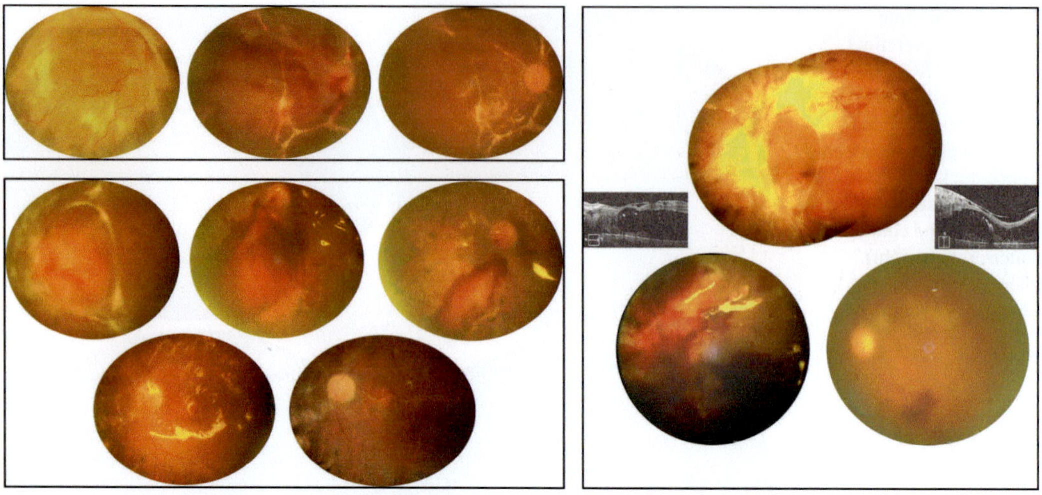

Fig. 6.3 Three examples of reabsorption of preretinal blood of different severity grades under SO. Thin and scattered blood is shown in the upper left panel; thick and localized blood is shown in the lower left panel; and thick and confluent blood is shown in the right panel. No significant complications developed during the reabsorption process in any of the three patients. (Courtesy of Dr. Chung-May Yang)

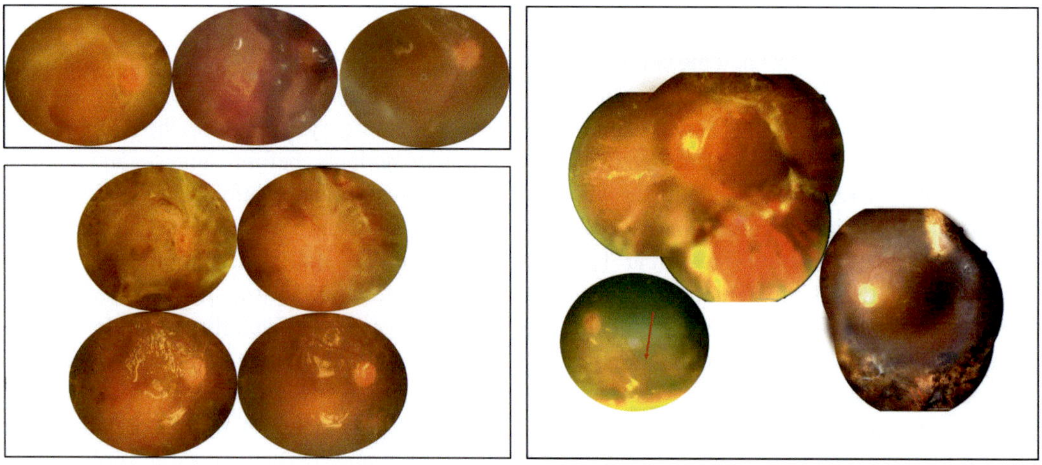

Fig. 6.4 Another three examples of reabsorption of preretinal blood of different severity grades under SO. Thick and localized blood is shown in the upper left panel and the right panel; thin and scattered blood is shown in the lower left panel. The red arrow in the right panel points to thick blood. However, no significant complications were noted during the blood reabsorption process. (Courtesy of Dr. Chung-May Yang)

that bevacizumab may induce new vessel constriction within 1 day after treatment. One week after injection, the proliferative tissue became fibrosis-like in appearance with a marked decrease in vascularity. In addition, the calibers of the major and secondary branches of the normal retinal vessels decreased (Fig. 6.4). This change indicates that decreased flow in the new vessels may slow the entire retinal circulation [6]. These hemodynamic changes in the retinal circulation greatly reduce the likelihood of intraoperative bleeding.[55] Anti-VEGF agents may also induce fibrovascular tissue contraction. Although this effect may not be obvious in eyes with mild to moderate proliferation, in severe active fibrovascular proliferation it may result in more severe RD. This complication especially tends to occur in eyes where the FVP forms a full

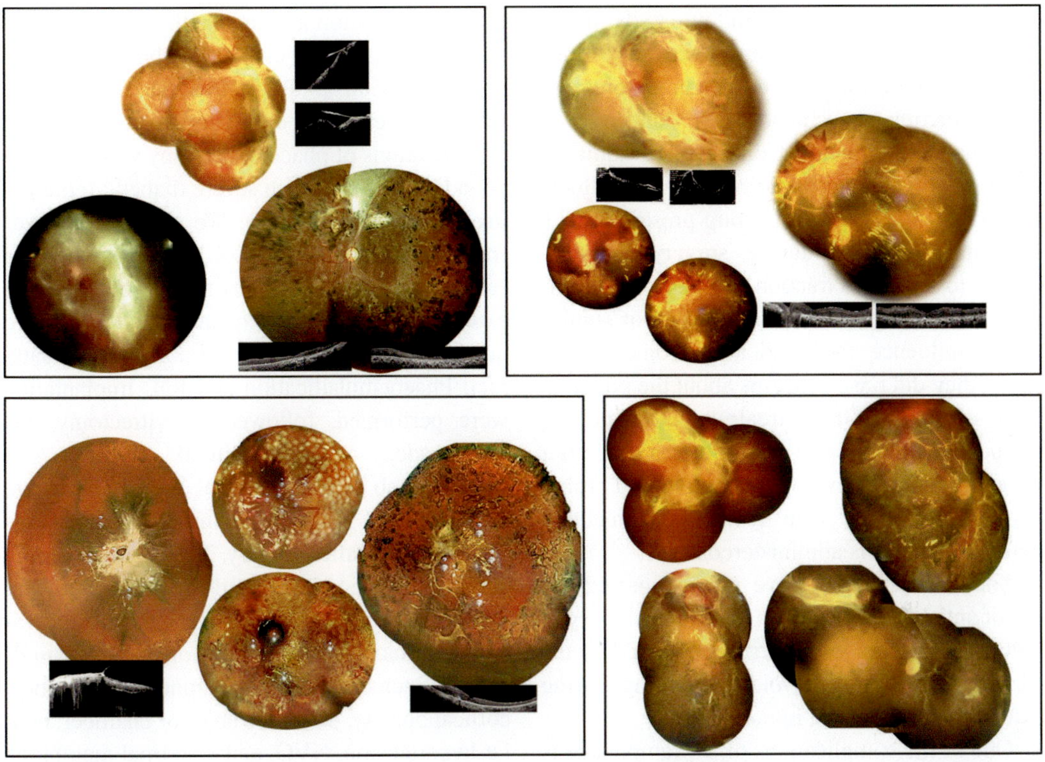

Fig. 6.5 Four examples of preretinal fibrosis after reabsorption of preretinal blood under SO. In the upper left panel, the preoperative composite color photo and OCT images are shown on the upper panel, and the intraoperative video image is shown on the lower left panel. A large fibrotic plaque was noted under the SO after preretinal blood reabsorption. Cataract surgery and SO removal were performed, and the retina remained attached (lower right wide angle color photo and OCT images). The other three panels show preoperative color images with or without OCT images, the evolution of blood and the development of preretinal fibrosis. In the lower right panel, the sequential composite color photos show the retinal changes before surgery (upper left), under SO (upper right and lower left), and after SO removal (lower right). (Courtesy of Dr. Chung-May Yang)

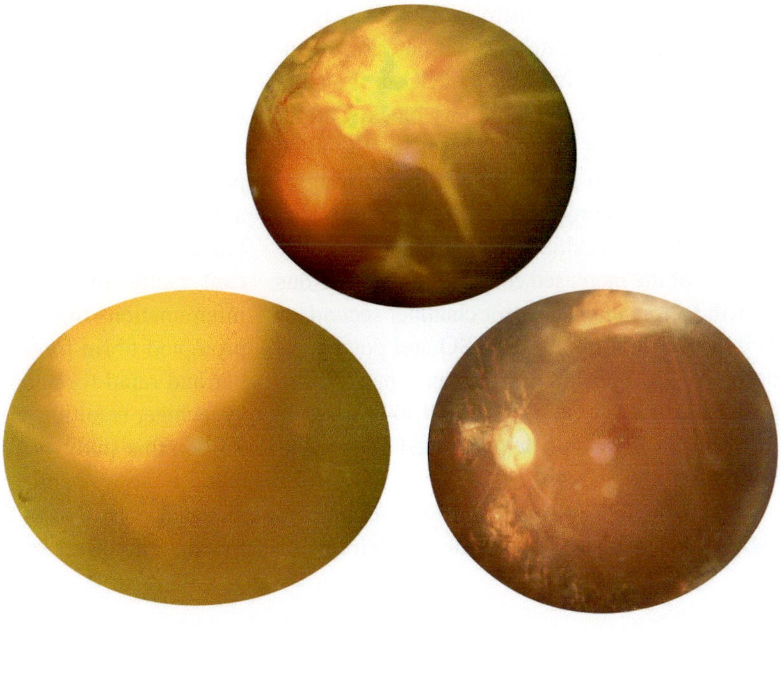

Fig. 6.6 This patient had CTRRD preoperatively (upper). After surgery with SO infusion, the preretinal blood changed to a large yellow fibrin-like clot/mass (lower left). SO removal, partial removal of the mass with scissors and cutters, and SO reinfusion were performed. Cataract surgery and SO removal were subsequently performed. The retina was reattached (lower left), but the BCVA was counting fingers at 50 cm. Please see Chap. 17, Fig. 17.8. (Courtesy of Dr. Chung-May Yang)

circle around the arcade. In our study of 22 patients in which vitrectomy was performed 7–9 days after intravitreal bevacizumab pretreatment, traction detachment was converted to combined detachment in one eye. In addition, more patients in the bevacizumab pretreatment group than in the control group presented with subretinal bleeding during surgery, possibly related to increased traction and microbreak formation. Although these changes did not significantly influence the surgical outcome in our study, they did raise concerns about the potential harm of anti-VEGF pretreatment. Considering the possible increase in traction over time after drug injection, in severe FVP, one should probably not wait more than 1 week postinjection before treatment is administered.

Some investigators have also suggested the use of anti-VEGF therapy at the end of surgery to reduce postoperative hemorrhage induced by the early growth of NV. Avoiding bucking during extubation is of utmost importance.

One of the complications of SO tamponade is increased IOP. An immediate postoperative increase in IOP may be related to SO overfill, choroidal thickening, and anterior rotation of the ciliary body as a result of postoperative inflammation. Choroidal thickening and the incompressible nature of SO, as opposed to long-acting gas tamponade, may result in anterior chamber shallowing and/or pupillary block, leading to a very high IOP. A late increase in IOP may be related to SO migrating into the anterior chamber, significant emulsification of SO in the anterior chamber, NVG, and pupillary block. Careful IOP monitoring is very important for SO-filled eyes. In eyes with pseudophakia, preexisting or created during combined cataract surgery and DV, posterior synechia occurs frequently, partly because of the increased concentration of various growth factors in the anterior chamber secondary to the sequestration effect of SO and postoperative face-down positioning. Because patent laser peripheral iridectomies (PIs) tend to close rapidly, surgical PI should be performed in the presence of pseudophakia.

Patients with PDR are likely to have visually significant cataracts. Because of the high rate of cataract formation and the challenges associated with cataract surgery after PPV, phacovitrectomy has become an attractive treatment option. We retrospectively studied the surgical outcomes and complications of phaco-vitrectomy with SO tamponade in patients with severe diabetic retinopathy (data not published). We enrolled 28 eyes from 28 consecutive PDR patients who had severe proliferation with fibrovascular tissue extending beyond the equator in at least two quadrants, tractional RD, and a significant cataract. Phacoemulsification and IOL implantation were performed, followed by vitrectomy, SO tamponade, and intravitreal injection of bevacizumab (1.0 mg/0.1 mL). The mean age was 53.1 ± 8.1 years. The retinas of all 28 patients were attached after surgery. The logMAR visual acuity improved significantly from 2.28 ± 0.62 preoperatively to 1.80 ± 0.77 1 year postoperatively. Intraoperative and postoperative complications included hyphema, zonule dehiscence, corneal opacity, SO in the anterior chamber, ocular hypertension, NVG, and epiretinal membrane (ERM). Intraoperative PI was performed in 22 eyes. Postoperative IOP increased in 18 eyes (64.29%). Among the five eyes with an IOP greater than 40 mmHg, four did not receive PIs. The percentage of patients with angle-closure glaucoma and postoperatively high IOP elevation was lower in patients who received PIs. The mean postoperative spherical equivalent from 23 available patients was +1.93 ± 2.47 D. Compared with the calculated target refractions, the postoperative refractions showed a hyperopic shift (+3.06 ± 2.36 D).

In this study, we found that the incidence of postoperative IOP elevation was high (>64%). In addition to the usual causes of increased IOP in SO-filled eyes, cataract surgery is another significant factor for increased IOP. The excessive inflammation from the combined procedures prompted fibrin formation in the anterior chamber and rapid formation of 360-degree posterior synechiae, resulting in pupillary block and high IOP. In this study, patients without PIs had difficulty treating pupillary blocks by LI due to repeated occlusion of the iridotomy from severe inflammation. In contrast, eyes with surgical PI had a lower chance of having a postoperative IOP greater than 40 mmHg and early postoperative IOP elevation. Therefore, surgical PI was mandatory in our later cases and is considered an important procedure for preventing pupillary block and reducing IOP elevation in combined surgery. Another important point is the refractive change after the combined procedures. The refractive changes were associated with the refractive index of the IOL material, the posterior radius of the IOL model, and the interface regularity between the posterior capsule and the SO. SO has a greater refractive index ($n = 1.405$) than does the vitreous ($n = 1.336$). A higher refractive index of the SO has a less convergent effect, and the concave SO-IOL interface diverges from the incoming light, leading to a hyperopic shift after surgery. Our previous study revealed a hyperopic shift (+2.89 ± +2.15 D) after cataract surgery in SO-filled eyes [20, 21]. Similarly, in the present study, the mean hyperopic shift was +3.06 ± 2.36 D compared with the predicted refraction. For patients with long-term SO tamponade, postoperative hyperopic shift with high variability should be taken into consideration when choosing the IOL power.

6.3 Indications for Silicone Oil Removal

The indications for SO removal were as follows: (1) massive preretinal blood or fibrin in the early postoperative period, (2) a significant preretinal membrane causing macular structural changes and affecting central vision, (3) a mature cataract or cataract causing a progressive vision decrease, (4) an IOP greater than 25 mmHg lasting for more than 4 weeks despite maximal antiglaucomatous eye drops, (5) progressive corneal endothelial cell loss, (6) significant emulsified SO in the anterior chamber causing decreased vision or increased IOP, (7) a macular hole, and (8) a patient's request in a stable condition [1, 2, 3]. In principle, unless early intervention within a short period of time was needed, at least 9 months were allowed before removing the SO [2, 3]. The main reason is that after surgery for severe PDR, postoperative inflammation is strong, and it usually takes a prolonged period of time to obtain a quiet eye without causing intraocular inflammation. Surgery on an inflamed eye increases the possibility of RI or NVG; hyphema or VH may be more frequent after SO removal.

SO removal is performed by using a standard three-port PPV. The anterior chamber, including the chamber angle, is irrigated to remove SO droplets if necessary. The visually significant cataract is removed, and an intraocular lens is implanted when indicated. Peripheral iridectomy is performed if no patent PI is present to avoid postoperative posterior synechia. The retina is carefully examined after SO removal, and supplemental endolaser is used if previous panretinal photocoagulation has been insufficient. The ERM and internal limiting membrane (ILM) in the macular area are removed to improve structural changes. Repeated air-fluid exchange is performed to remove residual SO, followed by a common dose of IVI anti-VEGF to counter possible early postoperative inflammation-induced RI.

Examples of SO infusion and removal are shown in Fig. 6.7.

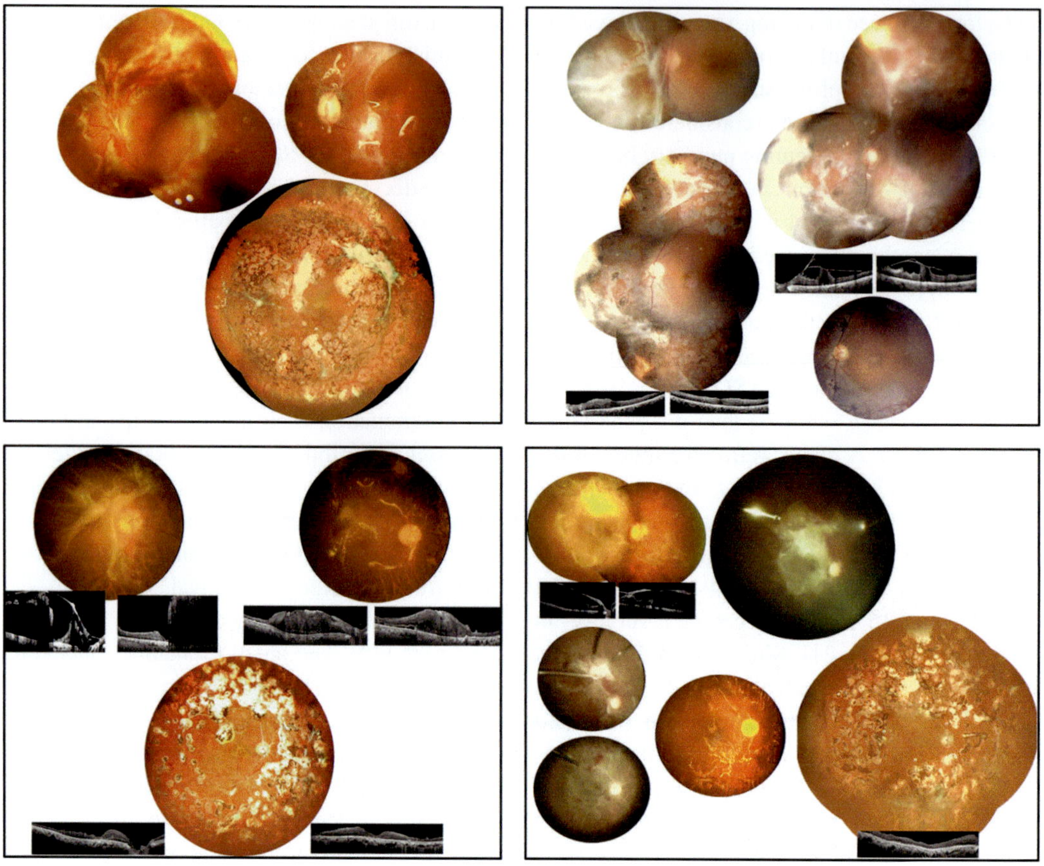

Fig. 6.7 Four examples of preoperative, SO-filled postoperative images, and post-SO-removed images (with or without OCT images). In the upper left, upper right, and lower left panels, preoperative images are shown on the upper left, and SO-filled postoperative images are shown on the upper right. In the upper left and lower left panels, ERM removal was performed during the SO removal surgery. In the lower right panel, 2 bimanual dissection intraoperative video images are shown on the left, and an SO-filled postoperative color image is shown in the lower center. (Courtesy of Dr. Chung-May Yang)

6.4 Complications of Silicone Oil Removal

Retinal redetachment is one of the most serious complications after SO removal. Improvements in surgical techniques and instruments, as well as the use of anti-VEGF agents, may play important roles in lowering the redetachment rate. Furthermore, we believe that SO removal surgery performed after an extended period of SO tamponade may have the advantages of stabilizing the retina, reducing the possibility of excessive postoperative inflammation, and rendering the residual fibrotic tissue less contractile. These advantages may decrease the likelihood of redetachment.

As noted before, one of the concerns of an extended period of SO tamponade in the vitreous cavity is the possibility of ocular hypertension secondary to SO droplets obstructing the trabecular meshwork. Careful monitoring of IOP after SO tamponade is very important.

Intraocular bleeding, including vitreous hemorrhage and hyphema, is an infrequent but significant complication after SO removal since it can affect IOP and markedly delay visual recovery. In our study with prolonged SO tamponade, approximately 5% of eyes had VH, and 3% had hyphema [3]. Patients with VH and hyphema after SO removal in our series had a significantly shorter duration of SO tamponade than those without. This suggests that an extended duration of SO tamponade may prevent postoperative hyphema and VH. As this intraocular bleeding may be related to the formation of NV, under careful IOP monitoring, an extended duration of SO tamponade should be considered for patients with high ischemic drive, which increases the likelihood of NV.

The formation of ERMs under oil is common after vitreoretinal surgery even in the absence of blood. An important feature of ERMs under oil associated with blood clots is the propensity for the formation of thick membranes, fibrotic bands, or plaques and their attachment to retinal blood vessels [2, 3, 7, 22]. Attempting to remove the tissue with forceps peeling at these sites was likely to cause vessel avulsion and bleeding, interfering with the adequate removal of the membrane. Even retinal tears may be created. It is better to partially peel the membrane in the area that is most likely to cause macular structural changes and leave the part untouched at a site close to the retinal vessels. Proper ERM removal may result in gradual normalization of the macular structure. However, we detected significant membrane recurrence in half of the patients who underwent surgery within 3 months, suggesting a persistent, strong, pro-proliferative microenvironment in these eyes. Please refer to Chap. 18 for more discussion of this complication.

References

1. Shen YD, Yang CM. Extended silicone oil tamponade in primary vitrectomy for complex retinal detachment in proliferative diabetic retinopathy: a long-term follow-up study. Eur J Ophthalmol. 2007;17(6):954–60. https://doi.org/10.1177/112067210701700614.
2. Chen SN, Chen SJ, Wu TT, Wu WC, Yang CH, Yang CM. Refining vitrectomy for proliferative diabetic retinopathy. Graefes Arch Clin Exp Ophthalmol. 2023;261:3659. https://doi.org/10.1007/s00417-023-06134-w.
3. Tsui MC, Hsieh YT, Yang CM. Silicone oil removal after extended tamponade in proliferative diabetic retinopathy-a long range of follow-up. Eye (Lond). 2020;34(12):2307–14. https://doi.org/10.1038/s41433-020-0815-2.
4. Yeo JH, Glaser BM, Michels RG. Silicone oil in the treatment of complicated retinal detachments. Ophthalmology. 1987;94(9):1109–13. https://doi.org/10.1016/s0161-6420(87)33328-7.
5. Yang CM. Surgical treatment for diabetic retinopathy: 5-year experience. J Formos Med Assoc. 1998;97(7):477–84.
6. Yeh PT, Yang CM, Lin YC, Chen MS, Yang CH. Bevacizumab pretreatment in vitrectomy with silicone oil for severe diabetic retinopathy. Retina. 2009;29(6):768–74. https://doi.org/10.1097/IAE.0b013e3181a3b7ef.
7. Yeh PT, Yang CM, Yang CH. Distribution, reabsorption, and complications of preretinal blood under silicone oil after vitrectomy for severe proliferative diabetic retinopathy. Eye (Lond). 2012;26(4):601–8. https://doi.org/10.1038/eye.2011.318.
8. Group. TSS. Vitrectomy with silicone oil or sulfur hexafluoride gas in eyes with severe proliferative vitreoretinopathy: results of a randomized clinical trial. Silicone study report 1. Arch Ophthalmol. 1992;110(6):770–9. https://doi.org/10.1001/archopht.1992.01080180042027.
9. Azen SP, Scott IU, Flynn HW Jr, Lai MY, Topping TM, Benati L, et al. Silicone oil in the repair of complex retinal detachments. A prospective observational multicenter study. Ophthalmology. 1998;105(9):1587–97. https://doi.org/10.1016/S0161-6420(98)99023-6.
10. Leaver PK, Gray RH, Garner A. Silicone oil injection in the treatment of massive preretinal retraction. II. Late complications in 93 eyes. Br J Ophthalmol. 1979;63(5):361–7. https://doi.org/10.1136/bjo.63.5.361.
11. Cox MS, Trese MT, Murphy PL. Silicone oil for advanced proliferative vitreoretinopathy. Ophthalmology. 1986;93(5):646–50. https://doi.org/10.1016/s0161-6420(86)33686-8.
12. Casswell AG, Gregor ZJ. Silicone oil removal. I. The effect on the complications of silicone oil. Br J Ophthalmol. 1987;71(12):893–7. https://doi.org/10.1136/bjo.71.12.893.
13. Casswell AG, Gregor ZJ. Silicone oil removal. II. Operative and postoperative complications. Br J Ophthalmol. 1987;71(12):898–902. https://doi.org/10.1136/bjo.71.12.898.
14. Huang CH, Hsieh YT, Yang CM. Vitrectomy for complications of proliferative diabetic retinopathy in young adults: clinical features and surgical outcomes. Graefes Arch Clin Exp Ophthalmol. 2017;255(5):863–71. https://doi.org/10.1007/s00417-016-3579-4.
15. Shih CW, Yang CM, Chen MS, Wang TJ. Intravitreal injection of bevacizumab and gas for diabetic premacular hemorrhage with active fibrovascular proliferation. Graefes Arch Clin Exp Ophthalmol. 2008;246(11):1547–51. https://doi.org/10.1007/s00417-008-0902-8.

16. Yang CM, Yeh PT, Yang CH, Chen MS. Bevacizumab pretreatment and long-acting gas infusion on vitreous clear-up after diabetic vitrectomy. Am J Ophthalmol. 2008;146(2):211–7. https://doi.org/10.1016/j.ajo.2008.04.028.
17. Oyakawa RT, Schachat AP, Michels RG, Rice TA. Complications of vitreous surgery for diabetic retinopathy. I Intraoperative complications. Ophthalmology. 1983;90(5):517–21. https://doi.org/10.1016/s0161-6420(83)34526-7.
18. Lewis H, Burke JM, Abrams GW, Aaberg TM. Perisilicone proliferation after vitrectomy for proliferative vitreoretinopathy. Ophthalmology. 1988;95(5):583–91. https://doi.org/10.1016/s0161-6420(88)33136-2.
19. Eliott D, Lee MS, Abrams G. Proliferative diabetic retinopathy: principles and techniques of surgical treatment. In: Ryan SJ, Hinton DR, Schachat AP, Wilkinson CP, editors. Retina. 4th ed. Philadelphia, PA: Elsevier Mosby; 2006. p. 2413–5.
20. Liu YL, Yang CM, Huang JY, Chen MS, Hou YC. Postoperative hyperopic shift after cataract surgery in silicone oil-filled eyes. Acta Ophthalmol. 2014;92(4):e334–5. https://doi.org/10.1111/aos.12264.
21. Smith RC, Smith GT, Wong D. Refractive changes in silicone filled eyes. Eye (Lond). 1990;4(Pt 1):230–4. https://doi.org/10.1038/eye.1990.32.
22. Hsu YR, Yang CM, Yeh PT. Clinical and histological features of epiretinal membrane after diabetic vitrectomy. Graefes Arch Clin Exp Ophthalmol. 2014;252(3):401–10. https://doi.org/10.1007/s00417-013-2479-0.

7 Premacular Fibrosis, Taut Posterior Hyaloid, and Epiretinal Membrane: General Consideration

Abstract

Premacular membranes with or without connections to the posterior hyaloid (PH) are very common in eyes with nonproliferative diabetic retinopathy (NPDR) or proliferative diabetic retinopathy (PDR). They may cause various macular structural changes, depending on the adhesion pattern and the traction force (Raymond, Ophthalmology 102:406–411, 1995; Carpineto et al., Retina 39:1061–1065, 2019, Tsui et al., Sci Rep 11:23839, 2021; Hsia et al., J Ophthalmol 2022:3156642, 2022; Pendergast et al., Am J Ophthalmol 130:178–186, 2000). The manifestations and optimal surgical approach have not been well investigated. Important features and treatment strategies are briefly discussed in this chapter.

7.1 Case Report

A 57-year-old woman had underlying acute promyelocytic leukemia with complete remission, hypertension, and hyperlipidemia. She also had suffered from type 2 DM for years with retinopathy and neuropathy. She had previously undergone cataract surgery in both eyes. The patient had progressive blurred vision in both eyes for 3–4 years and visited our clinic. On examination, best-corrected visual acuity (BCVA) was 0.05 in both eyes. Fundus examinations showed dense preretinal fibrosis around the disc, covering the nasal side of the macula area in a vertical fashion and extending toward the nasal periphery in the right eye. Subretinal patchy hard exudates were noted in the upper macula. A subretinal band was noted at the upper midperiphery. In the left eye, similar dense preretinal fibrosis was noted around the disc, extending broadly to the nasal side and forming a vertical band covering the nasal side of the macula area. Multiple subretinal fibrotic bands were observed in the upper and lower arcades and on the nasal side. Optical coherence tomography (OCT) revealed a premacular membrane with upper paramacular elevation in the right eye and irregular macular thickening, elevation, and central cysts in the left eye. She underwent vitrectomy with membrane removal in the right eye. The postoperative course was uneventful. Six months later, BCVA remained at 0.05 in both eyes. Fundus examinations revealed an attached retina with a fibrotic band in the upper part of the right eye and diffuse preretinal fibrosis as described above with an extramacular tractional retinal detachment (TRD) in the left eye. Multiple subretinal fibrotic bands persisted in the left eye. She underwent vitrectomy, subretinal band removal, and IVI of 3.5 mL of SO infusion in the left eye. The postoperative course was uneventful. However, BCVA was 0.05 in the right eye but decreased to HM/25 cm in the left eye 7 years later (Fig. 7.1).

C.-M. Yang, *Surgery for Complications of Diabetic Retinopathy*,
https://doi.org/10.1007/978-981-96-2848-3_7

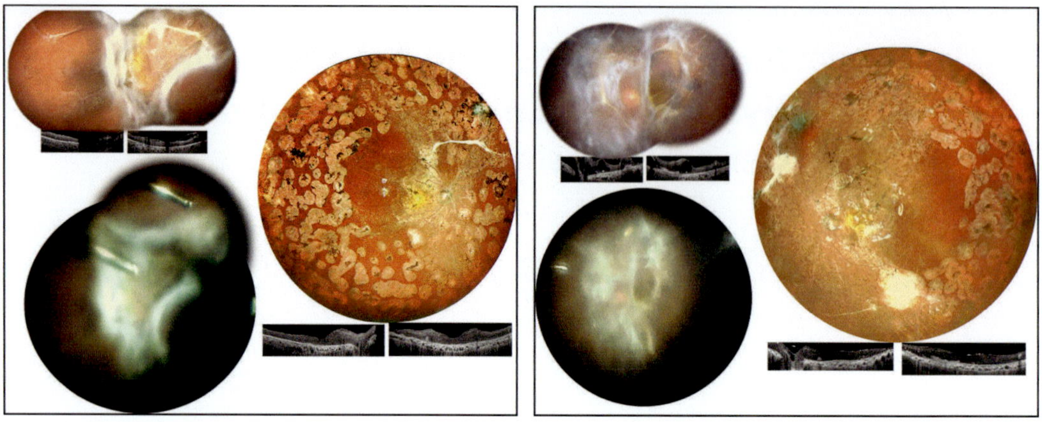

Fig. 7.1 Two sets of images showing pre- and postoperative retinal changes in both eyes of a patient with extensive preretinal fibrosis affecting the macula. In the left panel, dense preretinal fibrosis around the disc on the nasal side of the macula area extending toward the nasal periphery, forming a thick band, and a subretinal band in the upper retina were noted in the right eye. OCT revealed the ERM and paramacular tenting (upper left composite color photo and OCT images; lower left intraoperative composite video image). After surgery, the macular contour improved, the retina was attached, and the subretinal band persisted (right wide angle color photo and OCT images). In the right panel, severe predominantly fibrotic proliferation was observed around the disc, extending broadly to the nasal side and partially covering the nasal side of the macula area. Multiple subretinal fibrotic bands were observed in the upper and lower arcades and on the nasal side. Irregular macular thickening, elevation and central cysts were noted on the OCT images (left upper composite color photo and OCT images and left lower intraoperative video image). After surgery with SO, the retina was attached, and an improved macular structure was noted on the OCT images (right wide angle color photo and OCT images). (Courtesy of Dr. Chung-May Yang)

7.2 Premacular Fibrosis, Taut Posterior Hyaloid, and ERM

Preretinal fibrotic membranes, thickened PH, or epiretinal membranes (ERMs) in DR may cross the macula without causing macular structural changes. Some premacular fibrotic membranes or taut PHs may actually be positioned above the macular surface without any vitreomacular adhesion (VMA) (Fig. 7.2). However, in common scenarios, the membrane either has a VMA at multiple sites or is tightly adherent to the macular surface, causing various macular abnormalities. These changes include central and/or paracentral tenting or thickening with or without cysts; elevation or tenting at multiple points within the macular area; traction macular schisis or detachment; lamellar macular hole (LMH) with surrounding thickening, cysts, or schisis; and MH. It is not unusual to have subfoveal fluid pockets or even large areas of RD, especially in MH or TRD [1–5]. Taut PH- or ERM-associated diabetic macular edema (DME), tractional macular schisis (TMS), LMH, and MH are discussed in other chapters.

The macular abnormalities from traction of thickened preretinal tissue (including preretinal fibrotic membrane, thickened PH, and ERM) may be observed in NPDR or PDR. In PDR, these thickened membranes may be the major vitreoretinal abnormalities or may be associated with a widespread fibrovascular proliferation (FVP). In the latter condition, the FVP is usually long standing, predominantly fibrotic, and is situated either outside the arcade or distributed around the macula. Although DR may be chronic, macular changes may progressively worsen, from a normal contour to thickening and even to TRD (Figs. 7.3 and 7.4).

When structural changes are significant and visual function is impaired, surgery may be indicated. If the thickened preretinal tissue is the major abnormality, the surgical aim is to release the macular traction by PH and ERM removal. The operation is usually straightforward. After PH and ERM removal, ILM peeling should be performed to prevent membrane recurrence. In

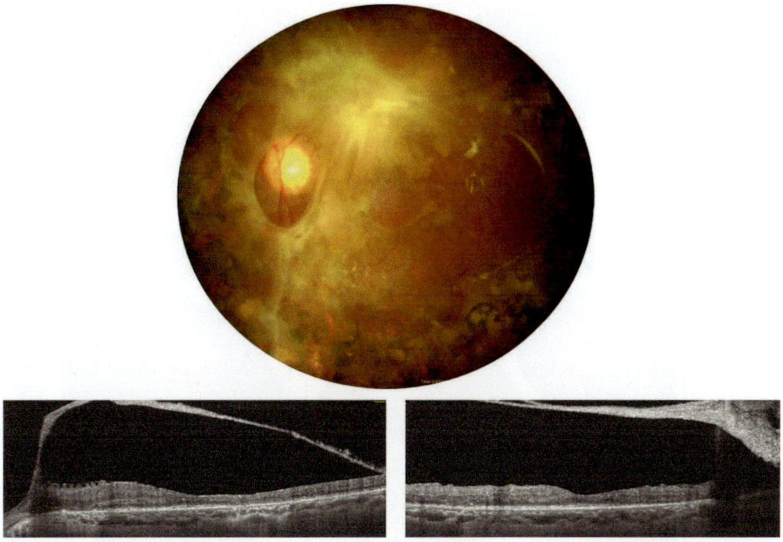

Fig. 7.2 This patient had moderate predominantly fibrotic proliferation around the disc and in the upper arcade. OCT images revealed a thick premacular membrane covering the macula without causing significant macular structural changes. (Courtesy of Dr. Chung-May Yang)

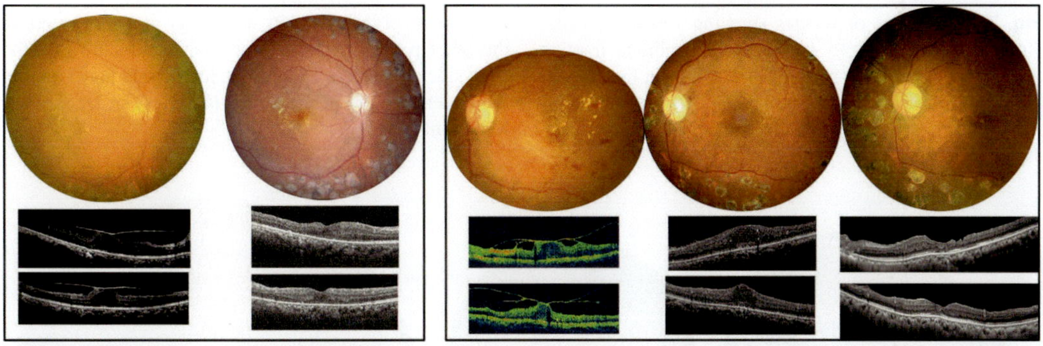

Fig. 7.3 Two examples of a premacular membrane as the major pathological change. In the two patients, no significant FVP was observed; paramacular hard exudates were noted on the right side. A thickened premacular membrane causes foveal tenting on the left side, and a multilayered membrane causes foveal and parafoveal tenting on the right side (left column in both panels). After surgery, the patient's condition greatly improved (right column in the left panel; center and right column in the right panel). (Courtesy of Dr. Chung-May Yang)

many cases, however, the PH remains attached to the midperiphery. Caution should be exercised when midperipheral PVD induction is attempted because unexpected VR adhesion may be encountered. Forceful suction may induce retinal breaks.

If the thickened premacular tissue is part of a more extensive FVP, whether the FVP outside the macular area should be removed is a judgment by the surgeon. If the FVP membranes are quiescent, in the midperiphery, and highly adherent, they should be left untouched even if there is TRD outside the macula caused by these membranes. Any break induced in the face of unreleased traction can cause severe postoperative complications (Fig. 7.5). On the other hand, if the FVP is prominent in or near the posterior retina, it should be removed. Nonetheless, if surgery to completely remove the proliferative tissue is too complicated, minimal manipulation to release the macular traction may be an option. For more detail on minimal membrane removal, please see Chap. 1. For other vitreomacular interface disorders observed in DR, please see other chapters.

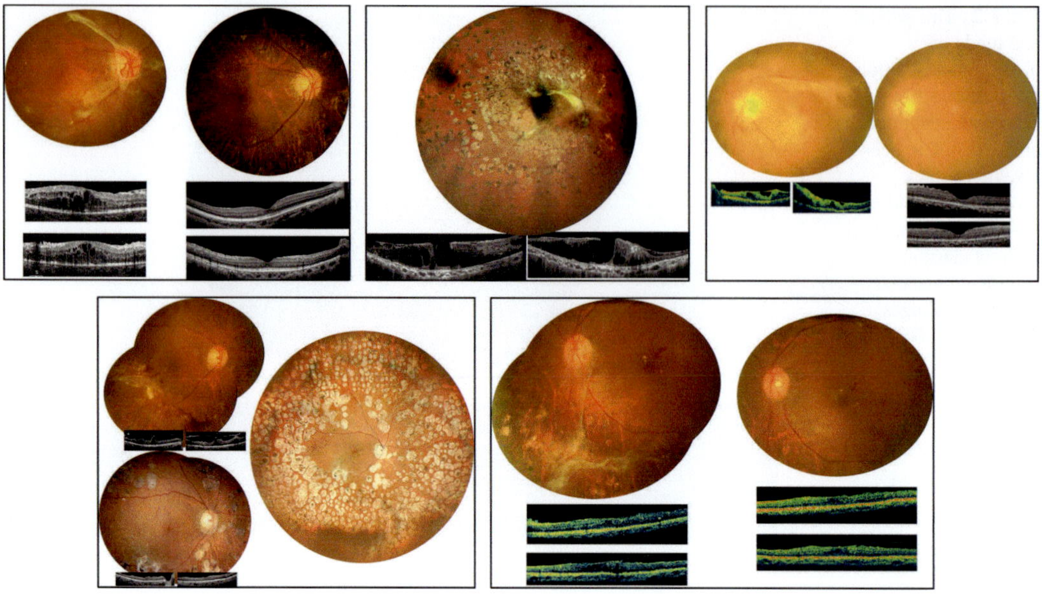

Fig. 7.4 Five sets of images showing various macular structural changes from premacular membrane traction associated with mild to moderate FVP. Except for the case in the lower left panel, all other patients had predominantly fibrotic proliferation. In the upper center panel, because of very poor vision, no surgery was performed. In the other panels, postoperative images are shown on the right side (upper left, upper right, lower right panels) or on the lower left (lower left panel). (Courtesy of Dr. Chung-May Yang)

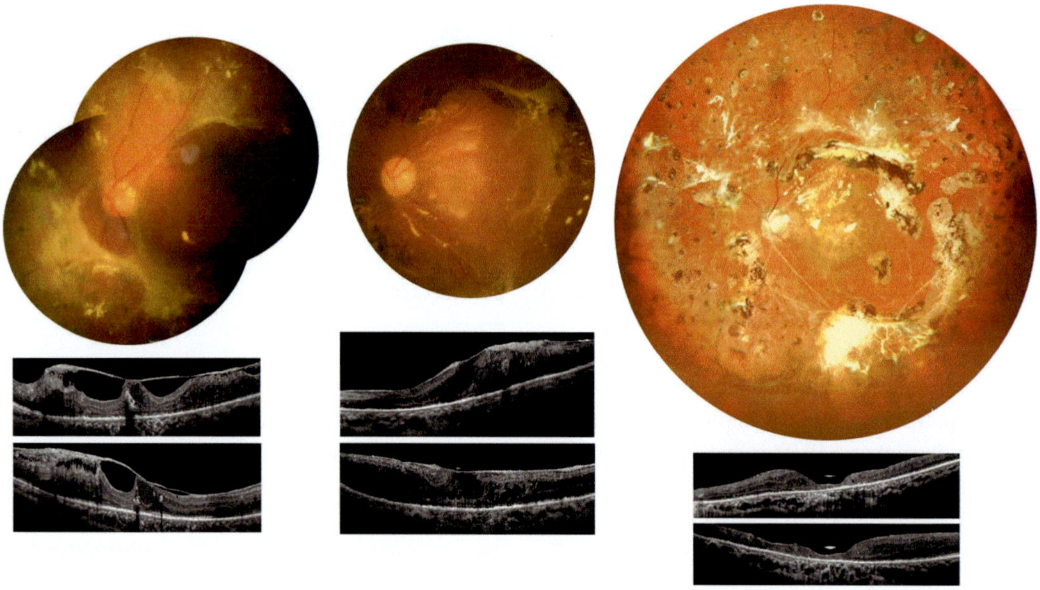

Fig. 7.5 This is a case of premacular membrane-induced macular and paramacular thickening and tenting in the left eye. Extensive fibrotic membranes were noted in the nasal and upper arcades (left color photo and OCT images). Her BCVA was 0.1. During surgery, total removal of FVP tissue was attempted, and retinal breaks at multiple sites were induced. To prevent postoperative RD, SO was injected. After surgery, reproliferation was noted under SO (center color photo and OCT images). Repeated surgery was performed. Although the macular contour improved, an atrophic fovea was noted (right wide angle color photo and OCT images). The BCVA remained at 0.05. (Courtesy of Dr. Chung-May Yang)

References

1. Duker JS, Kaiser PK, Binder S, de Smet MD, Gaudric A, Reichel E, et al. The international vitreomacular traction study group classification of vitreomacular adhesion, traction, and macular hole. Ophthalmology. 2013;120(12):2611–9. https://doi.org/10.1016/j.ophtha.2013.07.042.
2. Hsieh YT, Yang CM. Vitreomacular traction in diabetic retinopathy. Jpn J Ophthalmol. 2023;68(1):12–8. https://doi.org/10.1007/s10384-023-01034-2.
3. Panozzo G, Cicinelli MV, Augustin AJ, Battaglia Parodi M, Cunha-Vaz J, Guarnaccia G, et al. An optical coherence tomography-based grading of diabetic maculopathy proposed by an international expert panel: The European school for advanced studies in ophthalmology classification. Eur J Ophthalmol. 2020;30(1):8–18. https://doi.org/10.1177/1120672119880394.
4. Su CC, Yang CH, Yeh PT, Yang CM. Macular tractional retinoschisis in proliferative diabetic retinopathy: clinical characteristics and surgical outcome. Ophthalmologica. 2014;231(1):23–30. https://doi.org/10.1159/000355078.
5. Cheng CY, Hsieh YT, Yang CM. Broad vitreomacular attachment induced macular hole: structural changes and surgical outcome. Retina. 2023;44:627. https://doi.org/10.1097/IAE.0000000000004018.

8 Diabetic Macular Edema with or without Epiretinal Membrane

Abstract

The standard treatment for diabetic macular edema (DME) is medical treatment. The most widely performed modality is antivascular endothelial growth factor (anti-VEGF) injection alone or in combination with intravitreal or posterior subtenon steroids and/or lasers, either in a grid or focal pattern with regular or micropulse regimens (Schmidt-Erfurth et al., Ophthalmologica 237:185–222, 2017). Vitrectomy with membrane peeling for macular edema associated with a taut posterior hyaloid has been advocated and has become a consensus among retinal surgeons (Lewis et al., Ophthalmology 99:753–759, 1992; Harbor et al., Am J Ophthalmol 121:405–1413, 1996; Pendergast et al., Am J Ophthalmol 130:178–186, 2000; Kimura et al., Retina 25:454–461, 2005). Surgical treatment for intractable DME without visible epiretinal membranes (ERMs) on optical coherence tomography (OCT) has been debated (Kimura et al., Retina 25:454–461, 2005; Rosenblatt et al., Graefes Arch Clin Exp Ophthalmol 243:20–25, 2005; Yamamoto et al., Am J Ophthalmol 135:14–19, 2003; Ghassemi et al., J Curr Ophthalmol 28:199–205, 2016). The pathophysiology of ME caused by the vitreous and the indications and timing of surgery for eyes with DME unresponsive to anti-VEGF or steroids will be briefly discussed in this chapter.

8.1 Case Report

This patient was a 64-year-old man who had DM for 20 years. He also had HT and a history of cerebrovascular accidents. His latest HbA1c was recorded as 7%. His ophthalmic history revealed DR with macular edema in both eyes. He received 7 IVIs of anti-VEGF in both eyes, but vision did not improve. Panretinal photocoagulation (PRP) was administered during follow-up. Sequential OCT revealed persistent ME with ERM formation in the right eye and spontaneous partial ERM separation in the central macular area of the left eye. On examination, BCVA was 0.1 in the right eye and 0.16 in the left eye. The anterior segment was unremarkable in both eyes. Fundus examinations revealed artery attenuation, scattered hard exudates in the macular area, dot and blot hemorrhages mainly in the superior arcade in the right eye, and a 1× 1.5 disc diameter vertically oriented macular scar in the left eye. PVD was present, as evidenced by the presence of a Weiss ring and a scattered PRP scar at the periphery in both eyes. He underwent pars plana vitrectomy with ERM and ILM peeling in the right eye. After surgery, the ME improved. There was one episode of macular edema in the right eye, which was controlled by a single IVI Avastin injection. Follow-up OCT

C.-M. Yang, *Surgery for Complications of Diabetic Retinopathy*,
https://doi.org/10.1007/978-981-96-2848-3_8

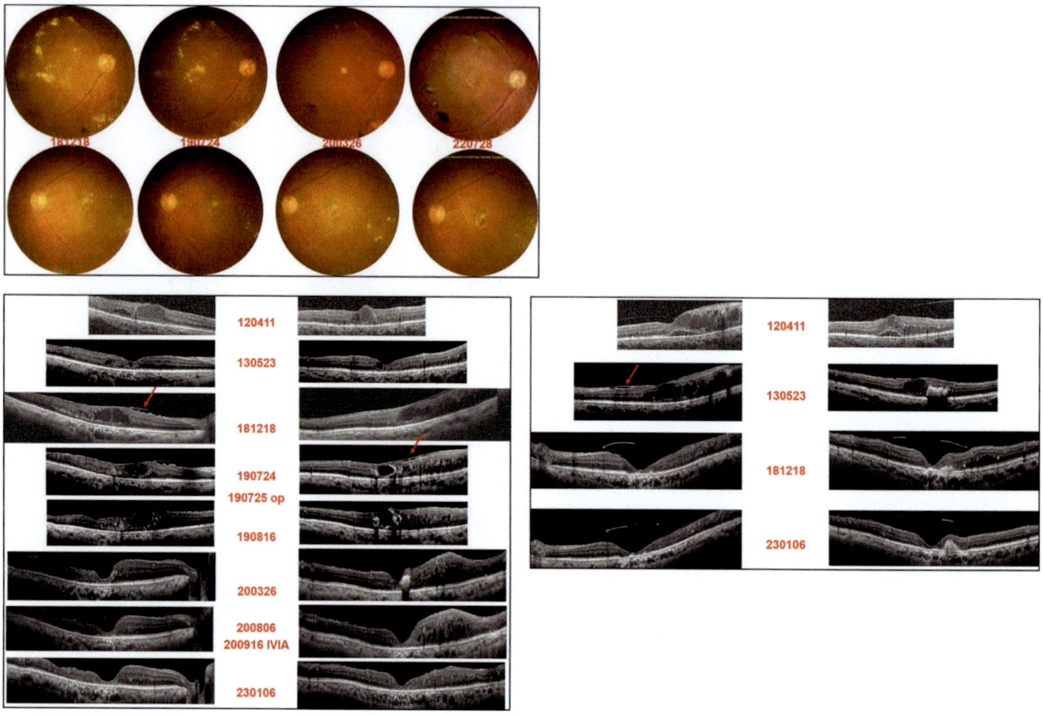

Fig. 8.1 This large image set contains three panels showing sequential color photographs (upper panel) and OCT images (lower two panels) of both eyes of the same patient. Macular edema with subsequent MA was noted in both eyes (upper sequential color photos). The sequential horizontal and vertical OCT images in the lower left and right panels show the evolution of macular edema before and after surgery in the right eye (lower left) and the natural course without surgery in the left eye (lower right). Red arrows point to the ERMs that developed during FU in both eyes. The numbers indicate the date the images were obtained. Please see Chap. 20, Fig. 20.9, right panel. (Courtesy of Dr. Chung-May Yang)

revealed macular atrophy with foveal thinning in the right eye and an ERM with central separation, as well as a para-foveal scar in the left eye. The latest BCVA was 0.1 in the right eye and 0.2 in the left eye (Fig. 8.1).

8.2 Surgical Intervention for DME

Despite the general consensus of IVIs of anti-VEGF as the first-line treatment of choice for DME, several reasons supporting surgical intervention are available. For instance, studies have indicated that diabetic eyes have a thickened ILM compared with nondiabetic eyes, which may cause structural and functional disturbances in water movement between the vitreous and retina [1]. In addition, the posterior hyaloid is thickened and abundant in cells such as fibrocytes, macrophages, and myofibroblast-like cells [2]. The hyalocytes can transform into myofibroblasts, causing the posterior hyaloid to become contractile [3, 4]. Moreover, the vitreous in diabetic eyes contains VEGF and other cytokines that may increase intraocular inflammation. An antiangiogenic shift in the vitreous was observed after vitrectomy in eyes with proliferative diabetic retinopathy (PDR) [5]. All the aforementioned changes are important factors in inducing macular thickening. Hence, some researchers consider pathologic diabetic eyes to be "diabetic vitreoretinopathy." [6] PPV can address these pathological processes in a single setting. Some eyes with DME also have a taut PH or an ERM, and in approximately 10–15% of DME eyes, an ERM may develop during the medical treatment course [7]. Standard treatment may still be initiated or continue since it may remain effective. However, if the DME showed no response after 3–4 IVI injections, surgery to remove the PH or ERM was considered. After surgery, DME usually improves or subsides. Recurrent DME or persistent minor DME may be observed in some patients. Our experience shows that such patients may achieve long-term edema-free status after a limited number of booster IVIs of anti-VEGF and/or steroid injections. In other words, DME may become easier to control after surgery. However, functional recovery may be less obvious than the degree of anatomical improvement. As mentioned, surgery may also be an option for intractable DME even without taut PH or ERMs according to OCT. During surgery, some ERM fragments are inevitably present. Vitrectomy along with ERM and ILM peeling may reverse DME [8] or at least make it easier to control with intravitreal anti-VEGF or steroid injection.

Case examples of pre- and postoperative macular changes are shown in Fig. 8.2.

Several OCT biomarkers indicate more severe DME and may warrant frequent anti-VEGF treatment or even surgery when the medical response is inadequate. These markers include excessive HE (this will be discussed in the next chapter), intracystic hyperreflective material, disorganized inner retinal layers, disruption of both the external limiting membrane (ELM) and the ellipsoid zone, and disrupted septa between cystic spaces [9, 10]. Other markers, such as the pearl necklace sign

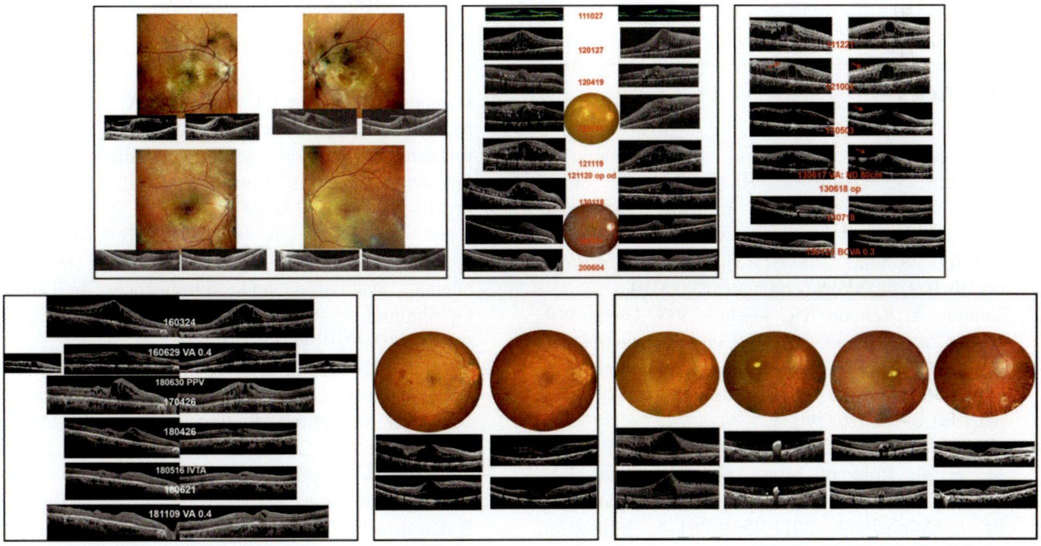

Fig. 8.2 Six sets of images showing good surgical response in DME patients. In the upper left panel, pre- and postoperative color images and OCT images of both eyes are shown. After removal of the taut PH and ILM peeling, the intractable DME improved substantially. In the upper center panel, pre- and postoperative sequential color photos and OCT images show ERM development before surgery, and DME subsided after surgery. In the upper right panel, sequential OCT images show taut PH/ERM development (red arrows) with intractable DME. After surgery, the patient's condition improved. In the upper center and right panels, the numbers in red are the dates of the examinations, procedures performed, or visual acuity level. In the lower left panel, DME with partial PH separation and mild ERM was noted initially (top OCT images). As the PH detached, the ERM became more prominent (second row of OCT images). After surgery, the DME improved but persisted (third and fourth row of OCT images). After IVI of triamcinolone acetonide (TA) once, long-term subsidence of the DME was achieved (in the last two rows of the OCT images). The numbers in white indicate the date of examinations, procedures performed, or visual acuity level. In the lower center panel, DME was associated with vitreomacular attachment without traction (left color photo and OCT images). After surgery, the ME subsided (right color photo and OCT images). In the lower right panel, preoperative color images and OCT images show ME and ERM (left); after anti-VEGF treatment, the ME decreased, but hard exudate accumulated in the central fovea (second column); after ERM and ILM peeling, the HE gradually subsided (two right columns). (Courtesy of Dr. Chung-May Yang)

(hyperreflective dots arranged in a ring-like fashion along the inner wall of the cysts) and cholesterol crystals or hyperreflective crystalline deposits, indicate chronic processes [11, 12]. Patients with these latter biomarkers may not achieve significant functional improvement after surgery.

Recently, pars plana vitrectomy with en bloc removal of the intracystic hyperreflective material has been reported. Mass spectrometry analysis revealed that the content within the cyst was composed of fibrinogen [13]. Macular thickness improved substantially after surgery. Whether a surgical approach can improve vision requires further study.

The effect of a surgically implanted port delivery system (PDS) for the sustained release of anti-VEGF medication on DME requires further study.

References

1. Matsunaga N, Ozeki H, Hirabayashi Y, Shimada S, Ogura Y. Histopathologic evaluation of the internal limiting membrane surgically excised from eyes with diabetic maculopathy. Retina. 2005;25(3):311–6. https://doi.org/10.1097/00006982-200504000-00010.
2. Kampik A, Kenyon KR, Michels RG, Green WR, de la Cruz ZC. Epiretinal and vitreous membranes. Comparative study of 56 cases. Arch Ophthalmol. 1981;99(8):1445–54. https://doi.org/10.1001/archopht.1981.03930020319025.
3. Hata Y, Nakao S, Kohno R, Oba K, Kita T, Miura M, et al. Role of tumor necrosis factor-alpha (TNFalpha) in the functional properties of hyalocytes. Br J Ophthalmol. 2011;95(2):261–5. https://doi.org/10.1136/bjo.2010.190322.
4. Sakamoto T, Ishibashi T. Hyalocytes: essential cells of the vitreous cavity in vitreoretinal pathophysiology? Retina. 2011;31(2):222–8. https://doi.org/10.1097/IAE.0b013e3181facfa9.
5. Yoshida S, Nakama T, Ishikawa K, Arima M, Tachibana T, Nakao S, et al. Antiangiogenic shift in vitreous after vitrectomy in patients with proliferative diabetic retinopathy. Invest Ophthalmol Vis Sci. 2012;53(11):6997–7003. https://doi.org/10.1167/iovs.12-9671.
6. Kroll P, Rodrigues EB, Hoerle S. Pathogenesis and classification of proliferative diabetic vitreoretinopathy. Ophthalmologica. 2007;221(2):78–94. https://doi.org/10.1159/000098253.
7. Kang YK, Park HS, Park DH, Shin JP. Incidence and treatment outcomes of secondary epiretinal membrane following intravitreal injection for diabetic macular edema. Sci Rep. 2020;10(1):528. https://doi.org/10.1038/s41598-020-57509-6.
8. Gandorfer A, Messmer EM, Ulbig MW, Kampik A. Resolution of diabetic macular edema after surgical removal of the posterior hyaloid and the inner limiting membrane. Retina. 2000;20(2):126–33.
9. Venkatesh R, Sangai S, Reddy NG, Sridharan A, Pereira A, Aseem A, et al. Intracystic hyperreflective material in center-involving diabetic macular edema. Graefes Arch Clin Exp Ophthalmol. 2021;259(9):2533–44. https://doi.org/10.1007/s00417-021-05083-6.
10. Campos A, Campos EJ, do Carmo A, Caramelo F, Martins J, Sousa JP, et al. Evaluation of markers of outcome in real-world treatment of diabetic macular edema. Eye Vis (Lond). 2018;5:27. https://doi.org/10.1186/s40662-018-0119-9.
11. Ajay K, Mason F, Gonglore B, Bhatnagar A. Pearl necklace sign in diabetic macular edema: evaluation and significance. Indian J Ophthalmol. 2016;64(11):829–34. https://doi.org/10.4103/0301-4738.195597.
12. Gelman SK, Freund KB, Shah VP, Sarraf D. The pearl necklace sign: a novel spectral domain optical coherence tomography finding in exudative macular disease. Retina. 2014;34(10):2088–95. https://doi.org/10.1097/IAE.0000000000000207.
13. Imai H, Otsuka K, Tetsumoto A, Miki A, Nakamura M. Effectiveness of en bloc removal of fibrinogen-rich component of cystoid lesion for the treatment of cystoid macular edema. Retina. 2020;40(1):154–9. https://doi.org/10.1097/IAE.0000000000002359.

9 Diabetic Macular Edema with Massive Hard Exudates

Abstract

Massive amounts of hard exudates result from severe retinal vascular leakage and may significantly affect vision if they occur in the macular area (Yang, Retina 20:121–125, 2000; Kumagai et al., Retina 29:464–472, 2009; Ferris and Patz, Surv Ophthalmol 28 Suppl:452–461, 1984). Any disease that causes vascular leakage, including hypertension retinopathy, central retinal vein occlusion (CRVO), branch retinal vein occlusion (BRVO), Coats disease, radiation retinopathy, vessel occlusion from autoimmune diseases, etc., may cause the development of massive amounts of exudates. Hard exudates are lipids and proteinaceous materials that deposit within the neurosensory retina and in the subretinal space (Fong et al., Arch Ophthalmol 115:873–877, 1997). In DR, massive HE is always associated with severe diabetic macular edema (DME). Whether medical treatment involving IVI of anti-vascular endothelial growth factor (VEGF)/steroid agents or surgical treatment should be used to treat this condition has not been investigated in depth. The manifestations, indications for surgery, and surgical outcomes will be discussed in this chapter.

9.1 Case Report

A 63-year-old female with hypertension and type 2 DM who had been receiving oral medication for 20 years complained of blurred vision in both eyes for 8 months. She underwent bilateral panretinal photocoagulation (PRP) for proliferative diabetic retinopathy (PDR) and several IVIs of anti-VEGF for DME in both eyes at another hospital; however, her vision did not improve. On examination, best-corrected visaul acuity (BCVA) was 0.1 in the right eye and 0.01 in the left eye. Fundus examinations revealed bilateral diabetic macular edema with massive hard exudates, which was more severe in the left eye. OCT revealed severe edema and macular thickening without taut posterior hyaloid. Pars plana vitrectomy with internal limiting membrane (ILM) peeling, macular focal laser, and supplementary PRP was performed on the left eye. During surgery, heterogeneous ICG staining, indicating the presence of ERMs, was noted. Eight months post surgery, hard exudates resorbed significantly, and VA improved to 0.2 in the left eye. VA of the right eye remained poor (BCVA 0.02) despite repeated IVI bevacizumab injections, posterior subtenon injections of triamcinolone, and macular laser photocoagulation. Hard exudates persisted but decreased in amount in the right eye (Fig. 9.1).

C.-M. Yang, *Surgery for Complications of Diabetic Retinopathy*,
https://doi.org/10.1007/978-981-96-2848-3_9

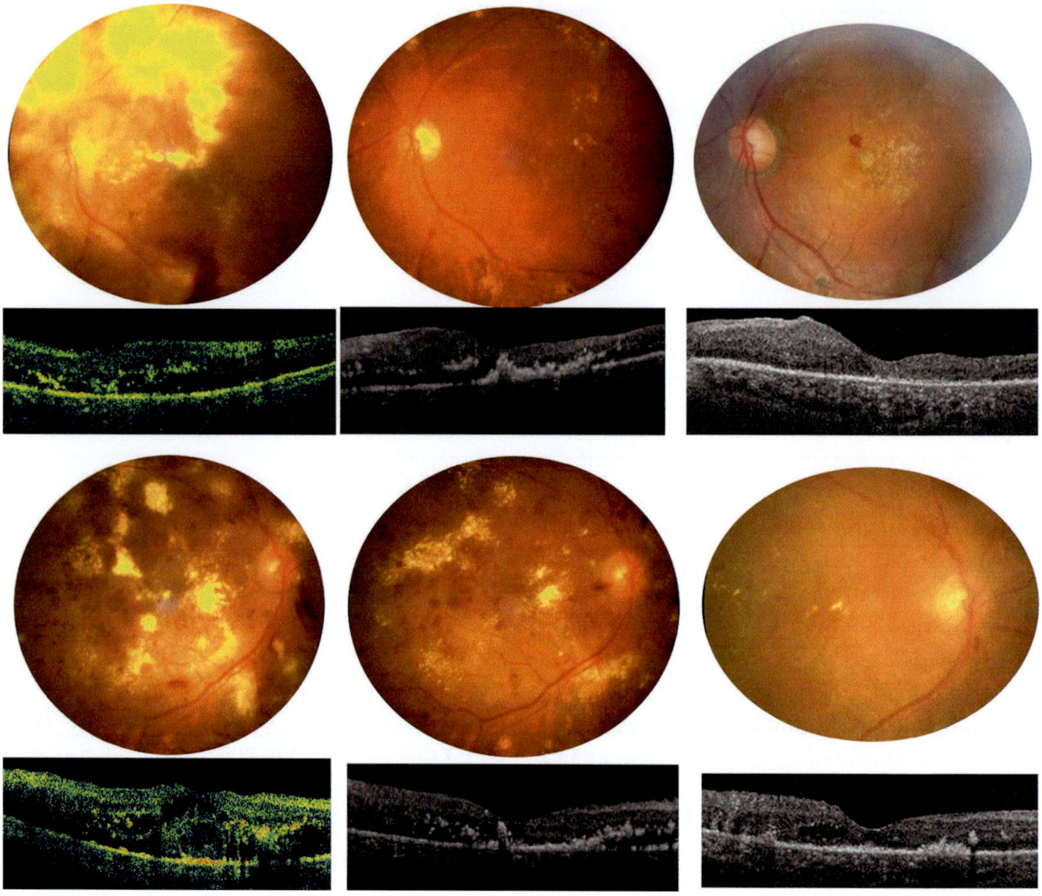

Fig. 9.1 One set of images showing the evolution of DME with massive hard exudates in the left eye (upper two columns) and the right eye (lower two columns). Sequential images were obtained at the same time for both eyes. Surgery was performed in the more severe left eye. OCT images showed severe edema and macular thickening without taut posterior hyaloid in both eyes (second and fourth rows). Postoperatively, hard exudates resorbed significantly in the left eye. Hard exudates persisted but decreased in amount in the right eye (lower two columns). The right eye developed VH later and eventually underwent surgery. (Courtesy of Dr. Chung-May Yang)

9.2 DME with Massive Hard Exudates

DME is a major cause of vision loss in patients with DR. Several treatment modalities, such as focal laser photocoagulation [3, 4], intravitreal or subtenon injection of triamcinolone [5], sustained-release corticosteroid implantation, and IVI of anti-VEGF agents, have been proposed to manage DME. Currently, IVI of anti-VEGF is considered the first-line treatment for DME, whereas IVI of corticosteroids may be considered for pseudophakic eyes or patients at high risk of thromboembolic events [6–8]. Laser treatment continues to play an important role in preventing moderate vision loss in non-center-involving DME patients. Surgical interventions are normally reserved for those with evidence of vitreoretinal traction. Studies have demonstrated that vitrectomy has long-term benefits for diffuse DME, even for those without a thickened and taut posterior hyaloid (please see Chap. 8). In addition, vitrectomy combined with ILM peeling has shown favorable anatomical and functional outcomes [9].

DME with massive hard exudates is a severe form of DME; it usually indicates excessive leakage and is considered a poor visual prognostic factor. Massive amounts of hard exudates tend to deposit in the foveal area and form submacular fibrotic plaques, causing damage to photoreceptors with irreversible central visual loss [2, 10]. Although medical and surgical treatments have been proposed for enhancing the resolution of exudates [11–17], this disease remains a major challenge. We have reported that pars plana vitrectomy (PPV) with posterior hyaloid removal, focal macular endolaser, and PRP can reduce massive amounts of macular exudates [1]. In addition, ILM peeling can remove the tangential traction exerted by the residual cortical vitreous and ILM, prevent postoperative epiretinal membrane (ERM) formation, and improve the oxygen supply by removing the diffusion barrier [9, 18]. After surgery, HE may initially increase in size as intra- and subretinal fluid is gradually reabsorbed. It soon decreases in size, indicating vessel permeability improvement. Unfortunately, subretinal fibrotic plaque may form in some patients, preventing visual improvement.

We conducted a retrospective study to evaluate the one-year anatomical and functional outcomes of DME patients with massive hard exudates managed by PPV with ILM peeling and compared them with those managed by nonsurgical treatments [19]. Patients showing evidence of taut and thick posterior hyaloid structures by OCT examinations were not included. Massive hard exudates were defined as fovea-involved, single or multiple patches of confluent hard exudates with a total area of >3 disc areas at the posterior pole confirmed by color fundus photography; (2) the presence of intraretinal and/or subretinal hyperreflective materials involving the fovea confirmed by optical coherence tomography (OCT); and (3) a BCVA ≤20/200.

For surgery, a standard microincision vitrectomy system was used. After core vitrectomy, triamcinolone acetonide was injected to identify and facilitate the removal of the PH if no posterior vitreous detachment (PVD) was observed. After complete vitrectomy, ICG (25 mg ICG in 15 mL of 5% glucose) was slowly injected above the macula. Excess ICG was immediately removed, and the ILM staining pattern was observed. Homogeneous staining indicated no ERMs, whereas scattered staining or poor staining indicated the presence of ERMs and/or residual vitreous remnants. ILM peeling was initiated at the site of positive ICG staining. The ILM and overlying ERM were peeled off the retinal surface in a circumferential manner for at least 3.5-disc diameters centered at the fovea. After a mild focal laser was applied to the extrafoveal microaneurysms within the arcade, a peripheral scatter laser was applied to the equator and slightly beyond the equator as complete PRP. Bevacizumab (1.25 mg) was injected into the vitreous cavity at the end of surgery.

After surgery, IVI of anti-VEGF was administered as needed. In addition, intravitreal triamcinolone acetonide (IVTA) at 4 mg/0.05 mL per dose or posterior subtenon injection of triamcinolone acetonide (PSTA) at 40 mg/0.5 mL per dose was administered as a supplementary treatment if needed.

During the operation in the vitrectomy group, 14 (67%) eyes had complete PVD, and 7 (33%) eyes had incomplete PVD or no PVD. Nonhomogeneous ICG staining of the macula before ILM peeling, which indicated the presence of an ERM/vitreous remnant, was noted in 16 (76%) eyes.

After treatment, CRT decreased steadily in the vitrectomy group but fluctuated in the nonsurgical group. Compared with eyes in the nonsurgical group, eyes in the vitrectomy group had better visual improvement ($P < 0.05$ at 6 and 12 months and at the final visit) and a greater decrease in CRT ($P < 0.05$ at 3 and 6 months and at the final visit) after adjustment for baseline BCVA. Hard exudates resolved more rapidly in the vitrectomy group than in the nonsurgical group, with 94.1% versus 47.4% of eyes showing significant absorption after 6 months of treatment ($P = 0.003$). Subfoveal plaque or nodule formation after treatment was observed in 33% (5/15) of eyes in the vitrectomy group and 37% (7/19) of eyes in the control group. In the vitrectomy group, 62% of the eyes did not require any further injections for treating DME after the operation (Fig. 9.2).

In DR, massive amounts of hard exudates tend to be associated with PDR. In the above study, 75% of the eyes had PDR. There are two possible

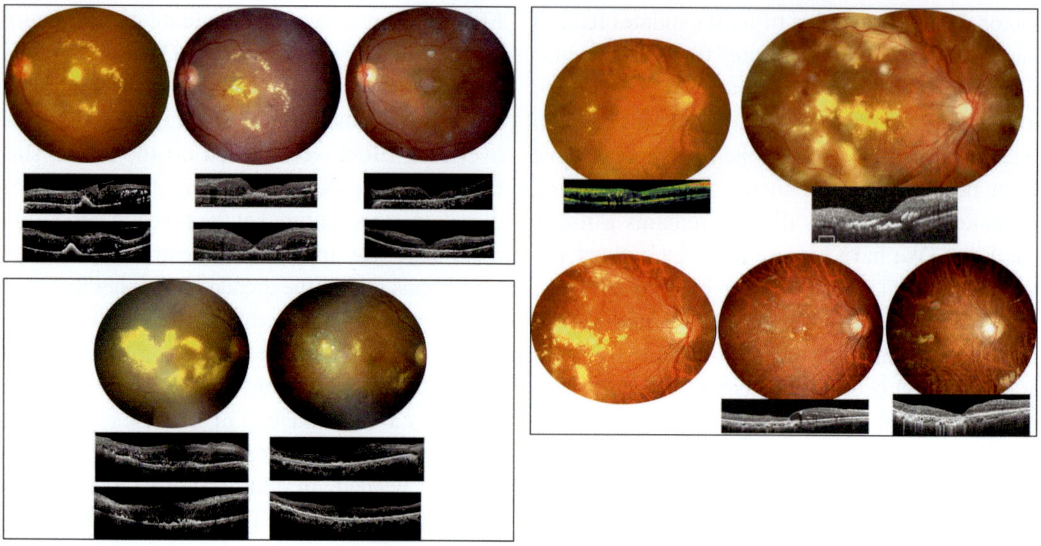

Fig. 9.2 Three examples of massive hard exudates responsive to vitrectomy with ERM and ILM peeling. In the upper left panel, preoperative OCT showed taut posterior hyaloid traction (left side color and OCT images). In the other two patients, preoperative OCT did not show premacular traction (left side in the lower left panel and the two upper images in the right side panel). After surgery, all patients showed resolution of macular edema and decreased amounts of hard exudates. (Courtesy of Dr. Chung-May Yang)

reasons for this close association. First, eyes with PDR usually have extensive nonperfusion areas and produce excessive VEGF, which in turn greatly increases vascular permeability and causes the outpouring and accumulation of hard exudates. Second, eyes with PDR are frequently treated with PRP. During PRP sessions, a laser can induce inflammation and a VEGF surge, resulting in severe macular edema with massive amounts of hard exudates. The strong association between PDR and massive HE is part of the reason we perform PRP during vitrectomy. Another reason is that in some cases, postoperative VH may develop, preventing adequate fundus examination and timely PRP. Although PRP may induce inflammation and potentially aggravate ME, simultaneous PH removal, ERM/ILM peeling, and the use of anti-VEGF agents during surgery may effectively prevent this side effect of PRP. In the long run, PRP may constrict retinal vessels and has a positive effect on reducing macular edema.

Severe hard exudates have been recognized to be the strongest risk factor for the development of subretinal plaque or fibrosis and are associated with poor visual outcomes. Although vitrectomy with ILM peeling and PRP may be a good option for treating DME with massive HE, approximately 1/3 of patients still have submacular plaque with unsatisfactory visual function. We found that the prolonged presence of HE within the submacular space is more likely to result in submacular fibrotic plaque (Fig. 9.3). Thus, early and proactive treatment of DME with or without HE is important to prevent prolonged accumulation of HE within the submacular space.

Subretinal removal of massive submacular hard exudates has been reported [15, 20–22]. However, visual improvement did not significantly differ between patients who received PPV alone and those who received PPV along with hard exudate removal. This was probably due to irreversible retinal atrophy and degenerative changes in the affected eyes. Macular holes, retinal breaks, submacular hemorrhage, and neurosensory retina degeneration may develop after subretinal removal of hard exudates.

The final BCVA was significantly better among those without subfoveal plaque/nodule formation than among those with subfoveal plaque/nodule

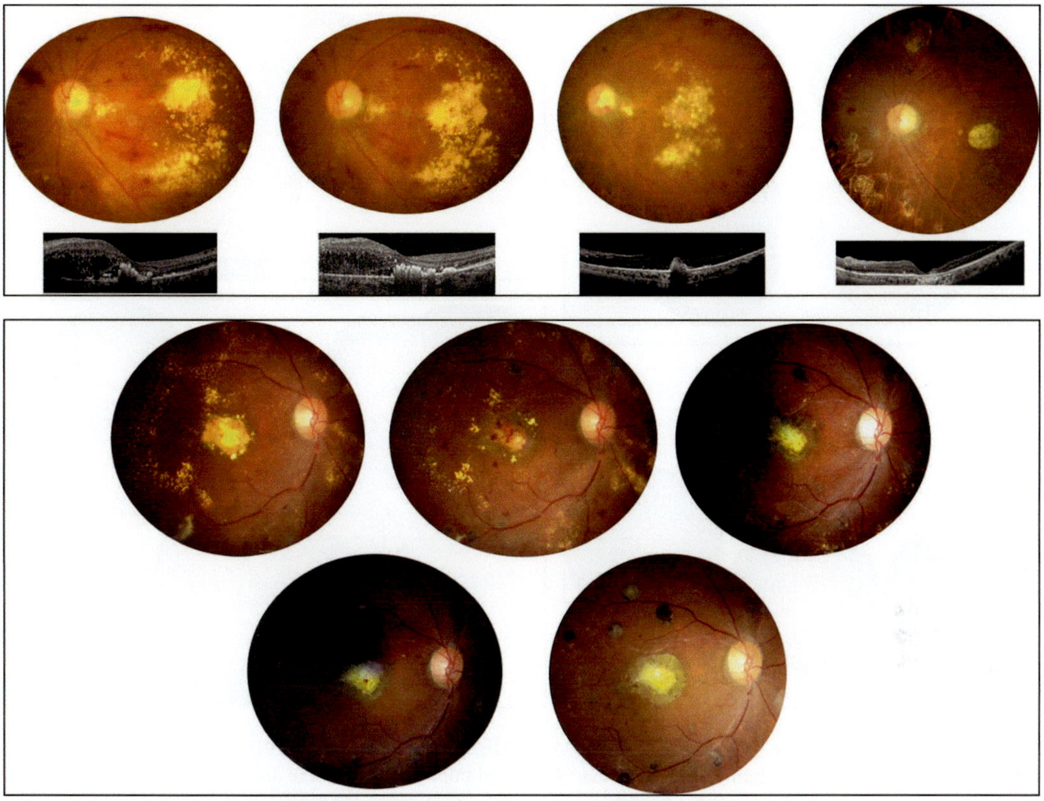

Fig. 9.3 Two examples of DME with massive hard exudates evolved to subfoveal fibrotic plaque after surgery. (Courtesy of Dr. Chung-May Yang)

formation in the vitrectomy group, indicating that DME should be managed promptly before massive hard exudate deposition in the macula.

In summary, PPV combined with ILM peeling may result in rapid resolution of hard exudates and provide long-term anatomical and functional benefits, avoiding possible complications related to multiple IVIs and a large treatment burden. Thus, PPV combined with ILM peeling may be a favorable alternative treatment option for DME patients with massive amounts of hard exudates (Fig. 9.4).

Massive amounts of hard exudates may be present outside the macular area. This condition develops from severe vascular leakage caused by the abnormal vascular permeability induced by strong vitreoretinal traction from FVP bands or membranes, which form broad adhesions with the retina. Exudates usually accumulate in the subretinal space, causing localized retinal detachment. After surgical release of vitreoretinal traction, the HE gradually resolved (Fig. 9.5). Because the adhesions are always along the retinal vessels, care should be taken to avoid bleeding and retinal break(s) during manipulation to release vitreoretinal adhesions. Iatrogenic breaks in the presence of subretinal exudate mounts make laser application and break sealing difficult and may result in retinal detachment after surgery.

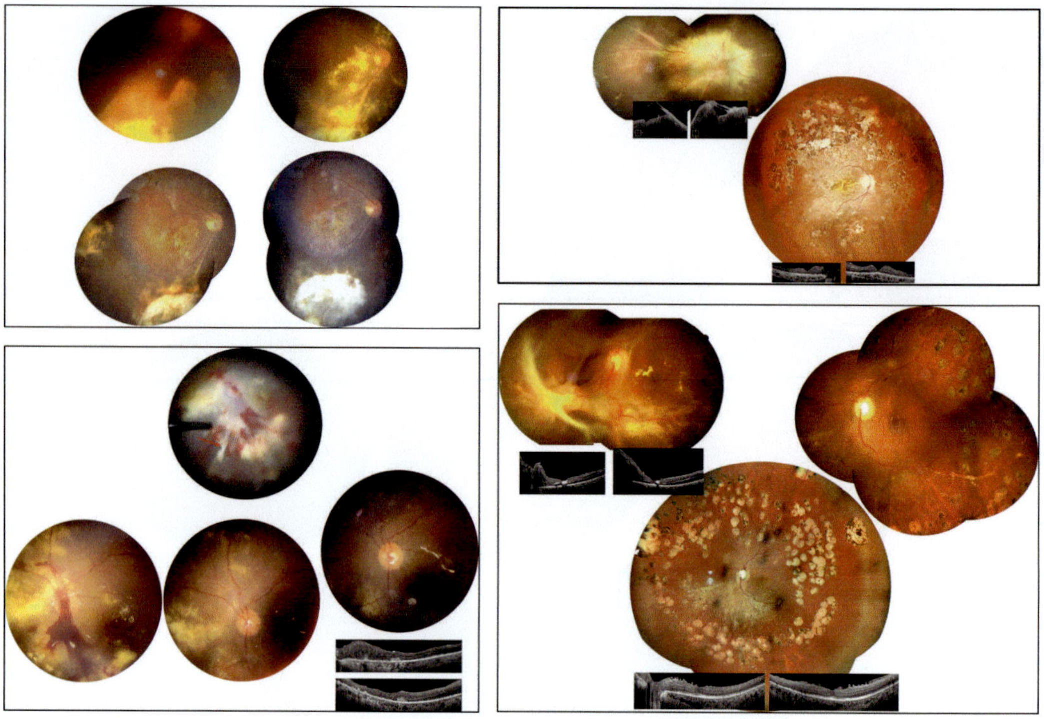

Fig. 9.4 Four sets of images showing FVP and DME with massive hard exudates extending outside the macula. The left side two panels show preretinal hemorrhage in addition to massive amounts of hard exudates. The right panels show prominent FVP traction with massive HE. After removal of the FVP, ERM, and ILM, all patients had improved anatomical and functional outcomes. In the left lower panel, the red arrow in the upper intraoperative video image points to the FVP. (Courtesy of Dr. Chung-May Yang)

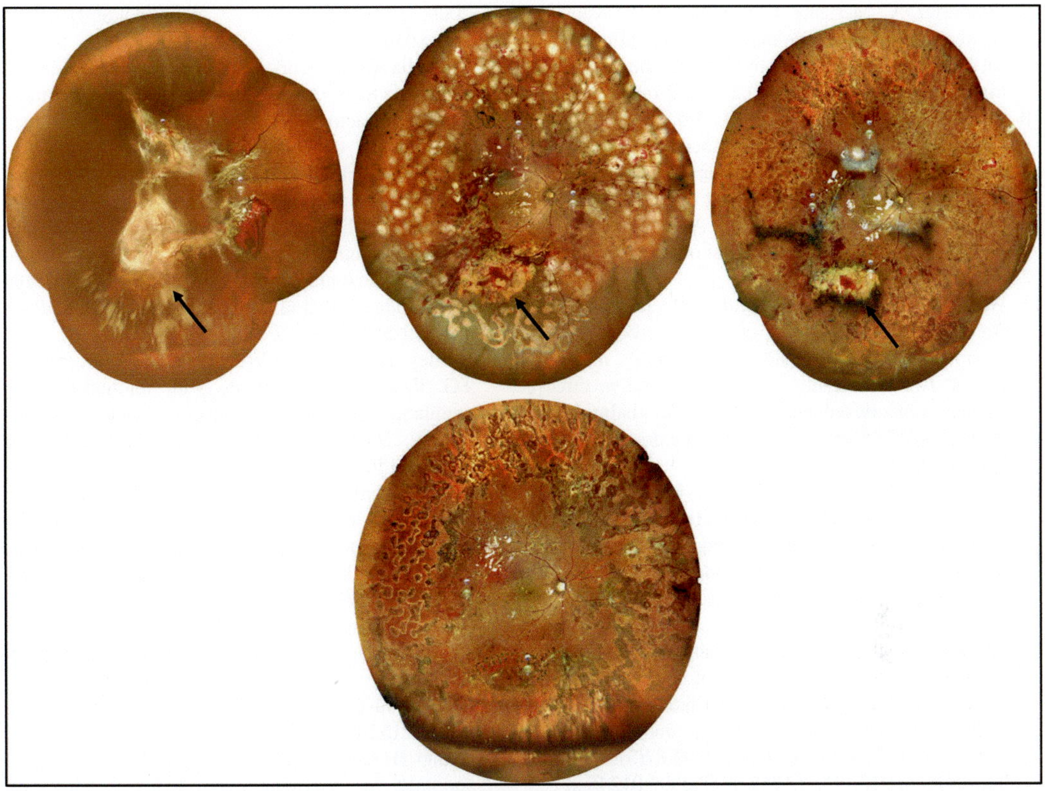

Fig. 9.5 One set of wide-angle images showing the FVP-induced massive amounts of hard exudates outside the macula. Preoperative image shows severe FVP around the arcade, which was most prominent in the temporal lower area (left upper). Massive amounts of HE were partially covered by the FVP membrane. Two weeks after surgery with SO infusion, massive HE became evident (upper center). The exudative patches decreased after 1 week (upper right) and disappeared 10 weeks after surgery (lower). The black arrow points to the massive HE patch. (Courtesy of Dr. Chung-May Yang)

References

1. Yang CM. Surgical treatment for severe diabetic macular edema with massive hard exudates. Retina. 2000;20(2):121–5.
2. Fong DS, Segal PP, Myers F, Ferris FL, Hubbard LD, Davis MD. Subretinal fibrosis in diabetic macular edema. ETDRS report 23. Early treatment diabetic retinopathy study research group. Arch Ophthalmol. 1997;115(7):873–7. https://doi.org/10.1001/archopht.1997.01100160043006.
3. Klein R, Klein BE, Moss SE, Davis MD, DeMets DL. The Wisconsin epidemiologic study of diabetic retinopathy. IV Diabetic macular edema. Ophthalmology. 1984;91(12):1464–74. https://doi.org/10.1016/s0161-6420(84)34102-1.
4. Group ETDRSr. Photocoagulation for diabetic macular edema. Early treatment diabetic retinopathy study report number 1. Early treatment diabetic retinopathy study research group. Arch Ophthalmol. 1985;103(12):1796–806.
5. Toda J, Fukushima H, Kato S. Injection of triamcinolone acetonide into the posterior subtenon capsule for treatment of diabetic macular edema. Retina. 2007;27(6):764–9. https://doi.org/10.1097/IAE.0b013e318030bfcd.
6. Ho AC, Scott IU, Kim SJ, Brown GC, Brown MM, Ip MS, et al. Anti-vascular endothelial growth factor pharmacotherapy for diabetic macular edema: a report by the American academy of ophthalmology. Ophthalmology. 2012;119(10):2179–88. https://doi.org/10.1016/j.ophtha.2012.07.058.
7. Schmidt-Erfurth U, Garcia-Arumi J, Bandello F, Berg K, Chakravarthy U, Gerendas BS, et al. Guidelines for the management of diabetic macular edema by the European society of retina specialists (EURETINA). Ophthalmologica. 2017;237(4):185–222. https://doi.org/10.1159/000458539.
8. Massin P, Audren F, Haouchine B, Erginay A, Bergmann JF, Benosman R, et al. Intravitreal triamcinolone acetonide for diabetic diffuse macular edema: preliminary results of a prospective controlled trial. Ophthalmology. 2004;111(2):218–24; discussion 24–5. https://doi.org/10.1016/j.ophtha.2003.05.037.

9. Gandorfer A, Messmer EM, Ulbig MW, Kampik A. Resolution of diabetic macular edema after surgical removal of the posterior hyaloid and the inner limiting membrane. Retina. 2000;20(2):126–33.
10. Chew EY, Klein ML, Ferris FL 3rd, Remaley NA, Murphy RP, Chantry K, et al. Association of elevated serum lipid levels with retinal hard exudate in diabetic retinopathy. Early treatment diabetic retinopathy study (ETDRS) report 22. Arch Ophthalmol. 1996;114(9):1079–84. https://doi.org/10.1001/archopht.1996.01100140281004.
11. Wells JA, Glassman AR, Ayala AR, Jampol LM, Bressler NM, Bressler SB, et al. Aflibercept, bevacizumab, or ranibizumab for diabetic macular edema: two-year results from a comparative effectiveness randomized clinical trial. Ophthalmology. 2016;123(6):1351–9. https://doi.org/10.1016/j.ophtha.2016.02.022.
12. Mello Filho P, Andrade G, Maia A, Maia M, Biccas Neto L, Muralha Neto A, et al. Effectiveness and safety of intravitreal dexamethasone implant (ozurdex) in patients with diabetic macular edema: a real-world experience. Ophthalmologica. 2019;241(1):9–16. https://doi.org/10.1159/000492132.
13. Larsson J, Kifley A, Zhu M, Wang JJ, Mitchell P, Sutter FK, et al. Rapid reduction of hard exudates in eyes with diabetic retinopathy after intravitreal triamcinolone: data from a randomized, placebo-controlled, clinical trial. Acta Ophthalmol. 2009;87(3):275–80. https://doi.org/10.1111/j.1755-3768.2008.01245.x.
14. Avci R, Kaderli B. Intravitreal triamcinolone injection for chronic diabetic macular edema with severe hard exudates. Graefes Arch Clin Exp Ophthalmol. 2006;244(1):28–35. https://doi.org/10.1007/s00417-005-0069-5.
15. Avci R, Inan UU, Kaderli B. Long-term results of excision of plaque-like foveal hard exudates in patients with chronic diabetic macular edema. Eye (Lond). 2008;22(9):1099–104. https://doi.org/10.1038/sj.eye.6702877.
16. Ciardella AP, Klancnik J, Schiff W, Barile G, Langton K, Chang S. Intravitreal triamcinolone for the treatment of refractory diabetic macular edema with hard exudates: an optical coherence tomography study. Br J Ophthalmol. 2004;88(9):1131–6. https://doi.org/10.1136/bjo.2004.041707.
17. Khairallah M, Zeghidi H, Ladjimi A, Yahia SB, Attia S, Zaouali S, et al. Primary intravitreal triamcinolone acetonide for diabetic massive macular hard exudates. Retina. 2005;25(7):835–9. https://doi.org/10.1097/00006982-200510000-00003.
18. Hartley KL, Smiddy WE, Flynn HW Jr, Murray TG. Pars plana vitrectomy with internal limiting membrane peeling for diabetic macular edema. Retina. 2008;28(3):410–9. https://doi.org/10.1097/IAE.0b013e31816102f2.
19. Lin HC, Yang CM, Chen SN, Hsieh YT. Vitrectomy with internal limiting membrane peeling versus nonsurgical treatment for diabetic macular edema with massive hard exudates. PLoS One. 2020;15(7):e0236867. https://doi.org/10.1371/journal.pone.0236867.
20. Naito T, Matsushita S, Sato H, Katome T, Nagasawa T, Shiota H. The results of submacular surgery to remove diabetic submacular hard exudates. J Med Investig. 2008;55(3–4):211–5. https://doi.org/10.2152/jmi.55.211.
21. Takagi H, Otani A, Kiryu J, Ogura Y. New surgical approach for removing massive foveal hard exudates in diabetic macular edema. Ophthalmology. 1999;106(2):249–56; discussion 56–7. https://doi.org/10.1016/S0161-6420(99)90054-4.
22. Takaya K, Suzuki Y, Mizutani H, Sakuraba T, Nakazawa M. Long-term results of vitrectomy for removal of submacular hard exudates in patients with diabetic maculopathy. Retina. 2004;24(1):23–9. https://doi.org/10.1097/00006982-200402000-00004.

10 Tractional Macular Schisis in Proliferative Diabetic Retinopathy

Abstract

Macular tractional retinal schisis (macular TRS) or tractional macular schisis (TMS) is a common type of macular elevation in PDR. It is characterized by bridging columnar tissues between the inner and outer retinal layers in the macular area (Imai et al., Am J Ophthalmol 132:81–84, 2001). Studies on the clinical manifestations and postoperative visual prognosis of macular TRS are limited. The clinical features, diverse patterns, and treatment results will be discussed in this chapter.

10.1 Case Report

This 57-year-old woman had a history of DM that had been diagnosed for 1–2 years after receiving oral medication for approximately half a year. She had experienced blurred vision in both eyes for 1 year. The patient visited an outside hospital where proliferative diabetic retinopathy (PDR) with fibrovascular proliferation (FVP) in both eyes was diagnosed. Panretinal photocoagulation (PRP) was performed in both eyes. She then underwent pars plana vitrectomy (PPV) for PDR with FVP in the left eye. Because of postoperative RD in the left eye, she was referred to our hospital. On examination, best-corrected visual acuity (BCVA) was 0.1 in the right eye, and counting fingers 70 cm in the left eye. She underwent phacoemulsification with posterior chamber intraocular lens (PCIOL) implantation and vitrectomy with an encircling scleral buckle and SO tamponade in the left eye. The retina reattached after surgery. During FU, her vision in her right eye worsened. On examination, BCVA was 0.03 in the right eye and 0.01 in the left eye. Fundus examination revealed a fibrotic membrane along the arcade and preretinal membrane in the right eye. OCT revealed a thick premacular membrane with traction macular schisis in the right eye. She underwent vitrectomy with epiretinal membrane removal and supplementary PRP in the right eye. After surgery, the macula flattened down, and the foveal contour was restored. A mild ERM was noted in the parafoveal area. Her BCVA improved to 0.15 (Fig. 10.1).

C.-M. Yang, *Surgery for Complications of Diabetic Retinopathy*,
https://doi.org/10.1007/978-981-96-2848-3_10

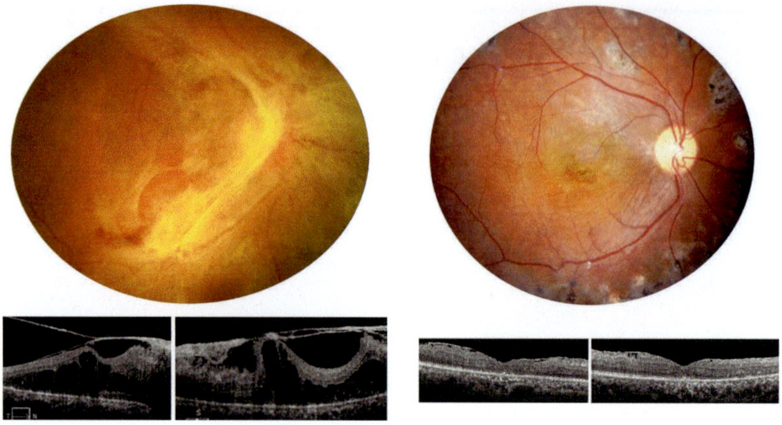

Fig. 10.1 Preoperative color photography revealed moderate fibrotic proliferation extending from the disc to the upper and lower arcades and to the nasal side; a condensed fibrotic band from the lower arcade to the macular area was also noted. (upper left) Preoperative OCT images showing the preretinal membrane, ERM, and diffuse traction schisis with irregular macular elevation (lower left). After surgery, the retina became flat (right color photo and OCT images). (Courtesy of Dr. Chung-May Yang)

10.2 Tractional Macular Schisis in PDR

There are three main types of traction-induced macular elevations in PDR: tractional macular thickening, TMS, and TRD. In TMS, OCT studies have shown that the inner retinal layer is normally reflective; the outer layer is less reflective but not optically empty. Bridging columnar tissues are frequently observed between the inner and outer layers [1]. In contrast, a well-demarcated outer surface of the neurosensory retina is found with an optically empty subretinal space in TRD [2, 3]. Histopathological studies have shown that the adherence of the PH membrane to the retina and vitreous body shrinkage might induce retinal elevation with splitting of the outer plexiform layer, leading to retinoschisis [4]. The bridging columnar tissues between the inner and outer layers of the split retina mainly consisted of Müller cells. Although TRS with or without retinal detachment has been suggested as the most frequent pattern of tractional macular elevation in eyes with PDR and peripheral retinoschisis is frequently found during surgery for complications of PDR, studies on the clinical manifestations and postoperative visual prognosis of macular TRS are limited. We studied the clinical characteristics and surgical outcomes of this specific entity [5]. We defined the OCT criteria for TMS as intraretinal splitting with vertical bridging columns of tissue in the macular region for at least 2 disc diameter areas and the presence of preretinal proliferative tissue adherent to the thickened retina, exerting tangential or oblique traction on the edge of the elevated retinal surface. Some patients demonstrated a small pocket of subfoveal fluid within or at the edge of retinal splitting. Three OCT patterns of schisis could be identified: (a) Localized elevation: the area of retinoschisis occurred locally within the parafoveal and foveal areas. (b) Eccentric elevation: the split or detached neurosensory retina was more prominent outside the parafoveal area and within the macular area. (c) Diffuse elevation: diffuse retinal splitting or detachment developed in the whole macular area, extending beyond the arcade (Figs. 10.2, 10.3, 10.4, and 10.5) In some cases, traction and retinal splitting may be predominantly situated outside the arcade, but the schisis extends all the way into the macular area (Fig. 10.6). All eyes with TMS involved the outer layer of the retina. Other macular abnormalities, including LMH or inner macular cysts, may be associated with TMS on OCT (Fig. 10.7).

In our study, the mean age of patients with TRS was greater than that of patients with TRD. The proportion of patients with inactive

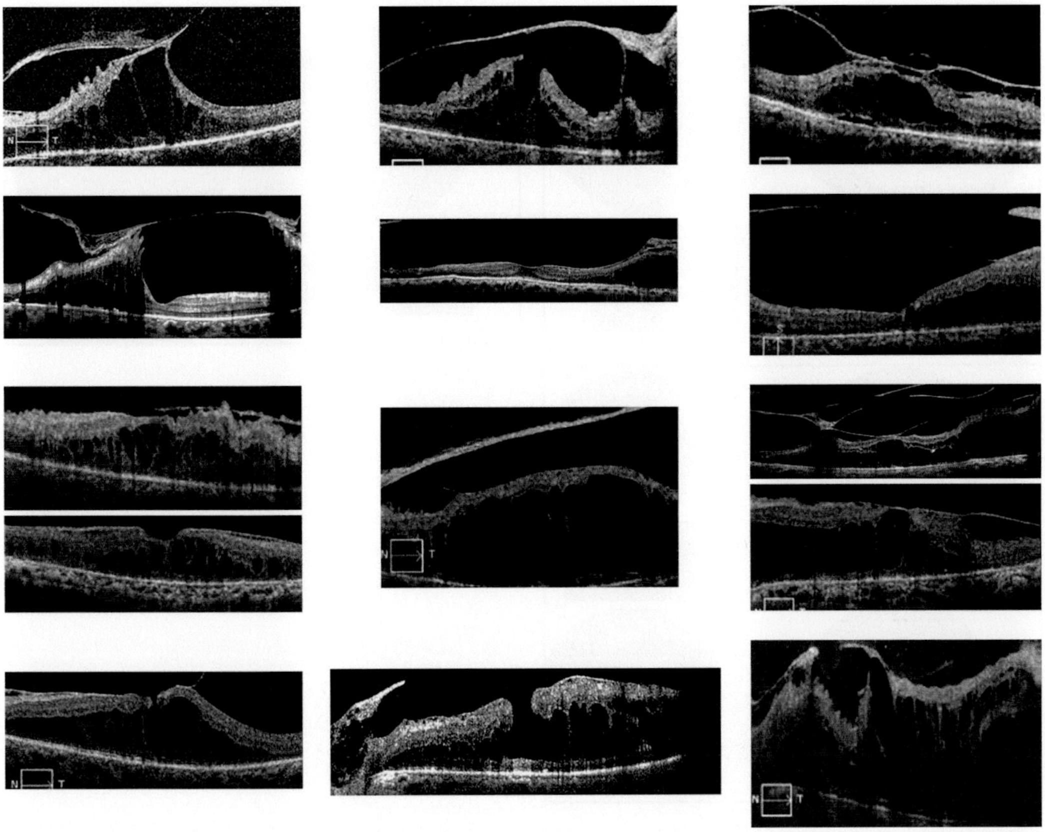

Fig. 10.2 One set of OCT images showing different patterns of TMS. Localized elevation is shown in the upper row; eccentric elevation in the second row; diffuse elevation in the third row; TMS with schisis in the left and center images of the bottom row; TMS with TRD in the right image of the bottom row. (Courtesy of Dr. Chung-May Yang)

fibrous proliferation was significantly greater in patients with TRS than in patients with TRD. All patients in the TRS group had grade 2 FVP severity, which was significantly lower than that of patients in the TRD group. In the TRS group, the FVP was centrally located in one-third of the eyes; the remaining eyes were evenly distributed among juxtapapillary, complete arcade, and incomplete arcade locations; however, in the TRD group, approximately two-thirds of the eyes were classified as complete arcade type. We postulated that in TRS, the traction force on the macular area gradually increases over time until it is strong enough to induce separation of the intraretinal layers but still not sufficient to induce tractional detachment. Depending on the major vector of the traction force, the schisis displays different morphologic patterns, as shown by the OCT findings. However, it has been reported that TRS may progress and result in combined TRD in some cases; thus, it should not be considered an abortive process of TRD (Fig. 10.8). As macular structural changes may worsen over time, the evolution process suggests that the schisis induced by proliferative tissue is a dynamic process even though the retina seems to be in a quiescent stage without active proliferation, indicating that a prolonged delay in surgery may result in further macular damage. On the other hand, on rare occasions, improvement of the macular structure may occur after spontaneous traction release (Fig. 10.4).

In our study, improvements in visual acuity after vitreoretinal surgery were observed in the TRS group. No significant difference in visual acuity gain after surgery was found between

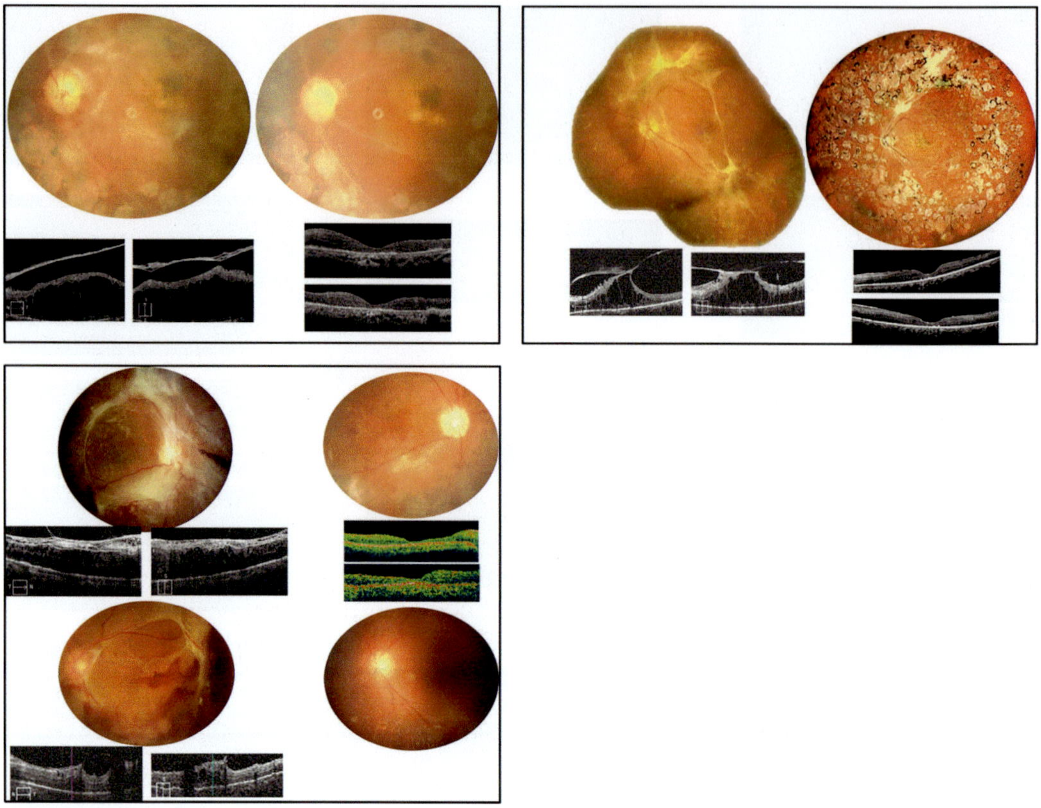

Fig. 10.3 Three sets of pre- and postoperative color photos and OCT images showing various structural changes in TMS associated with different severities of the FVP. In the upper two panels, the FVP seemed to be more severe in the upper right panel; however, TMS was diffuse in the upper left panel and localized in the upper right panel. In the lower panel, the right eye (upper left) had more severe FVP tissue than the left eye (lower left); accordingly, the right eye had diffuse TMS, and the left eye only had traction macular thickening, without definite schisis formation. Note that the left eye had an active FVP, while the FVP in the right eye was predominantly fibrotic. (Courtesy of Dr. Chung-May Yang)

patients with TRS and those with TRD. After surgery, in the TRS group, approximately 60% of patients achieved complete resolution of retinoschisis, and 40% experienced residual retinoschisis during a mean FU time of 2–2.5 years. We observed LMH formation after the operation (Fig. 10.4, lower left panel).

To summarize, macular TRS is frequently observed in patients with inactive, moderate fibrovascular proliferation on or adjacent to the macula. Various associated abnormalities can be detected. Surgery can improve visual acuity, although there may be residual macular changes.

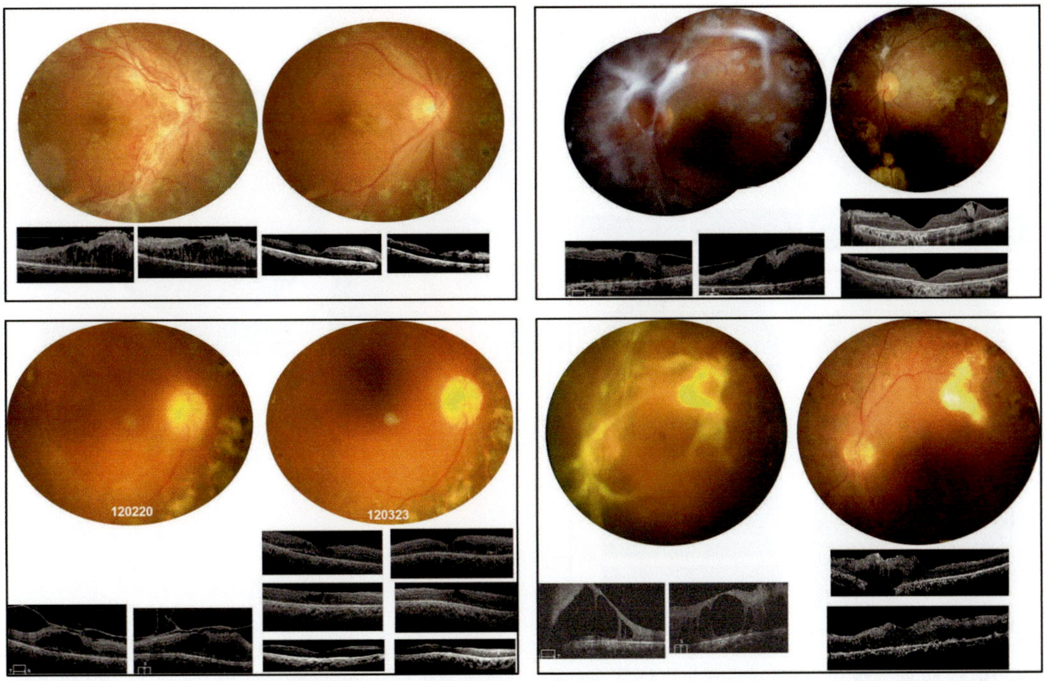

Fig. 10.4 Four sets of pre- and postoperative color photos and OCT images showing various structural changes in TMS associated with different severities of the FVP. Except for the upper left panel, which shows visible NV within the FVP tissue, all other patients had predominantly mild to moderate fibrotic proliferation. All panels show eccentric macular elevation in at least one OCT image before surgery (left lower OCT images in each panel). In the lower left panel, postoperative OCT images show that the macular structure changed from parafoveal cysts to cysts with LMH and then to spontaneous inner gap closure (lower right sequential OCT images). (Courtesy of Dr. Chung-May Yang)

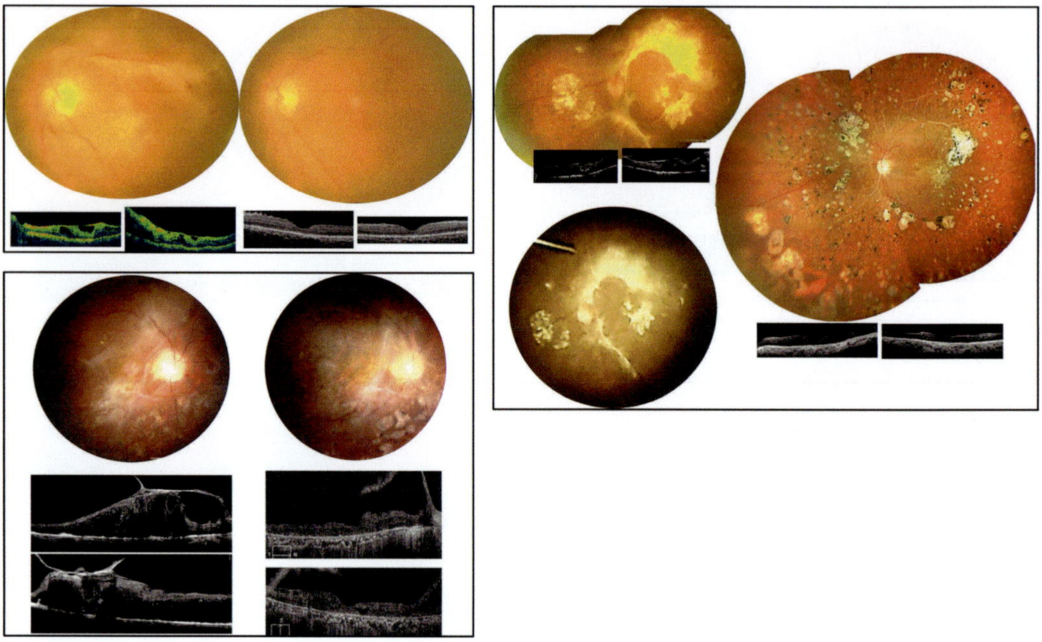

Fig. 10.5 Three sets of color photos and OCT images showing various structural changes in TMS associated with different severities of the FVP. Irregular and diffuse macular elevation was noted in all three patients. In the lower left panel, with thick preretinal tissue extending toward the macula, the TMS was more severe in this patient (left side color photo and OCT images) than in the other two patients. However, spontaneous detachment of the premacular tissue occurred, resulting in improved foveal contour (right side color photo and OCTs). Two patients in the upper left and right panels underwent surgery, and postoperative images are shown on the right side. (Courtesy of Dr. Chung-May Yang)

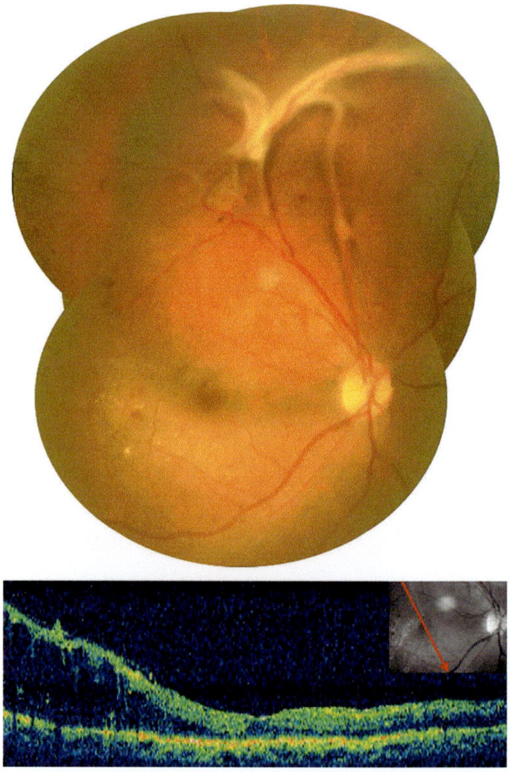

Fig. 10.6 Composite color photo and ICT image showing FVP bands and associated traction schisis situated mainly outside the arcade. The schisis extended to the parafoveal area. (Courtesy of Dr. Chung-May Yang)

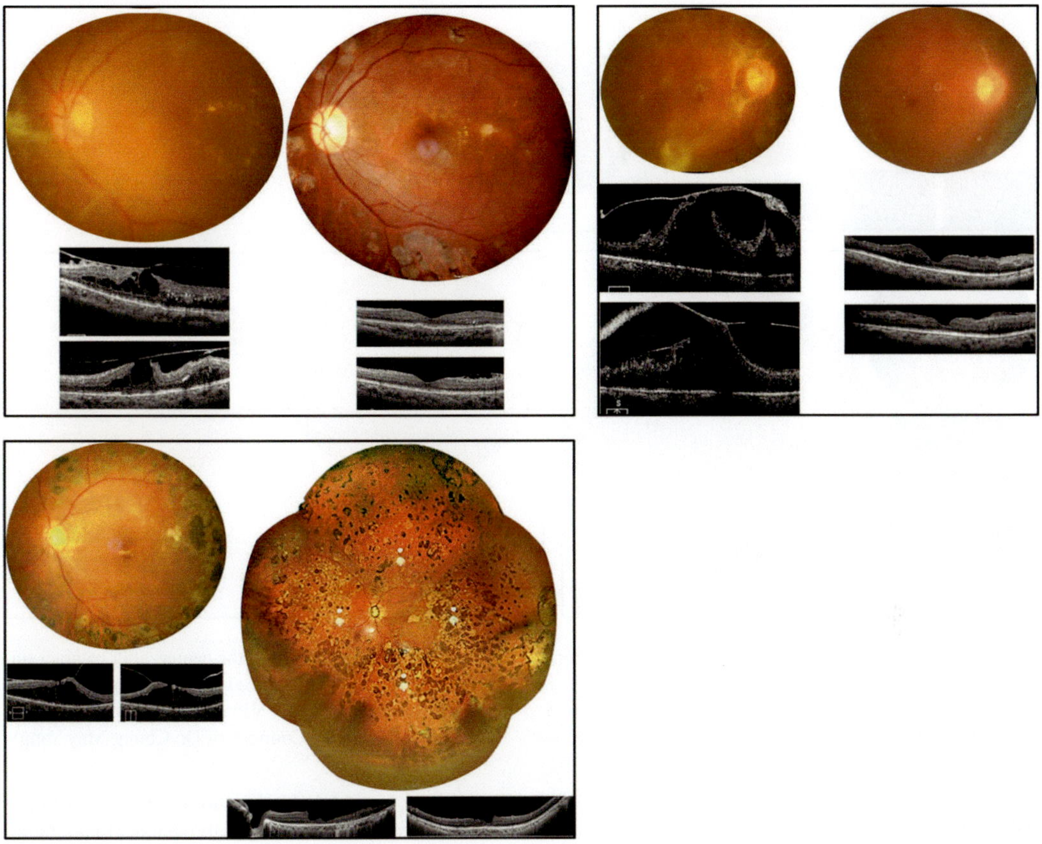

Fig. 10.7 Three sets of pre- and postoperative color photos and OCT images showing various structural changes in the LMH and TMS associated with different severities of the FVP. All patients showed foveal contour improvement after surgery (right side colors and OCT images in each panel). (Courtesy of Dr. Chung-May Yang)

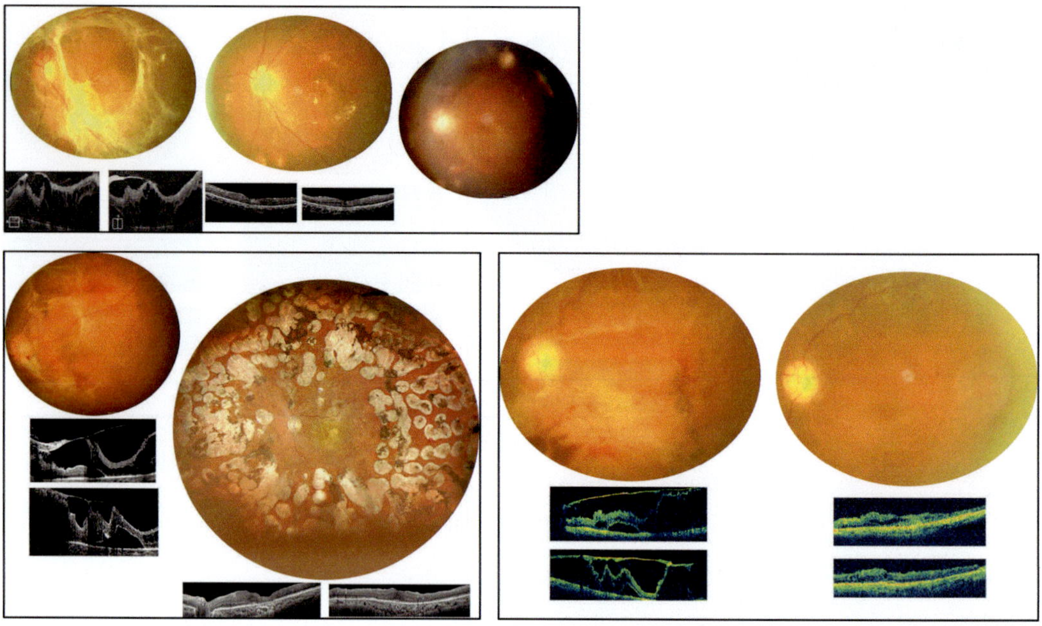

Fig. 10.8 Three sets of pre- and postoperative color photos and OCT images showing various structural changes in combined TMS and TRD associated with different severities of the FVP. In the upper panel, postoperative color photo and OCT images are shown in the center; after cataract surgery, HE subsided (right). In the lower two panels, TMS and TRD were associated with FVP activity before surgery (left images in each panel). (Courtesy of Dr. Chung-May Yang)

References

1. Imai M, Iijima H, Hanada N. Optical coherence tomography of tractional macular elevations in eyes with proliferative diabetic retinopathy. Am J Ophthalmol. 2001;132(1):81–4. https://doi.org/10.1016/s0002-9394(01)00910-2.
2. Lincoff H, Serag Y, Chang S, Silverman R, Bondok B, el-Aswad M. Tractional elevations of the retina in patients with diabetes. Am J Ophthalmol. 1992;113(3):235–42. https://doi.org/10.1016/s0002-9394(14)71573-9.
3. Iijima H, Imai M. Differentiation of retinal detachment from retinoschisis using optical coherence tomography. Am J Ophthalmol. 2003;136(3):577; author reply-8. https://doi.org/10.1016/s0002-9394(03)00439-2.
4. Faulborn J, Ardjomand N. Tractional retinoschisis in proliferative diabetic retinopathy: a histopathological study. Graefes Arch Clin Exp Ophthalmol. 2000;238(1):40–4. https://doi.org/10.1007/s004170050007.
5. Su CC, Yang CH, Yeh PT, Yang CM. Macular tractional retinoschisis in proliferative diabetic retinopathy: clinical characteristics and surgical outcome. Ophthalmologica. 2014;231(1):23–30. https://doi.org/10.1159/000355078.

11 Lamellar Macular Hole in Diabetic Retinopathy

Abstract

Lamellar macular holes (LMHs) are most commonly observed in otherwise healthy old-aged individuals, with the majority developing from the contraction of idiopathic epiretinal membranes (ERMs) (Gass, Arch Ophthalmol 94(5):793–800, 1976; Witkin et al., Ophthalmology 113(3):388–397, 2006; Parolini et al., Invest Ophthalmol Vis Sci 52:9074–9083, 2011). LMH may also be associated with other eye diseases, notably high myopia (Tanaka et al., Am J Ophthalmol 152(1):96–99.e1, 2011; Lai and Yang, Retina 38(7):1316–1323, 2018). LMH may be a vitreomacular interface disorder that is not infrequently encountered in patients with DR (Kuo et al., Eur J Ophthalmol 31:166–172, 2021). The specific features of LMH in DR patients compared with those in idiopathic patients have not been investigated. This issue will be addressed in this chapter.

11.1 Case Report

Patient 1: This 58-year-old woman had DM for more than 10 years. Her ophthalmic history revealed proliferative diabetic retinopathy (PDR) with fibrovascular proliferation in both eyes. She had undergone vitrectomy in her left eye for traction macular schisis 6 years before, followed by cataract operation in the same eye. The postoperative course was smooth. Regular FU revealed progressive VA worsening in the right eye. On examination, best-corrected visual acuity (BCVA) was 0.2 in the right eye and 0.1 in the left eye. Fundus examinations revealed a fibrotic band extending from the disc along the lower major vessels in the lower arcade. The left eye was flat with a PRP scar. OCT revealed a multilayered premacular membrane and LMH with epiretinal proliferation (EP). Vitrectomy with ERM/ILM peeling and EP embedding were performed. The foveal contour normalized to a certain extent. She underwent a cataract operation 22 months later. Her BCVA improved to 0.4 (Fig. 11.1).

Patient 2: This 64-year-old woman had DM, HTN, and coronary artery disease under medical control. The patient had suffered from decreased vision in both eyes for 2 years. The patient had PDR and PRP performed in both eyes during outpatient clinic FU. Cataract surgery was performed on the right eye. Although vision improved in the right eye, blurred vision persisted in the left eye. She was then referred to our clinic. On examination, BCVA was 0.5 in the right eye and 0.02 in the left eye. Moderate lens opacity in the left eye was observed. Fundus examinations revealed myelinated nerve fibers and PRP with minimal FVP in the left eye. OCT revealed a VMT with LMH and para-foveal schisis in the left eye. She underwent cataract surgery and vitrectomy with ERM/ILM peeling. The foveal contour greatly improved. Her BCVA was 0.5 and 0.05 2 years later (Fig. 11.2).

C.-M. Yang, *Surgery for Complications of Diabetic Retinopathy*,
https://doi.org/10.1007/978-981-96-2848-3_11

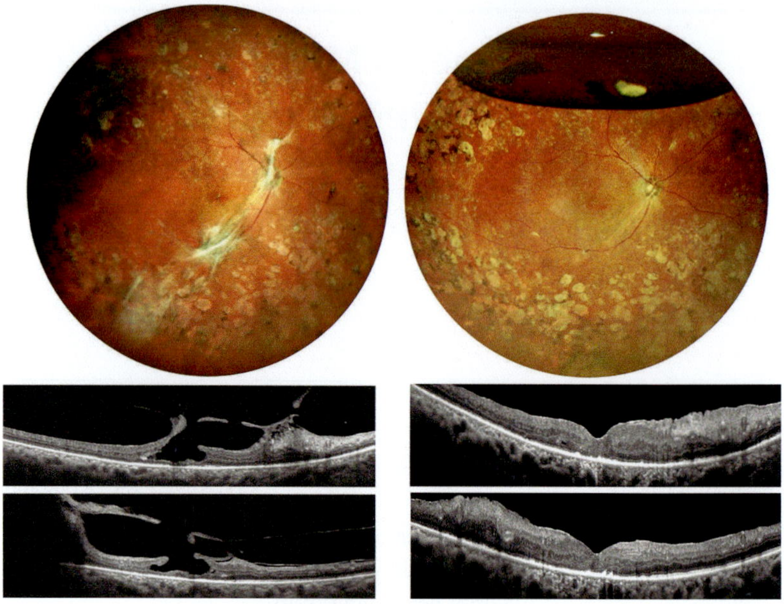

Fig. 11.1 Pre- and postoperative wide angle color photos and OCT images of the right eye of Patient 1. Before surgery, a fibrotic band extending from the disc along the lower major vessels in the lower arcade could be observed. OCT showed multilayer traction-induced LMH with EP at the edge (left). After surgery, the proliferative tissue was removed, and the macular contour improved (right). (Courtesy of Dr. Chung-May Yang)

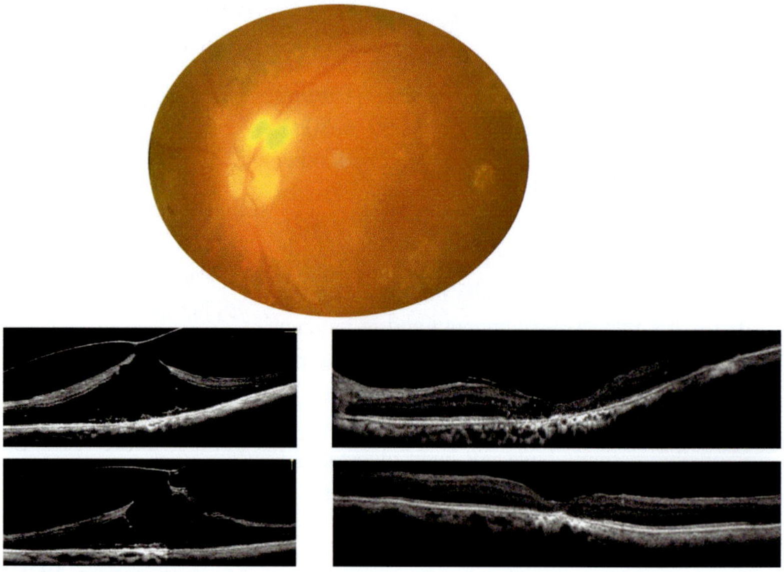

Fig. 11.2 Preoperative color photo (upper) and pre- and postoperative OCT images of the left eye of Patient 2. Before surgery, OCT revealed traction-induced LMH with a large central defect and parafoveal schisis (left). After surgery, the macular contour improved (right). (Courtesy of Dr. Chung-May Yang)

11.2 Lamellar Macular Hole in DR

In DR, excessive cytokines or growth factors secondary to vascular permeability alterations and/or retinal ischemia stimulate the formation of cystoid macular edema, ERMs, or fibrovascular membranes, causing various macular abnormalities. Because of the stronger traction force and more complex directions of traction, LMHs in eyes with DR have clinical features and surgical prognoses that are different from those of idiopathic LMHs. Since the lesions may develop in both eyes and cause marked loss of central vision, it is clinically relevant to recognize the clinical features and study the surgical outcomes of DR-associated LMH compared with those of idiopathic LMH.

Recently, a mound of homogenous material with medium reflectivity, named lamellar hole-associated epiretinal proliferation (LHEP) or simply EP, located on the epiretinal surface has been recognized in 30% of patients with LMH [3–5]. Previous studies have shown that LHEP occurs frequently in idiopathic LMH and high myopia-associated LMH [1, 3–5]. In our study [2], we demonstrated that LHEP was also present in DR-associated LMH patients, and the incidence of LHEP (47.1%) was comparable to that in idiopathic LMH patients (45.2%). However, DR-associated LMH showed some distinct characteristics. First, we found that DR-associated LMHs tended to have wider openings and deeper retinal defects than idiopathic LMHs. This may be related to more vitreomacular traction with multilayered ERMs/PHs in eyes with DR. Second, we also demonstrated that retinoschisis was more severe in the macular area of the DR group. This feature may also be strongly related to the significant traction forces from the ERM/PH. In fact, macular tractional retinoschisis or cysts may form first, and LMH may occur following the rupture of the thin inner lining at the fovea (Fig. 11.3, upper left panel). The visual function of eyes with LMH in DR may be disrupted by macular ischemia. This inadequate perfusion may result in poorer preoperative and postoperative vision even though the rate of ellipsoid zone disruption was not different from that of idiopathic LMH. In our study, we found that both the pre- and postoperative BCVA correlated with the height of the parafoveal schisis region at baseline. Preexisting macular tractional retinoschisis may have resulted in retinal tissue damage, which may not have resolved completely even after surgery. Therefore, we suggest that eyes with DR and macular tractional retinoschisis should be treated surgically if vision is affected. Delayed surgery may lead to more severe retinoschisis and LMH or full-thickness MH, which may result in poor visual recovery. Our study showed that visual improvement after timely surgery was comparable between DR-associated LMH and idiopathic LMH patients.

Recently, Govetto et al. described two different clinical entities for LMH: tractional type and degenerative type [6]. The degenerative type is characterized by the presence of a flat parafoveal contour, minimal vessel distortion, wide and deep foveal defects, the presence of EPs, and a lack of conventional ERMs. In our study, all patients had significant ERMs or VMTs. Although some patients in the DR group showed certain features of the degenerative type of LMH, such as a flat parafoveal contour, wide and deep foveal defects, or LHEPs, considerable overlap of characteristic changes of both types was observed. As all our patients had significant ERMs and/or VMTs, traction clearly played a major role in the formation of LMH in DR. Therefore, we believe that this classification cannot be adequately applied to DR-associated LMH.

The LMH in both the DR and HM usually has a wider and deeper retinal defect. One prominent feature of EP in highly myopic LMH patients is the significantly greater proportion of "broad" extension of EP than in nonhighly myopic eyes [1]. However, our study showed that the percentage of EPs in DR patients was comparable to that in idiopathic LMH patients. The formation of vitreomacular traction and LMH in highly myopic eyes usually progresses slowly without significantly affecting vision, which allows sufficient time for the development of a broad EP. In the DR group, however, the underlying vision may have been affected by DR itself, and the patients were more likely to seek help once the formation of LMH further worsened their vision. Therefore, we postulate that the lack of broad EP in the DR group may be due to the relatively shorter interval for the development of EP in diabetic eyes. In addition, the microenvironment in diabetic eyes often contains VEGF and inflammatory cytokines in the vitreous cavity, which is quite different from that in highly myopic eyes. Furthermore, TRD or full-thickness MH may develop from fibrovascular traction if diabetic patients are left untreated before there is enough time for LHM to develop widespread EP. These reasons may explain why LMH in DR patients has deeper and wider retinal defects but does not have more EP than idiopathic LMH patients and why this group had less extensive EP.

LMH may occur after the previous DV, even after the ERM and FVP tissue are removed during the initial surgery, and good

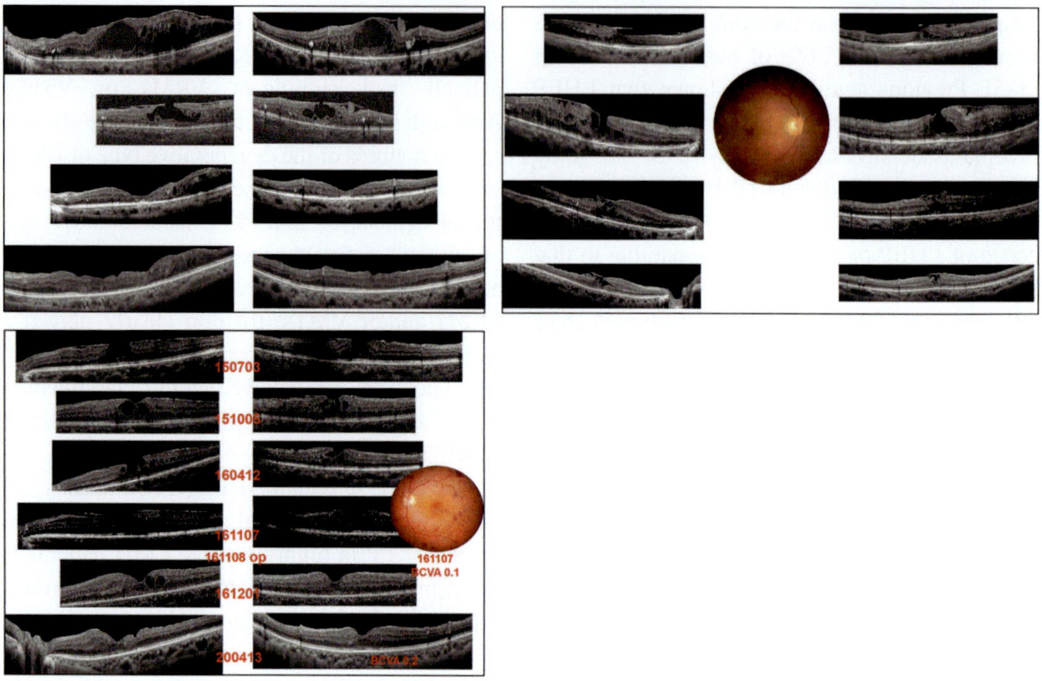

Fig. 11.3 Three examples of LMH formation/evolution in DR. In the upper left panel, sequential OCTs show DME with central cysts and ERM that changed to LMH after inner roof dehiscence; the foveal contour improved after surgery. In the upper right panel, the ERM induced LMH with a deep and narrow defect. Vitrectomy with an inverted ILM flap improved the structure. The lower panel shows the changes in the LMH and ERM configurations over time. After surgery, the foveal contour improved. The numbers in red indicate the date of examination or visual acuity. (Courtesy of Dr. Chung-May Yang)

anatomical and functional improvements are initially obtained. This is because ERMs tend to recur. Our previous study suggested that ILM peeling during vitrectomy for diabetic fibrovascular proliferative membranes may minimize postoperative ERM formation and improve visual prognosis [7]. We therefore suggest that ILM peeling should be considered in patients with DR complicated with ERM to reduce the rate of ERM recurrence and LMH formation.

Case examples of LMH formation and pre- and postoperative retinal changes are shown in Figs. 11.3, 11.4, and 11.5.

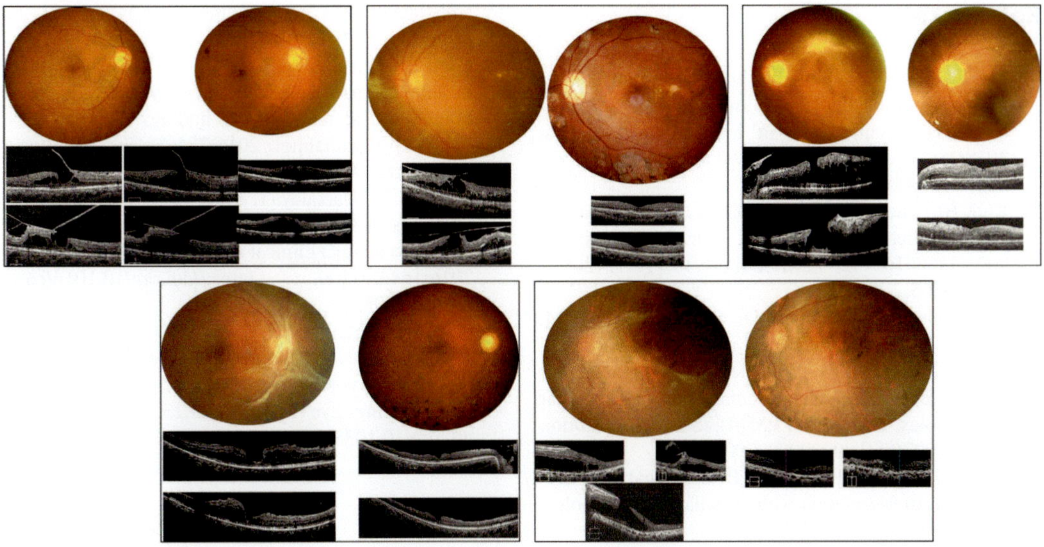

Fig. 11.4 Five examples of LMH with foveoschisis and macular traction. In each panel, the postoperative images are on the right side. The upper left panel shows the ERM and VMT; the upper central panel shows the taut posterior hyaloid/ERM traction; the upper right panel shows the disc and upper arcade fibrotic proliferation-induced LMH and schisis; the lower left panel shows the ERM-induced foveal thinning and parafoveal elevation and cysts/schisis; and the lower right panel shows the premacular fibrotic membrane-induced deep and wide LMH with EP. Except for the lower right panel, the other patients had no dense proliferative membrane on the macula. All patients had improved contours after surgery. (Courtesy of Dr. Chung-May Yang)

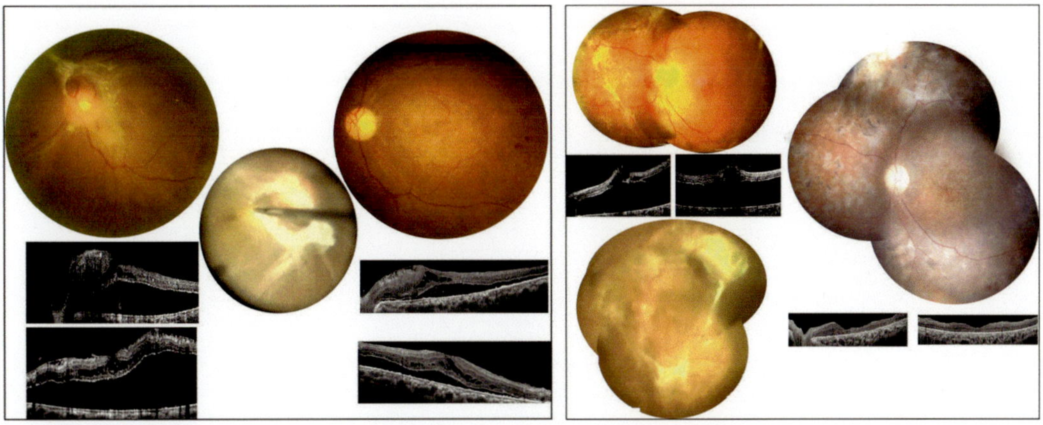

Fig. 11.5 Two examples of LMH with RD. In the left panel, the left fundus photo and OCT images show the FVP around the disc that caused LMH and TRD; FVP removal and ERM/ILM peeling were performed, as shown in the video image in the center; 4 months after surgery, the TRD improved, and the LMH disappeared, but the shallow subretinal fluid remained (right side images); the patient was then lost to FU. In the right panel, moderate FVP caused LMH and TRD, as shown in the left image and OCT images. Intraoperative composite video images are shown in the lower left. After surgery, the retina became flat, and the foveal contour improved, as shown in the right side composite color photo and OCT images. (Courtesy of Dr. Chung-May Yang)

References

1. Lai TT, Yang CM. Lamellar hole-associated epiretinal proliferation in lamellar macular hole and full-thickness macular hole in high myopia. Retina. 2018;38(7):1316–23. https://doi.org/10.1097/IAE.0000000000001708.
2. Kuo BI, Yang CM, Hsieh YT. Lamellar macular hole in diabetic retinopathy. Eur J Ophthalmol. 2021;31(1):166–72. https://doi.org/10.1177/1120672119879665.
3. Schumann RG, Compera D, Schaumberger MM, Wolf A, Fazekas C, Mayer WJ, et al. Epiretinal membrane characteristics correlate with photoreceptor layer defects in lamellar macular holes and macular pseudoholes. Retina. 2015;35(4):727–35. https://doi.org/10.1097/IAE.0000000000000375.
4. Pang CE, Spaide RF, Freund KB. Epiretinal proliferation seen in association with lamellar macular holes: a distinct clinical entity. Retina. 2014;34(8):1513–23. https://doi.org/10.1097/IAE.0000000000000163.
5. Lai TT, Chen SN, Yang CM. Epiretinal proliferation in lamellar macular holes and full-thickness macular holes: clinical and surgical findings. Graefes Arch Clin Exp Ophthalmol. 2016;254(4):629–38. https://doi.org/10.1007/s00417-015-3133-9.
6. Govetto A, Dacquay Y, Farajzadeh M, Platner E, Hirabayashi K, Hosseini H, et al. Lamellar macular hole: two distinct clinical entities? Am J Ophthalmol. 2016;164:99–109. https://doi.org/10.1016/j.ajo.2016.02.008.
7. Chang PY, Yang CM, Yang CH, Chen MS, Wang JY. Pars plana vitrectomy for diabetic fibrovascular proliferation with and without internal limiting membrane peeling. Eye (Lond). 2009;23(4):960–5. https://doi.org/10.1038/eye.2008.334.

Macular Hole in Proliferative Diabetic Retinopathy with Fibrovascular Proliferation

12

Abstract

A full-thickness macular hole (FTMH) most commonly appears in senile patients without apparent underlying disease. It may also occur after blunt ocular trauma or in the conditions of high myopia, rhegmatogenous retinal detachment (RD), or even macular dystrophy (Garcia-Arumi et al., Retina 17(5):372–377, 1997; Ho et al., Surv Ophthalmol 42(5):393–416, 1998; Kwok et al., Retina 20(5):439–444, 2000). Diabetic retinopathy (DR) is another disease entity that may be associated with macular hole (MH) (Yeh et al., Retina 29(3):355–361, 2009; Lai and Yang, Taiwan J Ophthalmol 5(2):85–89, 2015). An idiopathic FTMH may develop by oblique tractions from vitreomacular (VM) adhesion with visual field (VF) separation or from tangential epiretinal membrane (ERM)/thickened PH traction (Haouchine et al., Ophthalmology 108(1):15–22, 2001; Johnson, Curr Opin Ophthalmol 13(3):152–160, 2002; Hussain et al., Indian J Ophthalmol 51(4):353–355, 2003; Gass, Arch Ophthalmol 106(5):629–639, 1988; Tsai et al., Retina 36(9):1679–1687, 2016; Ang et al., Ophthalmologica 245(2):187–193, 2022; Uemura et al., Retina 43(2):215–221, 2023). In contrast, in eyes with proliferative diabetic retinopathy (PDR), a unique pro-proliferative microenvironment exists and promotes ERM and fibrovascular proliferation (FVP) formation, causing complex traction on the macula (Kase et al., Br J Ophthalmol 91(10):1376–1378, 2007; Iannetti et al. Invest Ophthalmol Vis Sci 52(8):5786–5789, 2011; Abu El-Asrar et al., Mol Vis 16:1098–1107, 2010; Abu El-Asrar et al., Clin Exp Ophthalmol 38(1):57–64, quiz 87, 2010). The development, configuration, and surgical results of FTMHs in PDR may differ from those in other conditions. However, there is little research on the mechanisms, features, and treatment methods of FTMH in PDR. In this chapter, these issues will be discussed.

12.1 Case Report

Patient 1: A 49-year-old man with DM and hypertension who was under oral medication control had progressive BV in both eyes for 2 years and received IVI Lucentis several times at an outside hospital under the impression of PDR with DME. He experienced sudden onset of blurred vision in the right eye and came to our clinic. On examination, BCVA was 0.05 in the right eye and 0.03 in the left eye. The anterior segment was unremarkable in both eyes. Fundus examination in the right eye revealed an attached retina, a large NV net on and around the disc, a panretinal photocoagulation (PRP)

C.-M. Yang, *Surgery for Complications of Diabetic Retinopathy*,
https://doi.org/10.1007/978-981-96-2848-3_12

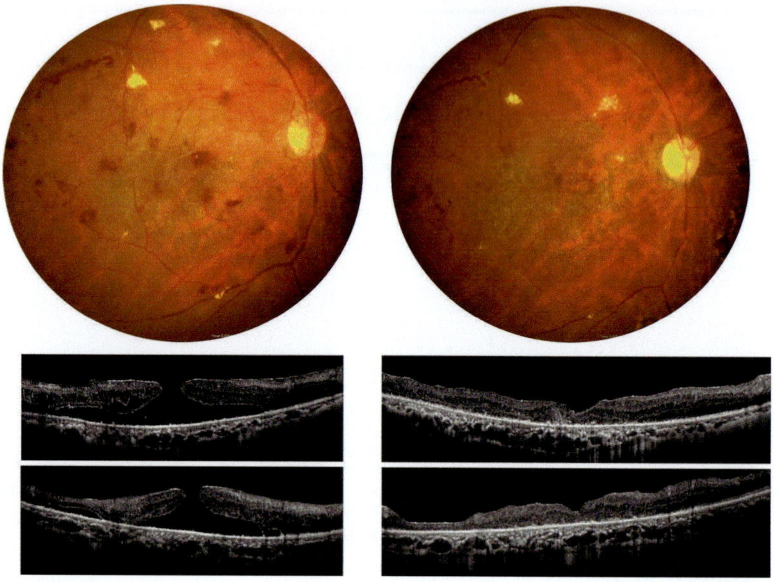

Fig. 12.1 Images showing pre- and postoperative retinal changes in the right eye in a patient with MH. Preoperative color photo and OCT images showing active NV and MH with localized shallow RD (left column). After surgery, the MH was sealed, and the retina was attached (right column). (Courtesy of Dr. Chung-May Yang)

scar, a small venous loop temporal lower to the macula, sausage-like tortuous vessels around the temporal upper area of the macula, soft exudate, and many hemorrhagic dots in the posterior pole. MH with localized RD was also noted. The left eye showed NV and collateral vessels on the disc, a PRP scar, vascular changes similar to those observed in the right eye, and artery sheathing. OCT revealed an ERM and MH with localized RD in the right eye and retinal thinning with cystic degeneration in the left eye. A diagnosis of PDR, MH with VH in the right eye, and PDR with old central retinal vein occlusion (CRVO) was made. ERM and ILM peeling, supplementary PRP, and gas infusion were performed on the right eye. The MH was sealed after surgery. Her BCVA improved to 0.1 (Fig. 12.1).

Patient 2: A 33-year-old man with DM, diagnosed 1 year before, developed PDR and was treated with PRP in both eyes. The patient underwent vitrectomy with SO infusion in the left eye for tractional retinal detachment (TRD). Blurred vision in the right eye was observed. On examination, BCVA was 0.04 in the right eye and 0.2 in the left eye. Fundus examination of the right eye revealed MH with localized RD, a dense FVP around the arcades extending to the equator, and mild VH. The left eye had an attached retina under SO. OCT revealed VM adhesion, ERM, MH with paramacular schisis, and RD in the right eye. Vitrectomy, ILM peeling with an inverted ILM flap, an endolaser, and intravitreal gas infusion were performed. The MH was sealed after surgery. Her BCVA improved to 0.2 with cataracts (Fig. 12.2).

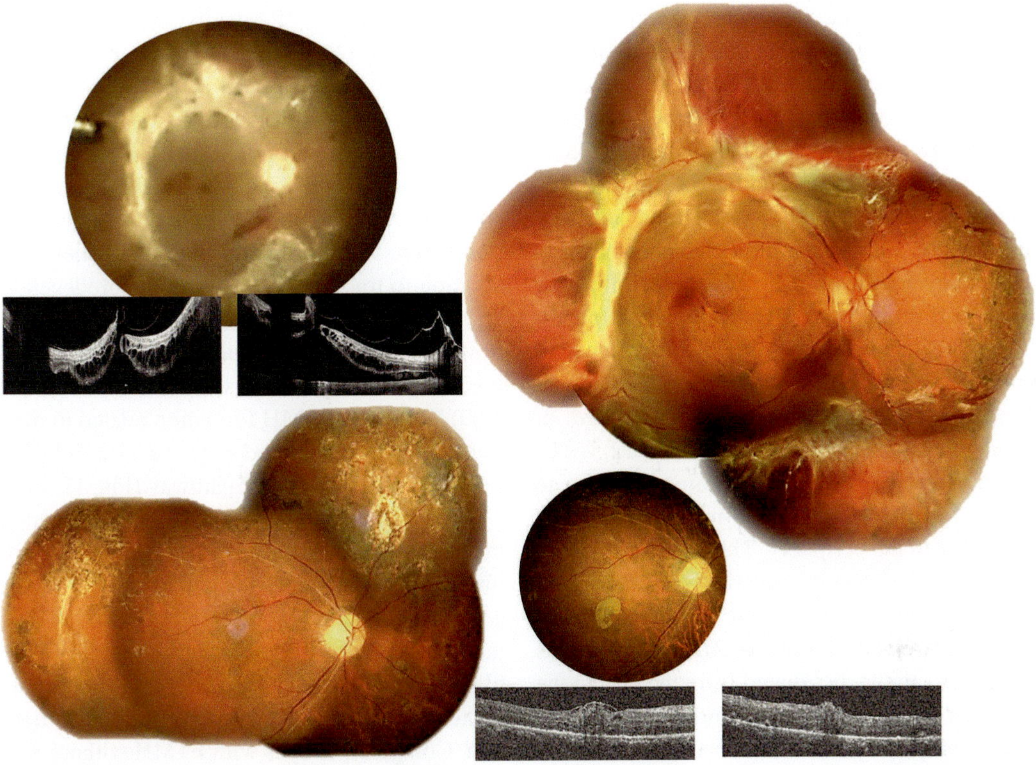

Fig. 12.2 One set of images showing pre- and postoperative retinal changes in a patient with MH with RD in PDR. Intraoperative video images and preoperative composite color photographs and OCT images are shown on the upper part; an active FVP around the arcade can be seen. Postoperative composite color images and OCT images are shown on the lower part; the MH was sealed with an ILM flap on the inner surface, and focal macular RPE atrophy was observed (color photo on the lower part). (Courtesy of Dr. Chung-May Yang)

12.2 Macular Hole in PDR with FVP

In PDR, MH may develop in eyes with minimal or no visible FVP. Alternatively, MH may be observed in conditions complicated by fibrovascular membranes, such as progressive fibrovascular proliferation, progressive disc or macular traction, and TRD or CTRRD [1, 2]. In eyes with PDR, complex traction on the macula may exist, rendering the configuration of the macula and mechanisms of FTMH formation likely to be distinct from those in idiopathic FTMHs [3].

We studied MH in PDR with FVP [1]. OCT and clinical observation pre- and intraoperatively suggested that the posterior hyaloids were usually adhered to or only partially separated from the macula. Even if significant vitreomacular separation has developed, connections frequently remain between the hyaloid and the hole edge. Two major patterns of the vitreomacular relationship can be identified: first, a thick and taut posterior hyaloid running parallel or oblique to the retinal surface, usually with multiple adhesion points on or close to the edge of the hole; the posterior hyaloid may or may not be detached. Second, the FVP tissue at the paracentral area, which may send the ERM to reach the hole edge, exerts considerable traction force on the hole. Several features unique to MH in PDR with FVP are noted. First, except at the hole edge, prominent cystoid changes are not typically observed. This finding suggested that cyst formation from severe macular edema does not play a major role in causing macular hole formation in diabetic FVPs. In addition, OCT shows that elevated or rolled-up edges are seen much less often than in idiopathic MH; rather, MH edges with flat surfaces are more common. Some even had slightly depressed edges. This finding may indicate that horizontally oriented traction, rather than vertical traction, contributes more to FTMH formation. The hole may assume a round, oval, or slit shape, depending on the direction and extent of traction forces. Strong adhesion and traction may cause the detachment area to extend beyond the border of the hole, unlike the small cuff around the MH in idiopathic conditions. The degree of traction and the presence of other breaks determine whether the retina is attached, shallowly or moderately detached, or highly elevated (Figs. 12.3, 12.4, and 12.5) The severity of FVP varied from point adhesion to broad proliferative tissue-retinal adhesion extending to the periphery. The location and distribution rather than the severity of FVP are usually used to determine the development of MH. In those with significant RD, many patients had fibrous tissue distributed from the disc to the arcade. The traction force around the arcade that exerts oblique traction on the macula, in addition to the adherent ERM usually found in such conditions, may be the primary force that induces RD when an MH forms.

In a study in which pre-MH and post-MH OCT were analyzed, four different types of FTMH formation pathways in PDR were identified [3]. Type 1 was characterized by ERM and/or vitreomacular traction (VMT) inducing foveoschisis, intraretinal cysts, or foveal detachment, followed by the formation of an FTMH or macular hole retinal detachment (MHRD). The majority of eyes had grade 2 FVP severity. This sequence is similar to that of idiopathic conditions, except that the tractions persist after MH formation. In this pathway, one unique condition is that traction may be attributed to sub-ILM hemorrhage leading to foveal structural changes and MH. In type 2, the ERM and/or FVP induced LMH with foveoschisis, followed by the formation of the FTMH or MHRD. LMH with or without schisis is a distinct feature before MH formation. The majority of eyes had grade 2 or 3 FVP severity. Type 3 was characterized by initial TRD with foveal cysts and/or foveoschisis and subsequent MHRD formation. The majority of eyes had grade 3 FVP severity. Type 4 was characterized by TRD associated with foveal thinning, followed by the formation of the MHRD. The macula could be on or off. The majority of eyes had grade 2 or 3 FVP severity. Both types 3 and 4 involved TRD, and both showed foveal structure abnormalities after traction before MH formation. In type 4 patients, in addition to traction, ischemia and neurodegeneration might also contribute to foveal thinning. Foveal thinning may occur before or after TRD involving the macula (Figs. 12.6, 12.7, 12.8, and 12.9) We observed MH formation related to traction from sub-ILM blood and the FVP band. This may be a type 1 or type 2 pathway (Fig. 12.10).

In our study, we found that FTMH formation might occur in either the active (38.1%) or fibrotic (61.9%) stage of the disease [3]. In the active stage, the traction force on the fovea may increase as the disease progresses, while in the fibrotic stage, the atrophic macula may contribute to the vulnerability of the structure to milder traction. Compared to eyes with FTMH without RD, those with MHRD had poorer BCVA, a shorter duration of FTMH formation, a greater proportion of Grade 3 and Grade 4 FVP, a greater percentage of active FVP, a lower percentage of ERM/VMT, and a greater percentage of TRD, all of which indicate that MHRD is more likely to occur in eyes with more severe PDR.

What is the best method of treatment? Because of the complex forces, varied severity of FVP, and different MH sizes and detachments involved, there is no standard treatment protocol. Adding to this complexity, spontaneous closure can occur (Fig. 12.11).

In one of our previous studies, we found that patients with shallow retinal elevation had persistent holes after vitrectomy when only the ERM but not the ILM was removed [1]. These findings indicate that ILM removal is crucial for hole closure, at least in shallowly detached retinas.

Summarized from our own practice and our experience in treating MH under various conditions, our treatment guidelines include simple ILM peeling for small to moderate MH with or without shallow RD and the use of ILM tissue for flap covering, flap insertion, or free fragment

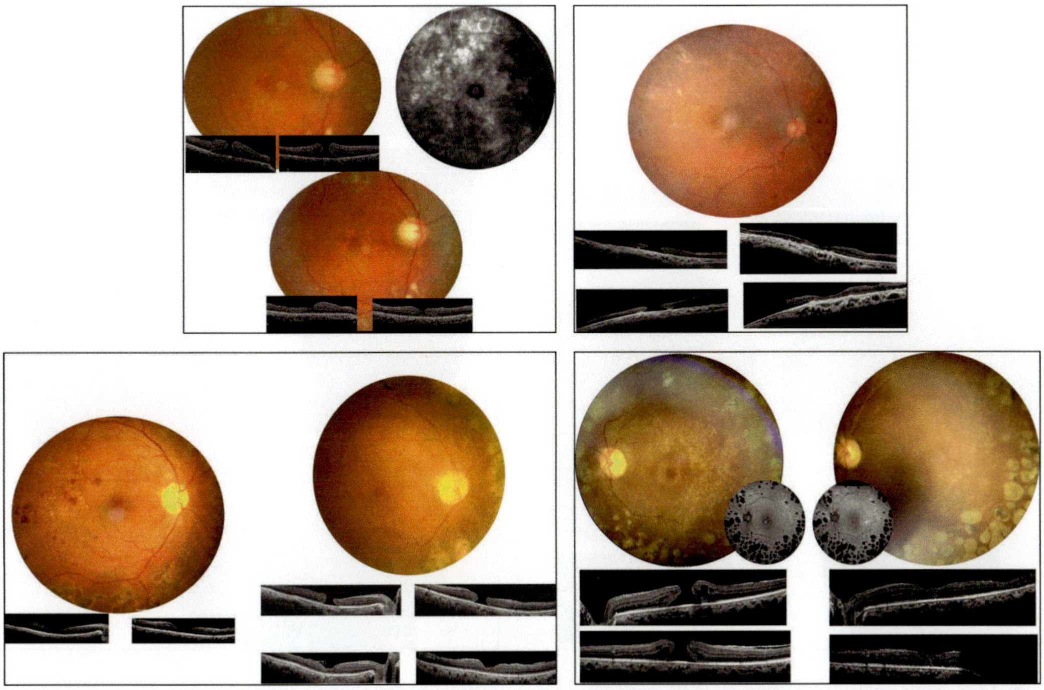

Fig. 12.3 Four sets of MHs without RD in PDR patients before and after surgery. In two sets (upper left and lower right), MH was associated with cystic changes at the hole edge; the other two sets showed no MH edge cysts. There was prominent vascular leakage in the macular area in the upper left panel, which may or may not contribute to MH formation and cystic changes. (Courtesy of Dr. Chung-May Yang)

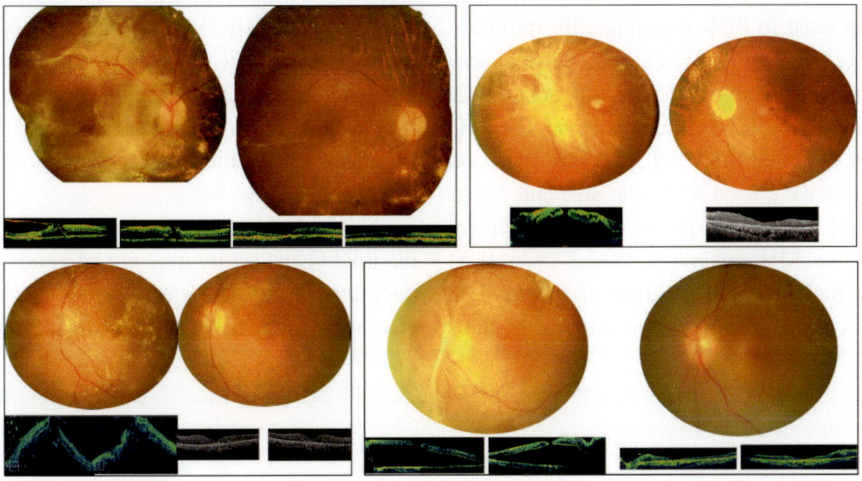

Fig. 12.4 Four sets of shallow to moderate elevations of the MHRD in PDR patients with FVP before and after surgery. The distribution and severity of FVP tissue vary in each set. Premacular membranes were present in each case, with a tightly adherent membrane in the lower right set. (Courtesy of Dr. Chung-May Yang)

insertion, depending on the intraoperative conditions, in patients with MHRD [4]. When using an ILM tissue flap or fragment, the initial choice to close the macular hole was always the inverted epiretinal ILM flap technique because this approach interferes least with photoreceptor regeneration and best avoids possible dye toxicity to retinal pigment epithelial cells after sur-

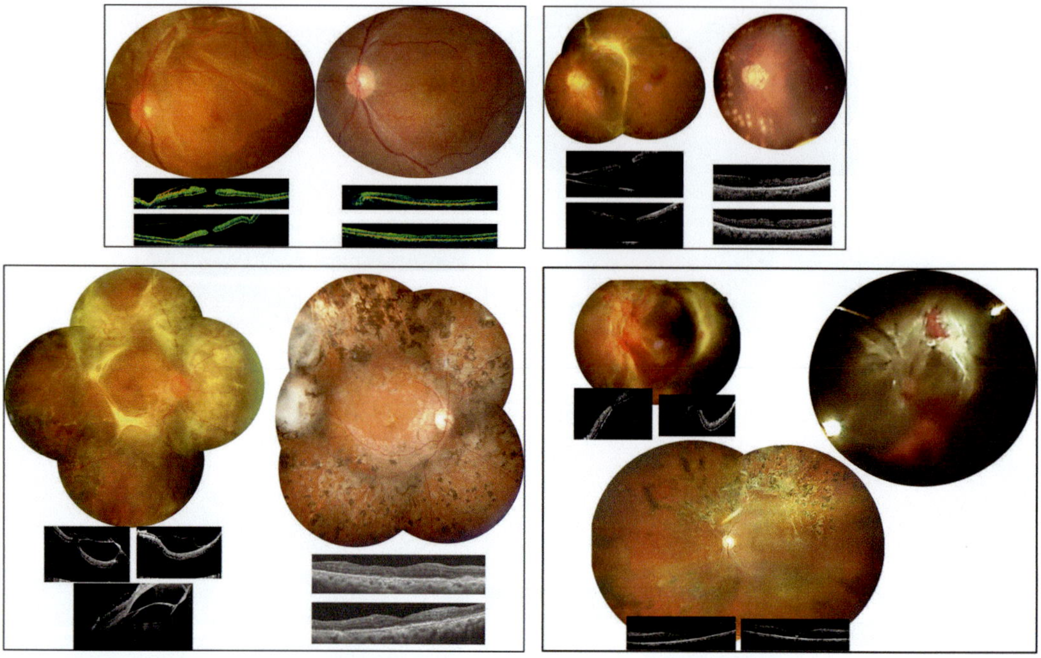

Fig. 12.5 Four sets of MHRDs in PDR patients with FVP before and after surgery. As the severity of FVP increased, RD became more prominent. Except for the lower left panel, in which the premacular membrane was attached to the central fovea before surgery (lower left OCT images), the MH edges in the other panels were flat without prominent cysts. (Courtesy of Dr. Chung-May Yang)

gery. However, because complex traction conditions exist in PDR patients, with multilayered ERMs adhering to and exerting vertical and/or horizontal traction on the macula, adequately large amounts of ILM tissue to cover the MH cannot be obtained. Inverted ILM flap insertion or free flaps were used when the size and integrity of the ILM flap were judged to be insufficient for adequate MH coverage. When even ILM insertion, including the addition of a free ILM flap, could not be performed, multiple ILM flaps were used. Indeed, in one of our case series, ten patients with MHRD were treated. Only two had inverted epiretinal ILM flaps; the others had either inverted ILM insertions (five patients) or free ILM flaps (three patients). Eventually, all ten of our patients achieved MH closure with a reattached retina [4].

Although the anatomical success rate is high, the final visual acuity may not be good; only preoperative visual acuity and the submacular fluid level were found to be associated with final vision.

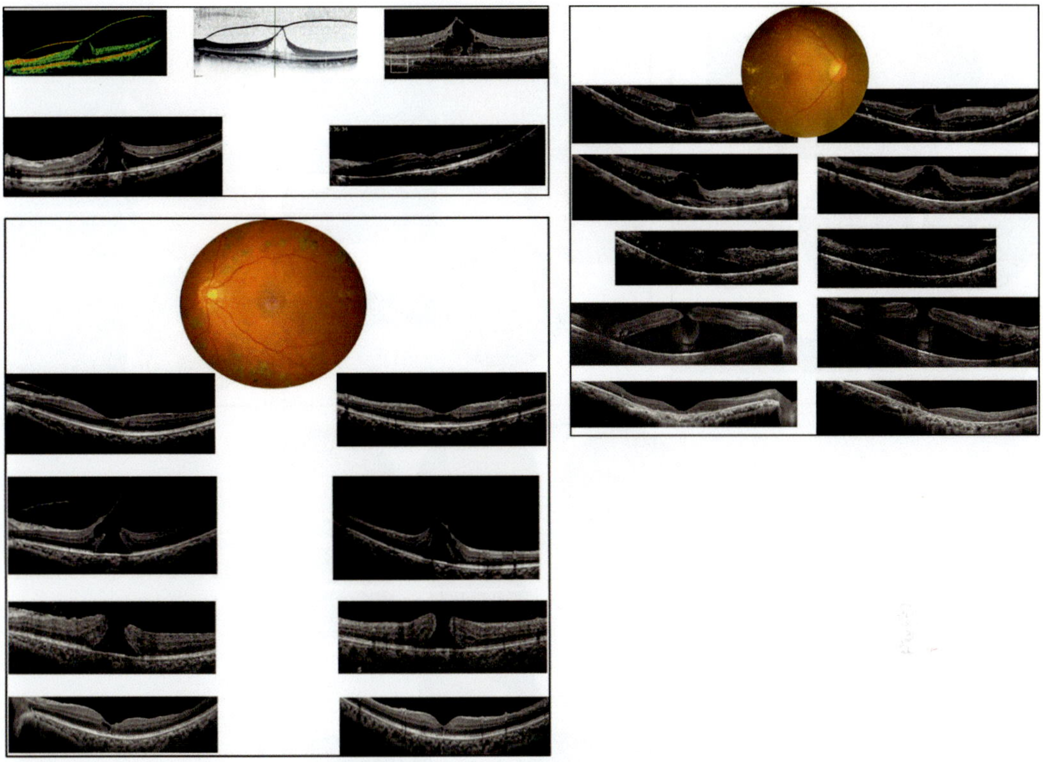

Fig. 12.6 Three sets of type 1 MH formation pathways and postoperative OCT images. Sequential preoperative OCT images show that ERM traction and/or VMT led to foveoschisis, cysts, or foveal detachment. Full-thickness MHs (upper left and lower left panels) or MHRDs (right panel) subsequently developed. All patients achieved MH closure after surgery. (Courtesy of Dr. Chung-May Yang)

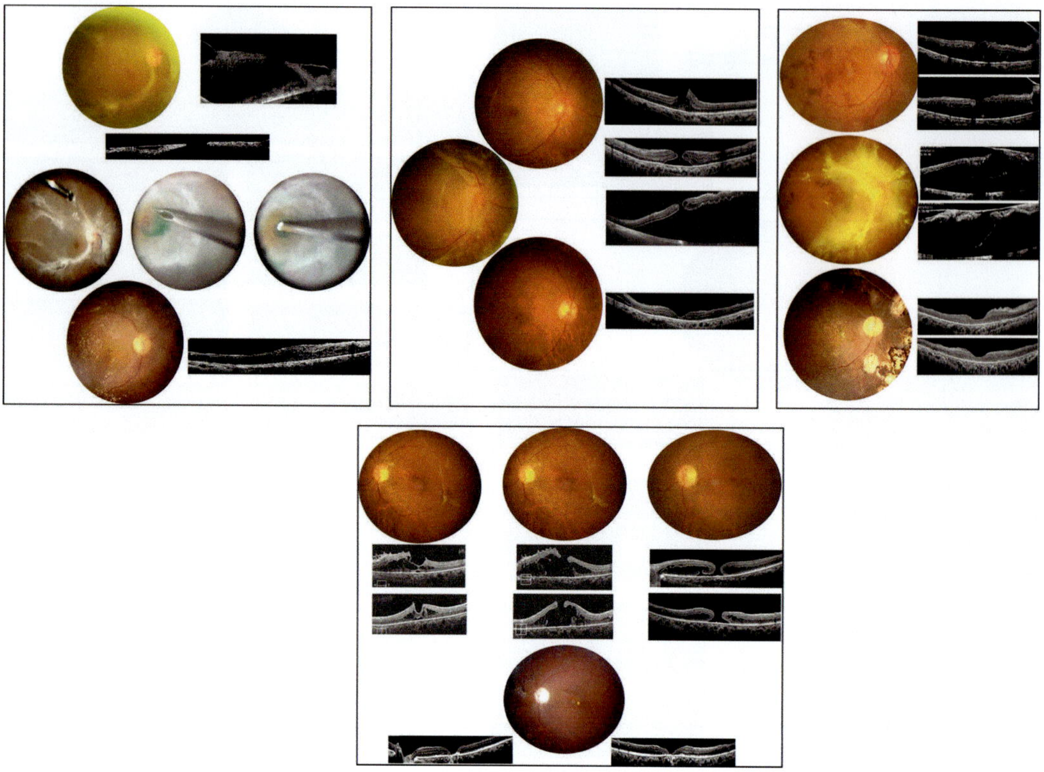

Fig. 12.7 Four sets of type 2 MH formation pathways and postoperative OCT images. Traction with or without schisis led to LMH with foveoschisis. FTMHs or MHRDs subsequently developed. LMH is a distinct feature of this type before MH formation. The upper right panel shows the same case as in Fig. 25.6, lower right panel, right eye. (Courtesy of Dr. Chung-May Yang)

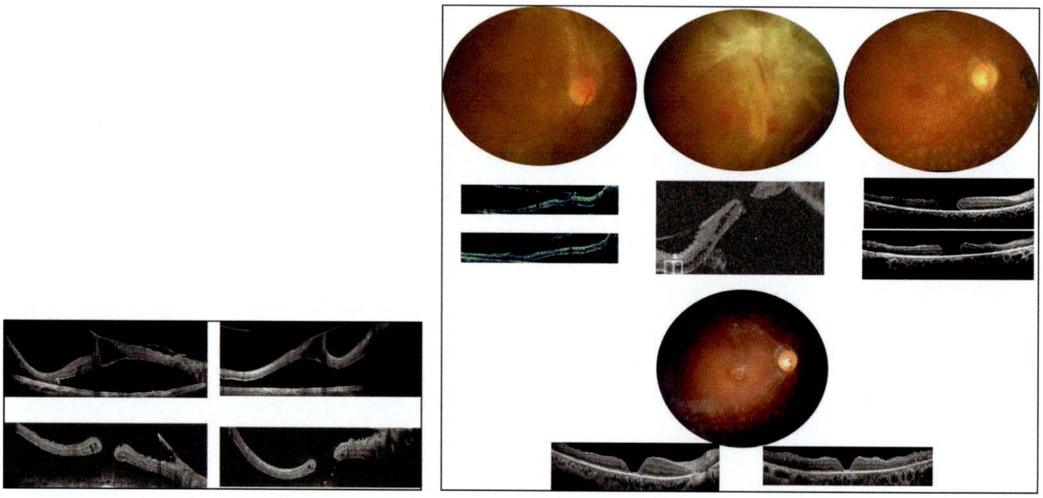

Fig. 12.8 Two sets of type 3 MH formations. The major feature is TRD with foveal cysts or schisis. MHRDs develop due to continuous traction on the abnormal foveal structure. The right panel also shows postoperative persistent MH (upper right), which eventually closed after lens capsular fragment insertion (lower color and OCT). (Courtesy of Dr. Chung-May Yang)

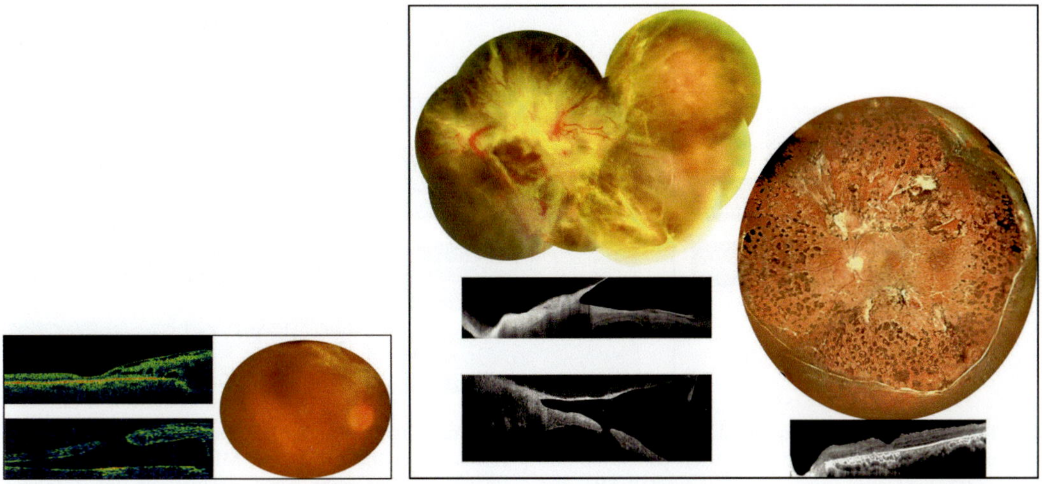

Fig. 12.9 Two sets of type 4 MH formation. The major feature is foveal thinning in the presence of TRD. The macula was attached to the left panel and detached from the right panel before MH formation. MHRD developed by continuous traction on this thin fovea. The right panel also shows postoperative images (right wide angle color photo and OCT) showing the attached retina and a closed MH. (Courtesy of Dr. Chung-May Yang)

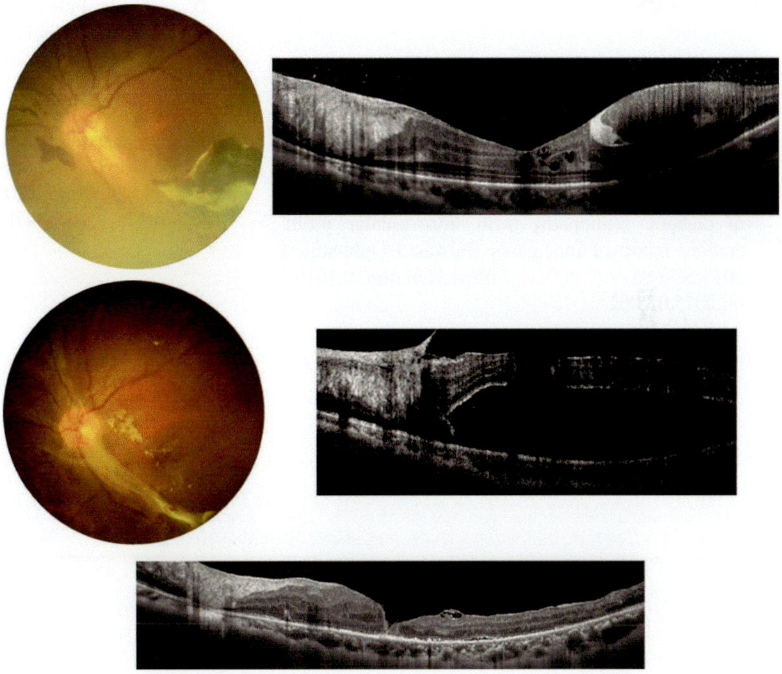

Fig. 12.10 Sequential pre- and postoperative images of a patient with MH formation. This case is unique because of the traction from sub-ILM blood and the lower arcade FVP band associated with parafoveal cysts. Within 1 month, MH developed. No intermediate stage of LMH was found. This may be a type 1 or type 2 pathway. (Courtesy of Dr. Tso-Ting Lai)

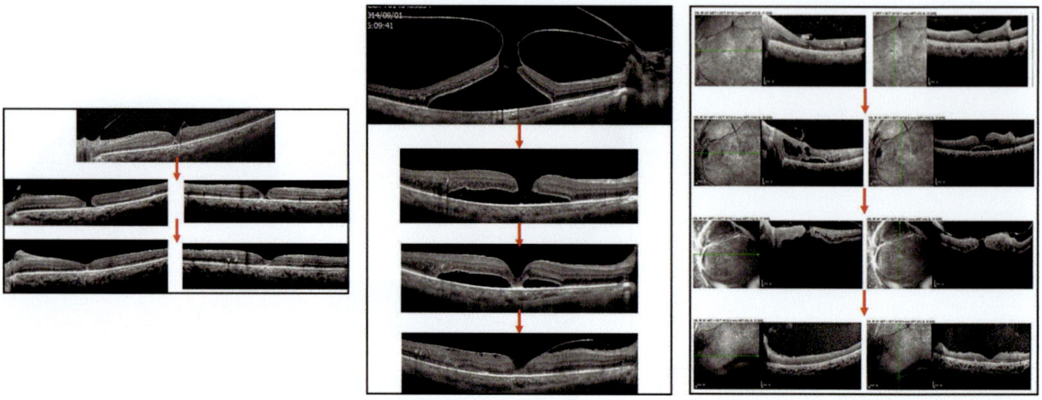

Fig. 12.11 Three sets of sequential OCT images showing spontaneous MH closure. In the left panel, the predominantly tangential traction caused a small MH, and spontaneous MH was noted at 3 months. In the center panel, multilayer traction induced MH with RD. Spontaneous MH closure with the attached retina occurred 6 months after the release of the VMT. Note the formation of the ERM after MH closure (bottom OCT image). In the right panel, traction on the localized detached macula induced MH with RD. Spontaneous retinal reattachment and MH closure were noted after traction release for 20 months. (Courtesy of Dr. Chung-May Yang)

References

1. Yeh PT, Cheng CK, Chen MS, Yang CH, Yang CM. Macular hole in proliferative diabetic retinopathy with fibrovascular proliferation. Retina. 2009;29(3):355–61. https://doi.org/10.1097/IAE.0b013e31818c3251.
2. Lai CT, Yang CM. Development of macular holes in diabetic retinopathy with fibrovascular proliferation: report of four cases. Taiwan J Ophthalmol. 2015;5(2):85–9. https://doi.org/10.1016/j.tjo.2015.03.002.
3. Tsui MC, Hsieh YT, Lai TT, Lai CT, Lin HC, Ho TC, et al. Full-thickness macular hole formation in proliferative diabetic retinopathy. Sci Rep. 2021;11(1):23839. https://doi.org/10.1038/s41598-021-03239-2.
4. Chen SN, Yang CM. Internal limiting membrane flaps for coexistent macular hole and retinal detachment in eyes with proliferative diabetic retinopathy. J Ophthalmol. 2018;2018:3470731. https://doi.org/10.1155/2018/3470731.

13 Vitreomacular Traction in Diabetic Retinopathy

Abstract

In the previous chapters, several vitreomacular interface disorders (VMIDs), including preretinal fibrosis, macular hole (MH), and lamellar macular hole (LMH), were discussed. VM traction (VMT) is another major category of VMID that warrants investigation.

13.1 Case Report

A 69-year-old woman had DM for more than 30 years. Blood sugar was fairly controlled with oral medication. Her ophthalmic history revealed a history of cataract operation in the right eye and proliferative diabetic retinopathy (PDR) with macular edema in the right eye, which had been treated with panretinal photocoagulation (PRP) and IVI anti-VEGF injections three times. The patient came to our clinic due to blurred vision in both eyes for several months. On examination, BCVA was 0.063 in both eyes; lens status showed posterior chamber intraocular lens (PCIOL) in the right eye and moderate cataract in the left eye. Fundus examinations and OCT revealed epiretinal membranes (ERMs) with lamellar macular holes (LMHs) in the right eye and ERMs and VMTs with broad adhesion, central foveoschisis, and mild foveal detachment in the left eye. Phacoemulsification with PCIOL implantation, vitrectomy with PH and ERM removal, and internal limiting membrane (ILM) peeling were performed on the left eye. The postoperative course was uneventful. Two months later, vitrectomy was also performed in the right eye. One and a half years later, the macular contour was smooth with a preserved foveal pit in both eyes. Her BCVA was 0.4 in the right eye and 0.7 in the left eye (Fig. 13.1).

C.-M. Yang, *Surgery for Complications of Diabetic Retinopathy*,
https://doi.org/10.1007/978-981-96-2848-3_13

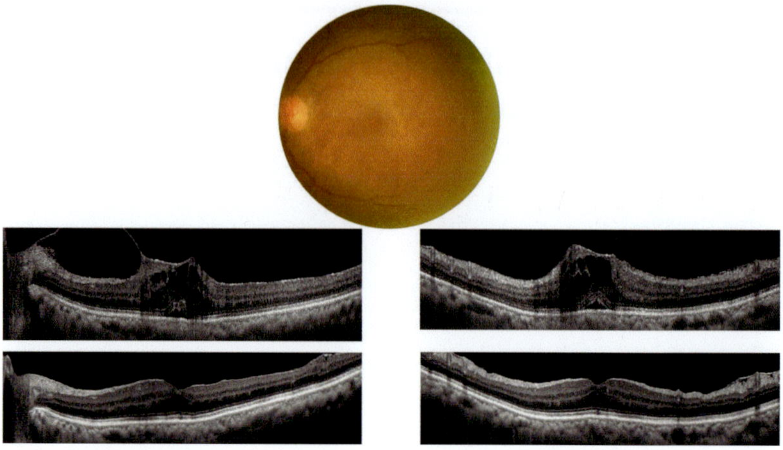

Fig. 13.1 Preoperative color photo (upper) and OCT images (middle row) showing ERMs and VMTs with broad VM adhesion, central cysts/schisis, and small subfoveal fluid pockets in the left eye. After surgery, OCT images show recovery of the foveal contour (lower row). (Courtesy of Dr. Chung-May Yang)

13.2 Vitreomacular Traction in DR

VMT, defined as incomplete posterior vitreous detachment (PVD)-induced macular traction that causes changes in the macular microstructure, has been proposed as a notable finding of the vitreoretinal relationship in DR [1]. In eyes with DR, the PH is thickened and contractile; the vitreous gel contains many cytokines as well as VEGF, which increases intraocular inflammation. These factors may render vitreomacular adhesions and traction more severe than those of idiopathic VMT [2]. Although fibrovascular traction-induced vitreomacular abnormalities in eyes with PDR have been reported [3, 4], macular changes from VMT unrelated to the posterior pole FVP have not been specifically described in the literature, even though they may have unique features. We conducted a retrospective study to investigate the morphological changes, clinical course, and anatomical and functional results after surgery for VMT in eyes with DR [2]. The recognition of this entity may extend our understanding of the various VMIDs in DR.

To observe the direct effect of uncomplicated VMT on other pathological changes, we excluded patients whose FVP was located along the arcades or posterior to the equator. All patients had an FU period of more than 6 months. For those who underwent surgery in both eyes, only the first operated eye was included in the study. In total, 30 eyes of 30 patients were included.

The mean age of the 30 patients was 69.5 ± 8.1 years, and 16 of them were female. Among the 30 eyes, 24 (80%) had PDR with PRP, and 6 (20%) had nonproliferative diabetic retinopathy (NPDR). The PH was thickened in all patients, and multilayered traction from different directions was noted in 14 eyes (46.7%). The proportion of multilayered traction was 50% in the PDR and 33.3% in the NPDR ($p = 0.66$) (Figs. 13.2 and 13.3). Furthermore, 21 eyes (70%) had tractional retinoschisis (Fig. 13.4), 7 (23.3%) had foveal detachment (Fig. 13.5), 5 (16.7%) had LMH (Fig. 13.4), and 3 (10%) had full-thickness macular hole (FTMH), including 2 with macular hole retinal detachment (MHRD) (Fig. 13.6). Macular thickening with edema was observed in one eye (Fig. 13.7).

Our study [2] showed that eyes with FTMH or ellipsoid zone disruption tended to have poorer visual acuity at baseline. A greater central retinal thickness (CRT) and foveal detachment at baseline were also associated with poorer vision, with borderline significance.

Clinical course examinations revealed that among the 30 eyes, 2 had PVD and spontaneous release of VMT within 3 months of observation. Both patients showed improved vision after PVD. One patient with MHRD also experienced spontaneous resolution of the VMT with closure of the MH and subsequent resolution of RD without surgical intervention (Fig. 13.8). The remaining 27 eyes underwent vitrectomy, ERM peeling,

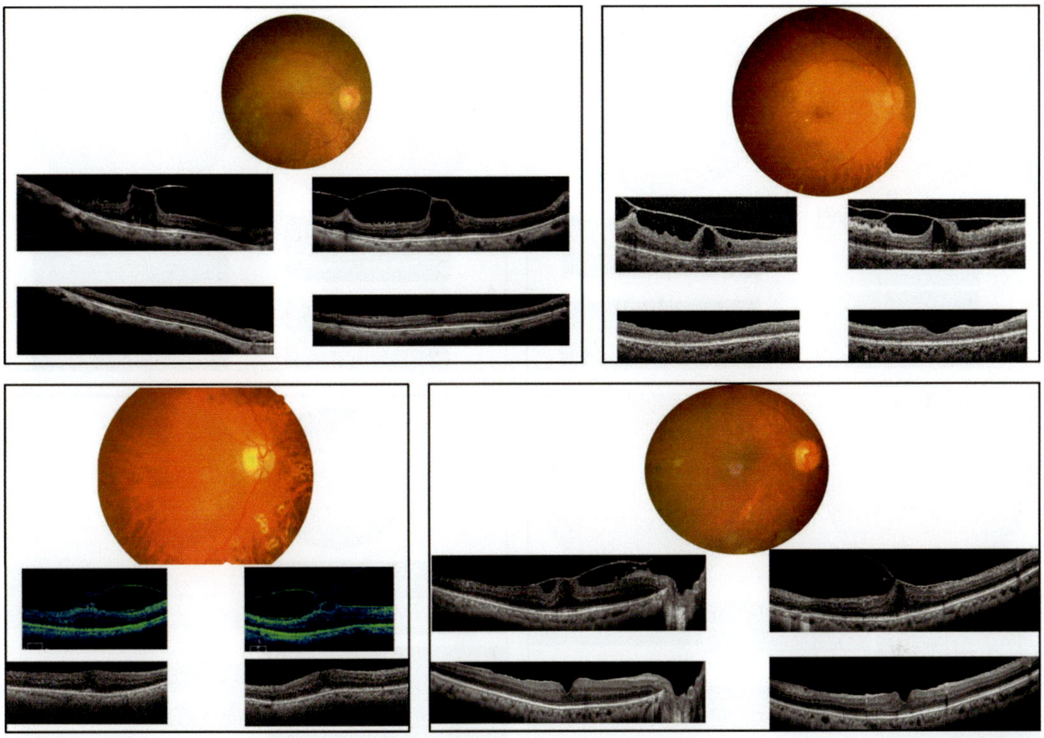

Fig. 13.2 Four examples of VMT in DR patients. In each panel, preoperative color images and OCT images are shown in the upper and middle rows, respectively, and postoperative OCT images are shown in the bottom row. Multiple adhesion sites, multilayered traction membranes, and multidirectional traction were observed preoperatively in each patient. After surgery, all patients had improved macular contours. (Right upper panel: courtesy of Dr. Chang-Hao Yang)

ILM peeling, and C_3F_8 tamponade. Postoperatively, the mean BCVA significantly improved from 1.02 ± 0.41 at baseline to 0.59 ± 0.36 at the final visit ($p < 0.001$). No patient experienced visual deterioration after the operation. However, one-third of the patients had disorganization of the retinal inner layers (DRIL), and ellipsoid zone disruption at the fovea was noted in more than 50%.

Only poorer preoperative vision was found to be associated with poorer postoperative visual outcome, while the severity of DR and baseline characteristics on OCT were not associated with postoperative visual outcome. After the operation, both DRIL and ellipsoid zone disruption were associated with poorer vision.

In the above study [2], we found that although pure VMT in DR induces less severe retinal structural changes than does VMT affected by the FVP, where extensive traction macular detachment or combined tractional and rhegmatogenous retinal detachment (CTRRD) may occur, the traction forces of the VMT in DR remain strong and complex. Studies have shown that PVD occurs later in eyes with DR than in nondiabetic eyes [5]. The anteroposterior or oblique traction forces from the incomplete PVD, as well as the strict tangential force from the ERM, may act synergistically. The PH in DR frequently attaches to the macula at multiple sites; it is also prone to attach to the midperipheral retina by abnormal vitreoretinal adhesion or fibrovascular tufts.

We found vitreoschisis with multilayered VMT not only in PDR patients (50%) but also in NPDR patients (33.3%) [2]. Complex traction and strong vitreomacular adhesion also contribute to the greater incidence of macular retinoschisis and concurrent macular holes in diabetic

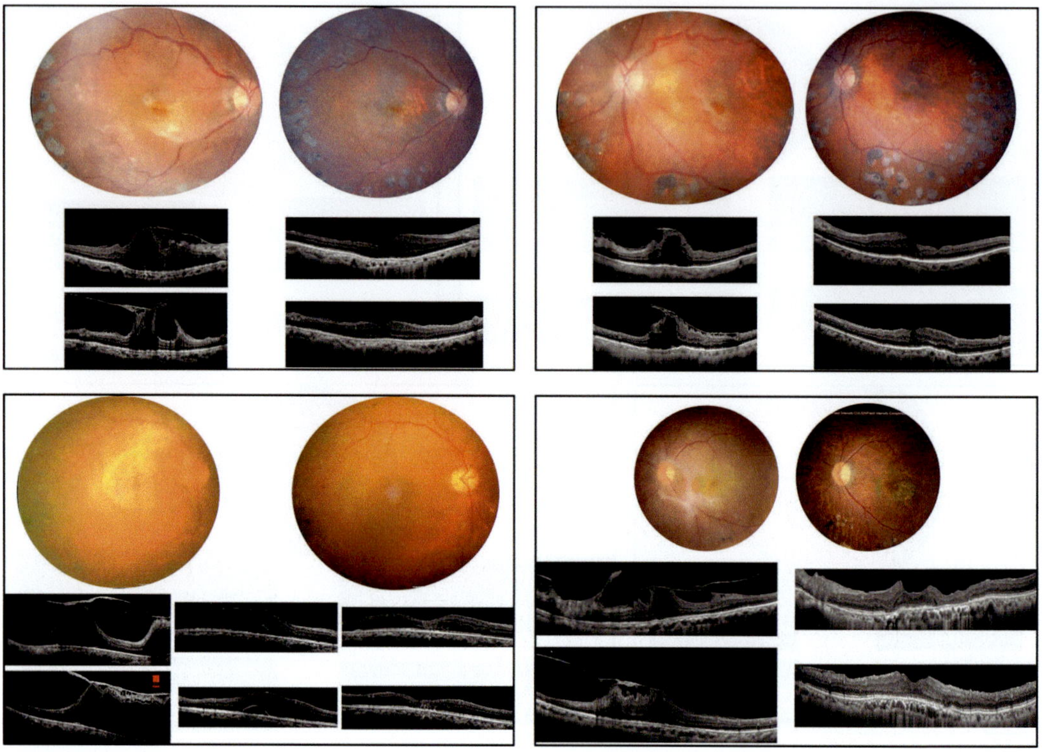

Fig. 13.3 Four sets of VMTs in the DR with a condensed premacular membrane. Images from the upper two panels were obtained from two eyes of the same patient. In each panel, preoperative color images and OCT images are shown on the left side, and postoperative images are shown on the right side. All patients had elevated central retina and multilayered traction (tangential ERM and more obliquely oriented vitreous membrane) preoperatively. The lower left panel shows traction macular schisis on the upper macular area preoperatively (bottom left OCT images). Structural improvement was noted in all patients (right images in all panels). (Courtesy of Dr. Chung-May Yang)

eyes than in nondiabetic eyes with VMT. After surgery, most patients (77.8%) had a faster and greater proportion of complete resolution of macular schisis than macular schisis caused by active fibrovascular traction or fibrotic tractional tissues in PDR patients.

The VMT is an important contributor to LMH in DR patients. In our study, 16.7% of patients with VMT in DR patients had LMH [2]. Our previous study revealed that in patients with LMH in DR, almost half of them had concurrent VMT [6]. In contrast, only 10% of patients with idiopathic LMH had concurrent VMT. Multidirectional vitreomacular traction in eyes with DR causes the formation of an LMH, and the connection between the vitreous and retina persists even after lamellar or full-thickness macular holes are formed [2].

MHRD is the most serious complication of VMT in DR; however, recovery from structural changes may occur after spontaneous release of the VMT, as found in the above study. We postulate that once vitreomacular traction is released, the macular hole may be sealed by gliosis because of the pro-proliferative microenvironment and minimal tissue loss from the VMT. In PDR with an active FVP, the macular hole is more difficult to seal even after ILM peeling because of possible residual fibrovascular tissues and contracture of the underlying retinal tissues [7].

In summary, our study revealed that the VMT in DR patients had a thicker posterior hyaloid, and many of them had multiple layers of vitreomacular traction and/or concurrent tractional macular retinoschisis. Some of these patients

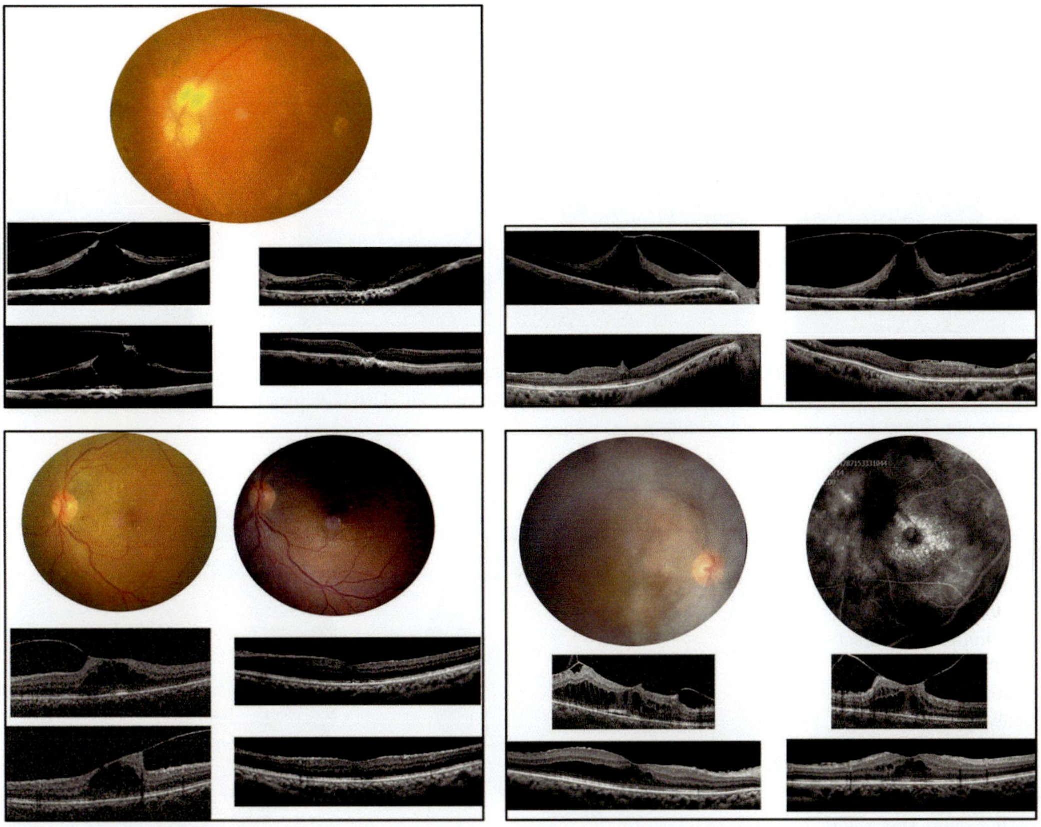

Fig. 13.4 Four sets of foveoschisis from the VMT before surgery. In the left two panels, the preoperative OCT images are on the left side, and the postoperative OCT images are on the right side. In the two patients in the left panels, disruption of the inner lining with the formation of LMH was also noted before surgery. In the two right panels, postoperative OCT images are shown at the bottom. All patients had improved macular structures after surgery. (Right upper panel: courtesy of Dr. Tzyy-Chang Ho)

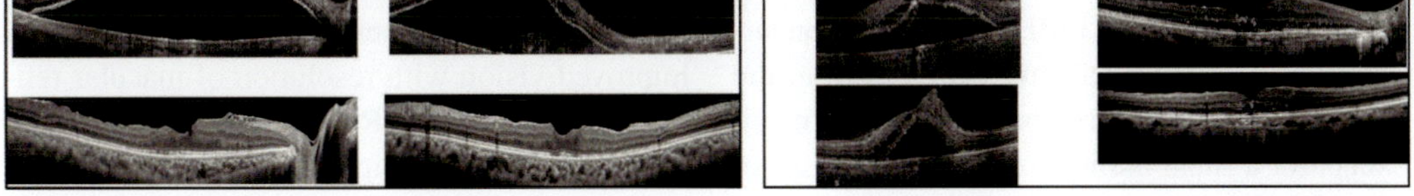

Fig. 13.5 Two sets of images showing posterior RD from the VMT in the DR. Both patients had intraretinal cysts before surgery (upper and middle rows in the left panel; left column in the right panel). The patients in the right panel also had asteroid hyalosis. After surgery, both patients showed recovery of the foveal contour. (Bottom row in the left panel; right panel; left panel: courtesy of Dr. Tzyy-Chang Ho)

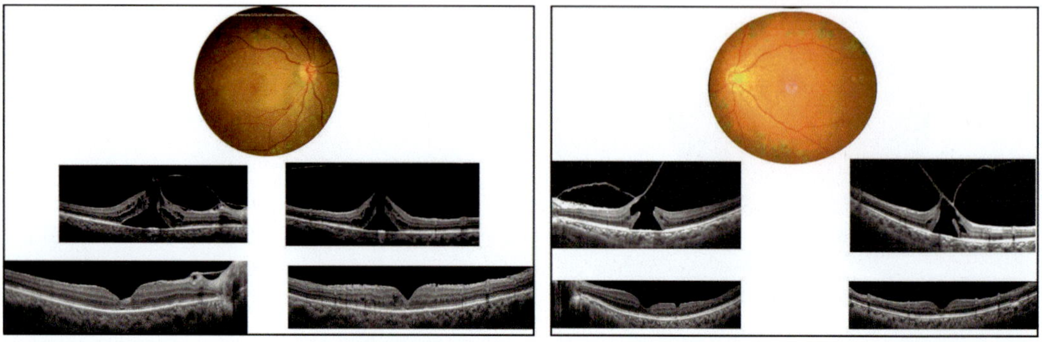

Fig. 13.6 Two sets of MHRDs from the VMT in the DR. In each panel, preoperative color images and OCT images are shown in the upper and middle rows, respectively, and postoperative OCT images are shown in the bottom row. (Left side panel: courtesy of Dr. Tzyy-Chang Ho)

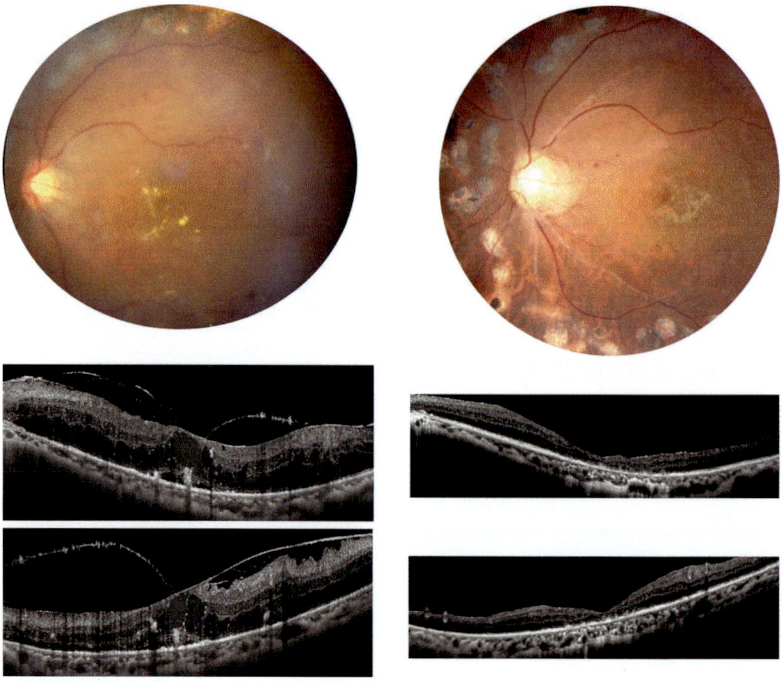

Fig. 13.7 A case of VMT associated with ME and HE (left side color photo and OCT images). After vitrectomy and cataract surgery, the foveal contour improved, but localized macular atrophy was noted (right side color photo and OCT images). (Courtesy of Dr. Chung-May Yang)

were complicated with LMH, FTMH, or concurrent RD. In general, patients with VMTs in the DR are good candidates for surgical treatment. Except for a small number of patients who experienced spontaneous resolution of VMT, all other patients who underwent surgery for VMT had improved vision with resolution of macular retinoschisis, MH, and RD. Persistent DRIL and ellipsoid zone disruption, however, were associated with poorer final vision.

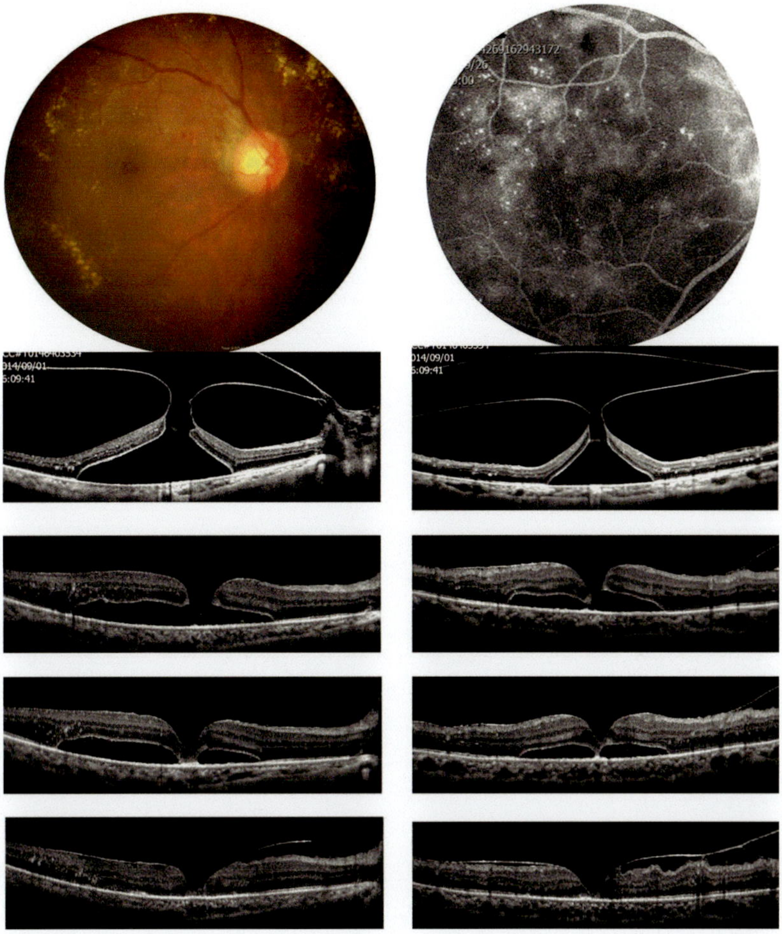

Fig. 13.8 Spontaneous MH closure and reattachment in the case of VMT-induced MHRD. After the release of the VMT, the ERM became obvious (bottom OCT images). (Courtesy of Dr. Yi-Ting Hsieh)

References

1. Panozzo G, Cicinelli MV, Augustin AJ, Battaglia Parodi M, Cunha-Vaz J, Guarnaccia G, et al. An optical coherence tomography-based grading of diabetic maculopathy proposed by an international expert panel: the European School for Advanced Studies in Ophthalmology classification. Eur J Ophthalmol. 2020;30(1):8–18. https://doi.org/10.1177/1120672119880394.
2. Hsieh YT, Yang CM. Vitreomacular traction in diabetic retinopathy. Jpn J Ophthalmol. 2024;68(1):12–8. https://doi.org/10.1007/s10384-023-01034-2.
3. Muqit MM, Stanga PE. Swept-source optical coherence tomography imaging of the cortical vitreous and the vitreoretinal interface in proliferative diabetic retinopathy: assessment of vitreoschisis, neovascularisation and the internal limiting membrane. Br J Ophthalmol. 2014;98(7):994–7. https://doi.org/10.1136/bjophthalmol-2013-304452.
4. Su CC, Yang CH, Yeh PT, Yang CM. Macular tractional retinoschisis in proliferative diabetic retinopathy: clinical characteristics and surgical outcome. Ophthalmologica. 2014;231(1):23–30. https://doi.org/10.1159/000355078.
5. Hayashi K, Sato T, Manabe SI, Hirata A, Yoshimura K. Posterior vitreous detachment in patients with diabetes mellitus. Jpn J Ophthalmol. 2020;64(2):187–95. https://doi.org/10.1007/s10384-020-00720-9.
6. Kuo BI, Yang CM, Hsieh YT. Lamellar macular hole in diabetic retinopathy. Eur J Ophthalmol. 2021;31(1):166–72. https://doi.org/10.1177/1120672119879665.
7. Yeh PT, Cheng CK, Chen MS, Yang CH, Yang CM. Macular hole in proliferative diabetic retinopathy with fibrovascular proliferation. Retina. 2009;29(3):355–61. https://doi.org/10.1097/IAE.0b013e31818c3251.

14 Vitreopapillary Traction in Proliferative Diabetic Retinopathy

Abstract

Vitreopapillary traction (VPT) may occur in eyes with or without DR (de Bustros et al., Arch Ophthalmol 105(2):196–199, 1987; Katz and Hoyt, Ophthalmology 102(2):349–354, 1995; Wisotsky et al., Am J Ophthalmol 126(1):137–139, 1998). It is characterized by vitreous traction on the disc margin through the fibrocellular membrane or an incompletely detached posterior hyaloid (Sebag, Eye (Lond) 6(Pt 6):541–552, 1992; Karatas et al., Eye (Lond) 19(6):676–682, 2005; Gabriel et al., Neuroophthalmology 44(4):213–8, 2020). The changes caused by prolonged traction on the disc were called "pseudopapilledema" by Schepens (Am J Ophthalmol 38(1:2):8–21, 1954). Diagnosis is based on clinical examination and/or OCT (Gabriel et al., Neuroophthalmology 44(4):213–218, 2020). VPT may damage the anterior optic nerve and cause visual function disturbance. Although the effect appears to be reversible, it might lead to irreversible optic nerve atrophy if left untreated. The possibility of visual function disturbance in the VPT was raised by De Bustros and associates in 1987 (de Bustros et al., Arch Ophthalmol 105(2):196–199, 1987). Kroll and associates further showed fundus photo, visual acuity, and VEP evidence of visual function improvement after traction release in isolated VPT patients in PDR (Kroll et al., Ophthalmologe 92(5):687–691, 1995; Kroll et al., Br J Ophthalmol 83(3):261–264, 1999). Early diagnosis and treatment of VPT can improve visual acuity and visual-evoked potentials and prevent progressive optic atrophy in diabetic eyes (Gabriel et al., Neuroophthalmology 44(4):213–218, 2020; Kroll et al., Ophthalmologe 92(5):687–691, 1995; Meyer et al., Acta Ophthalmol Scand 85(2):221–222, 2007). The clinical manifestations, disc changes, and surgical procedures will be discussed in this chapter.

14.1 Case Report

A 47-year-old woman had DM for several years. She had bilateral panretinal photocoagulation (PRP) for proliferative diabetic retinopathy (PDR). She came to our clinic complaining of blurred vision in the right eye. Her best-corrected visaul acuity (BCVA) was number of digits (ND) in the right eye and 0.7 in the left eye. Fundus examination revealed a wide area of preretinal hemorrhage. The hemorrhage reabsorbed within 2.5 months. After 1 year of follow-up, fundus examinations and optical coherence tomography (OCT) showed traction from the disc extending toward the macula, causing localized subretinal fluid (SRF) in the nasal paramacular and the submacular area. One year later, the SRF subsided, but the patient had persistent VF defects. On examination, BCVA was

C.-M. Yang, *Surgery for Complications of Diabetic Retinopathy*,
https://doi.org/10.1007/978-981-96-2848-3_14

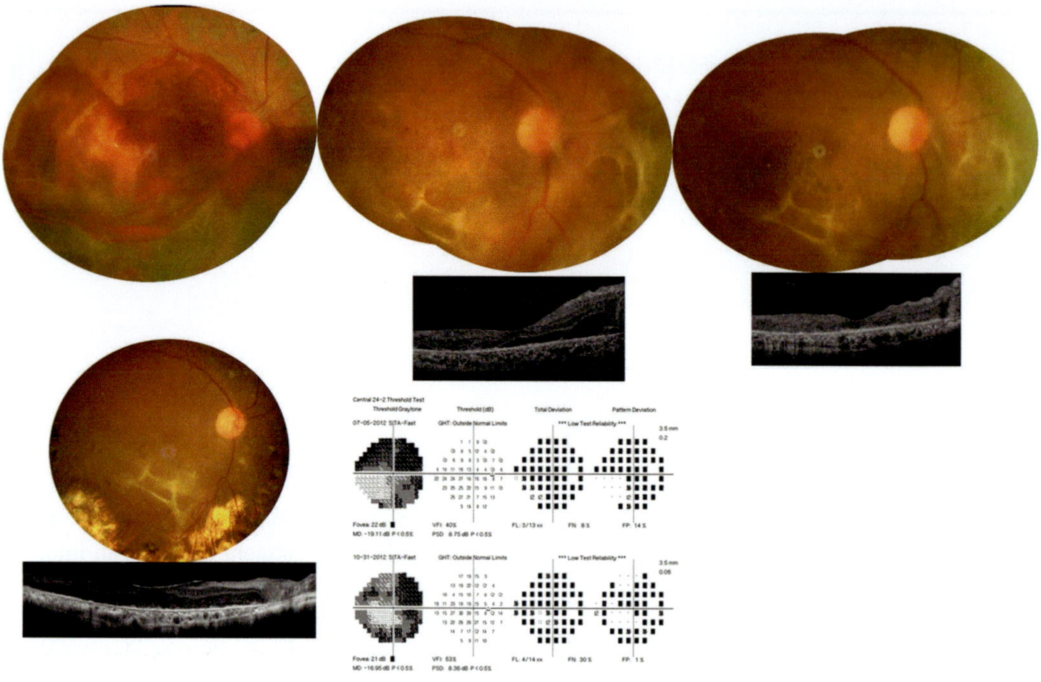

Fig. 14.1 The upper three composite color images and OCT images show the evolution of PDR from preretinal hemorrhage (upper left) to disc traction from the nasal and disc FVP membrane, causing macular detachment (upper center) to the VPT and a flat macula (upper right). Temporal pallor of the disc was observed. The lower left images show a pink disc and a flat macula with subretinal bands after surgery. The subsequent VF examination results on the lower right showed improvement of the VF defect at 3 months after surgery. (Courtesy of Dr. Chung-May Yang)

0.15 in the right eye. Fundus examinations revealed optic disc head traction from the fibrovascular proliferation (FVP) membrane along the lower part of the disc and in the nasal juxtapapillary area. The disc temporal pallor was noted. Subretinal fibrotic bands were observed in the lower macular area. OCT revealed a flat macula without edema. Visual field examination revealed defects in the upper and outer fields. Under the diagnosis of vitreopapillary traction (VPT) syndrome, she underwent vitrectomy to remove the fibrotic membrane. After surgery, the disc color improved, and BCVA improved to 0.4, with improved VF examination results (Fig. 14.1).

14.2 Vitreopapillary Traction in PDR

VPT is caused by strong adhesions at the margin of the optic disc and may occur in a number of different diseases, including DR, central retinal vein occlusion, Toxocara, PVD, and inflammatory diseases such as chronic uveitis [1, 3, 4]. Contracted fibrocellular vitreous membrane or incomplete detached posterior hyaloid may be the underlying cause; alternatively, FVP tissue growing on the disc may be the source of traction.

In DR, VPT is caused by the traction of the FVP on the disc, resulting in decreased vision and/or VF defects. This condition is unique in having a characteristic fundus feature, and if early treatment is given, visual function may be restored to a certain extent.

In a broad sense, any NVD combined with a fibrotic component may exert traction on the disc and cause neurotransmission or hemodynamic changes. These alterations, in turn, may affect visual function. However, disc traction is usually not a great concern compared with the more severe vitreoretinal abnormalities in DR. During surgery in PDR, the FVP on the disc is usually removed or isolated, resulting in the simultaneous release of disc traction. However, if one fails to recognize the potential effect of disc traction on visual function and leaves the FVP tissue on the disc and its connection with the nasal FVP tissue untreated during surgery, postoperative visual function may be compromised.

In a more specific sense, VPT in PDR is characterized by the traction of the FVP on the disc, usually from the nasal side, causing elevation and hyperemia of the nasal disc and temporal-side pallor; through altering neurotransmission and vascular perfusion around the disc, traction leads to visual field and/or visual function abnormalities. The pale color of the temporal disc is mainly caused by decreased perfusion from traction. The macular structures are not significantly affected. However, traction extending to the parapapillary region contributing to macular edema has been reported [2]. The temporal-side vessels on the disc may first bend toward the nasal side and then curve back. Macular OCT reveals a normal macular contour, but disc OCT reveals a protruded FVP with irregular elevation, usually peaking toward the nasal side (Fig. 14.2). Although the tissue is usually dragged toward and peaked at the nasal side, temporal side thickening and traction are usually present as well (Fig. 14.3).

Most FVP membranes that cause VPT in DR predominantly exhibit fibrotic features. They may be limited in extent or widespread in the nasal upper or lower quadrants (Fig. 14.3). Although nasal traction is most common, central disc traction or temporal traction may occasionally occur (Fig. 14.4). The BCVA usually decreases to approximately 0.05–0.2.

Fundus changes in the VP usually appear at the chronic stage of PDR when FV activity becomes rather quiescent, but an active FVP may also cause VPT (Fig. 14.5).

Although VPT may be an isolated phenomenon, without associated macular changes, many patients have macular lesions, and visual function changes are the combined effect of macular and disc abnormalities.

Treatment of VPT in PDR usually involves surgery, which aims to achieve traction release from the optic disc. The severity of FVP is mostly grade 2 or less. However, nasal proliferation is sometimes widespread, even beyond the equator. In such cases, to reduce the possibility of complications, one may just disconnect the disc and the FVP membrane without removing the other part of the FVP membrane.

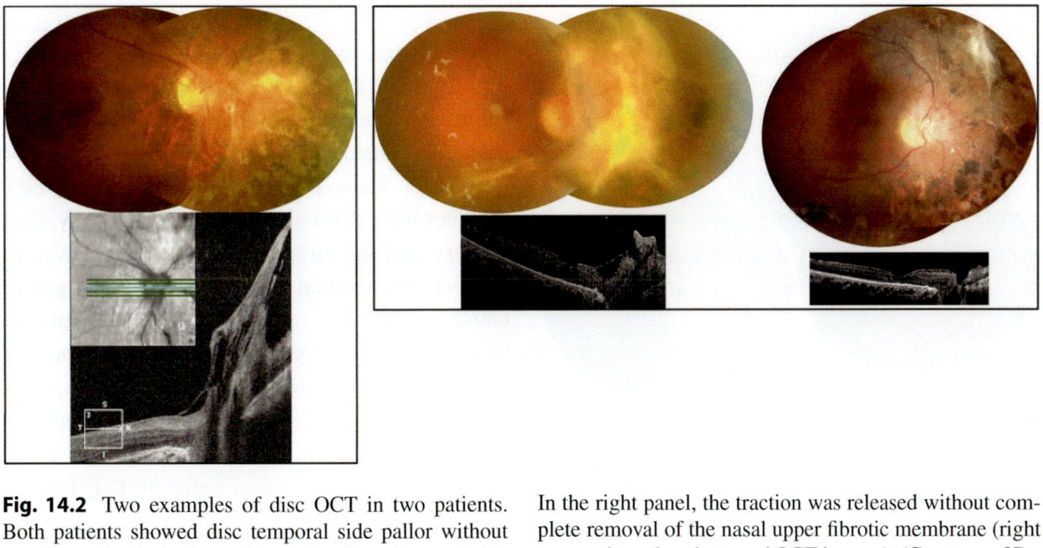

Fig. 14.2 Two examples of disc OCT in two patients. Both patients showed disc temporal side pallor without actual atrophy. In both panels, traction from the nasal side causes the disc tissue to be dragged toward the nasal side. In the right panel, the traction was released without complete removal of the nasal upper fibrotic membrane (right composite color photo and OCT images). (Courtesy of Dr. Chung-May Yang)

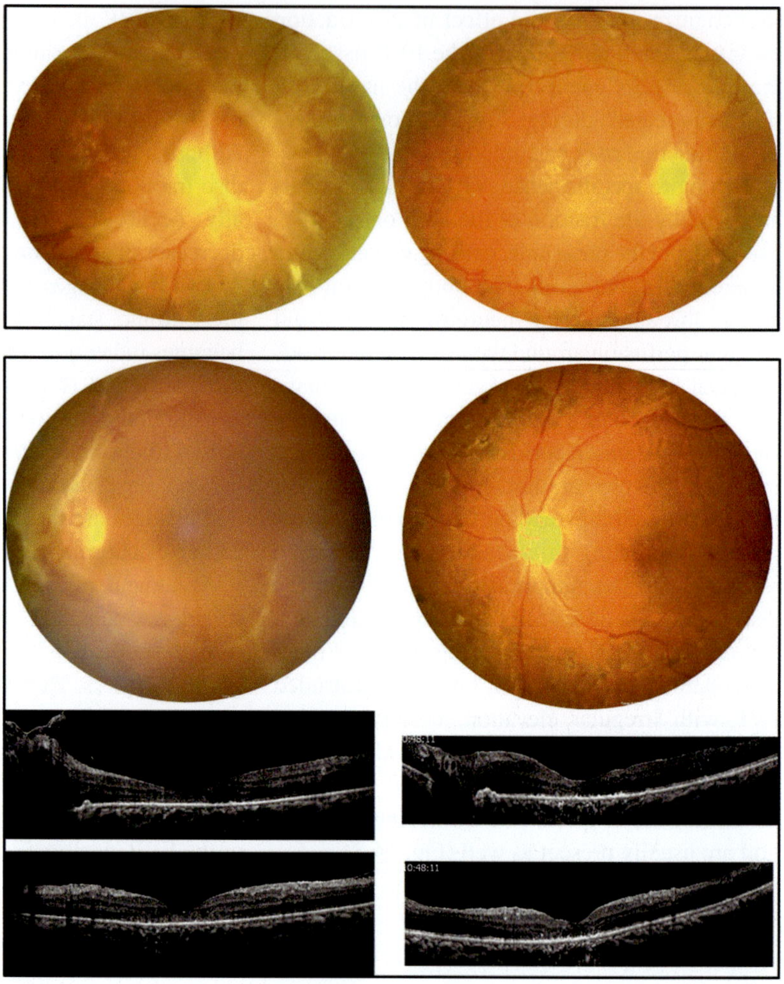

Fig. 14.3 Two examples of VPT in PDR. In the upper panel, the preoperative color photo shows macular atrophy, indicating a chronic PDR process. In the lower panel, despite the disc temporal pallor, the disc temporal side still showed elevation (lower left OCT horizontal image). (Courtesy of Dr. Chung-May Yang)

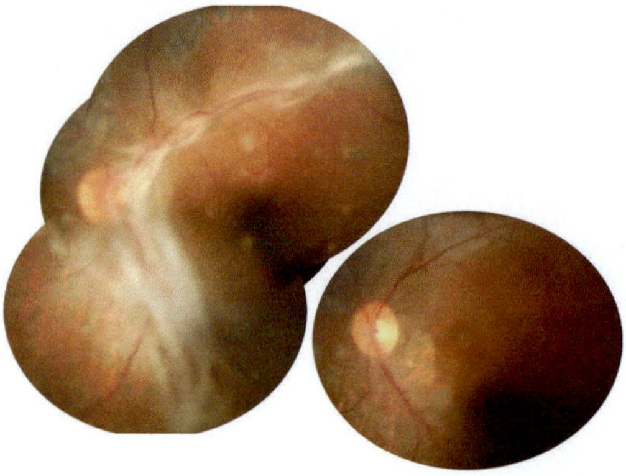

Fig. 14.4 An example of a VPT with disc traction from the temporal-side FVP. The nasal side disc showed some pallor changes (left composite color photo). After surgery, the disc returned to a pink color (right color photo). (Courtesy of Dr. Chung-May Yang)

After successful surgery, the disc color may rapidly turn pinkish. VA and VF also gradually improve. Even if BCVA does not change, patients may experience improved contrast sensitivity or a brighter view. Patients with prolonged VPT may not have good visual function recovery after surgery, and disc atrophy may eventually develop.

Post-DV residual FVP on the disc may also cause VPT and warrants further surgery (Fig. 14.6). However, visual function recovery may be less satisfactory.

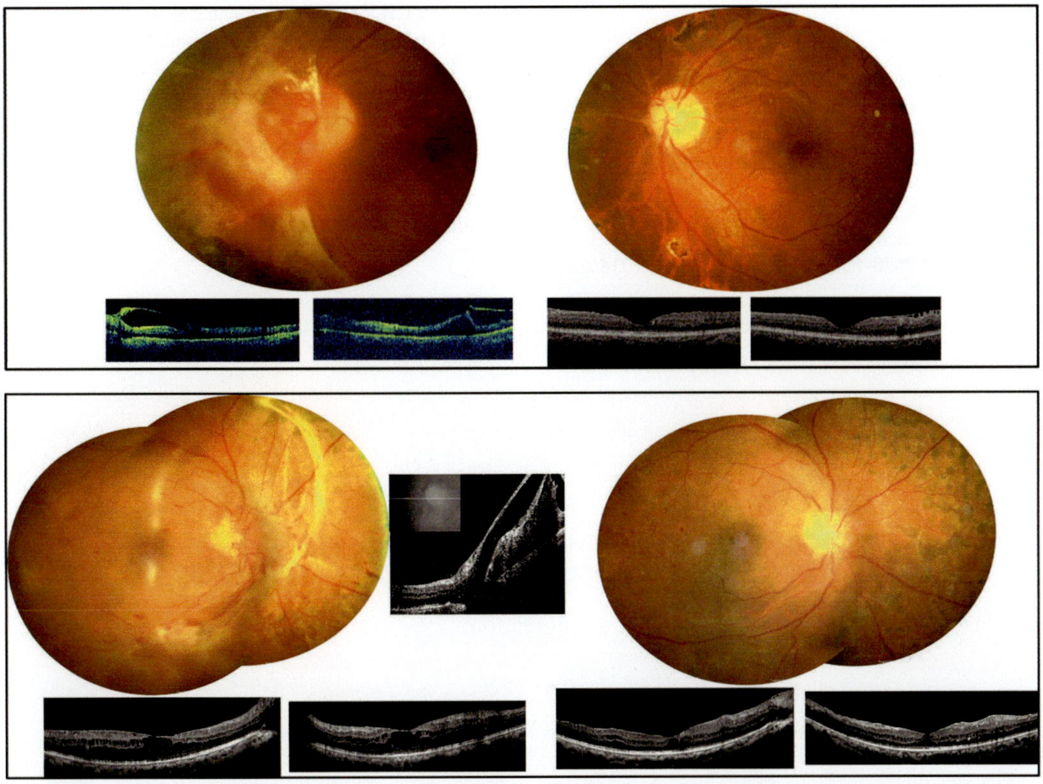

Fig. 14.5 Two sets of images showing VPT with active FVP. In the upper panel, traction on the temporal disc was visible from the OCT (left lower horizontal OCT image). In the lower set, disc OCT shows traction on the temporal and nasal discs, causing tissue thickening and nasal peaking (upper center OCT image). The disc color improved after surgery in both patients (right color photos and OCT images in each panel). (Courtesy of Dr. Chung-May Yang)

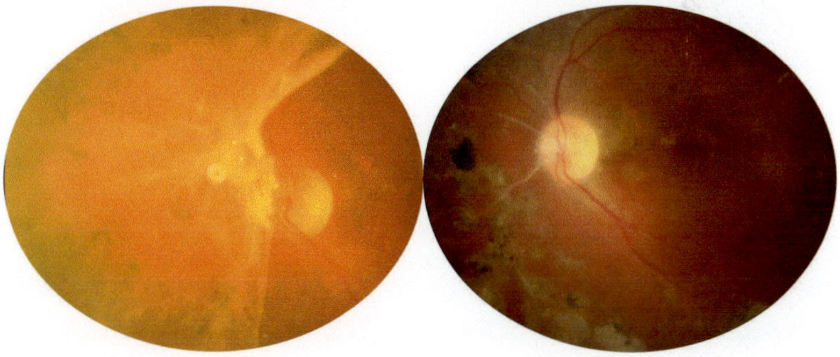

Fig. 14.6 The left color photograph shows the residual FVP membrane after surgery causing VPT. After further surgery to remove the membrane, the disc traction was released, but there was only limited VA improvement. (Courtesy of Dr. Chung-May Yang)

References

1. de Bustros S, Thompson JT, Michels RG, Rice TA. Vitrectomy for progressive proliferative diabetic retinopathy. Arch Ophthalmol. 1987;105(2):196–9. https://doi.org/10.1001/archopht.1987.01060020050026.
2. Karatas M, Ramirez JA, Ophir A. Diabetic vitreopapillary traction and macular edema. Eye (Lond). 2005;19(6):676–82. https://doi.org/10.1038/sj.eye.6701622.
3. Meyer CH, Schmidt JC, Mennel S, Kroll P. Functional and anatomical results of vitreopapillary traction after vitrectomy. Acta Ophthalmol Scand. 2007;85(2):221–2. https://doi.org/10.1111/j.1600-0420.2006.00792.x.
4. Rumelt S, Karatas M, Pikkel J, Majlin M, Ophir A. Optic disc traction syndrome associated with central retinal vein occlusion. Arch Ophthalmol. 2003;121(8):1093–7. https://doi.org/10.1001/archopht.121.8.1093.

15 Macular Hole During Diabetic Vitrectomy

Abstract

Intraoperative FTMHs most likely occur after vitrectomy for myopic traction maculopathy (Ho et al., Retina 34(9):1833–1840, 2014; Lin and Yang, Graefes Arch Clin Exp Ophthalmol 260(2):489–496, 2022). The DV for FVP may be another condition predisposing the eye to MH during surgery. Most previous studies focused on preexisting FTMHs in PDR patients before surgery (Lai and Yang, Taiwan J Ophthalmol 5(2):85–89, 2015; Tsui et al., Sci Rep 11(1):23839, 2021; Shukla et al., Eye (Lond) 20(12):1386–1388, 2006; Mason et al., Ophthalmic Surg Lasers Imaging 39(4):288–293, 2008; Yeh et al., Retina 29(3):355–361, 2009; Chen and Yang, J Ophthalmol 2018:3470731, 2018; Karimov et al., Clin Ophthalmol 14:4125–4133, 2020; Babu et al., Indian J Ophthalmol 69(11):3302–3307, 2021; Kumar et al., BMJ Case Rep 14(2):e240730, 2021). A literature search revealed no previous research describing the characteristics and treatment of FTMHs created during vitrectomy for PDR. Because an unsealed MH may significantly affect visual function and MH may lead to retinal detachment in postoperative eyes with PDR if traction release has not been thorough enough, it is important to investigate the clinical features, management, and prognosis of FTMHs created during surgery for PDR.

15.1 Case Report

A 57-year-old man with well-controlled DM and proliferative diabetic retinopathy (PDR) received panretinal photocoagulation (PRP) and intravitreal anti-vascular endothelial growth factor (VEGF) agents several times in both eyes. He complained of progressive blurred vision in the left eye for several months. On examination, best-corrected visual acuity (BCVA) was 0.125 in the right eye, and counting fingers 50 cm in the left eye. Fundus examinations revealed flame-shaped hemorrhage in the lower retina, a PRP scar, and mild VH in the lower vitreous cavity in the right eye; examination of the left fundus revealed that the fibrovascular proliferation (FVP) was distributed in the juxtapapillary area and PRP scar. OCT demonstrated tractional retinal detachment (TRD) and lamellar macular hole (LMH) in the left eye. Vitrectomy was performed in the left eye. During operation, full-thickness macular hole (FTMH) was created during the removal of FVP. The MH was covered by an inverted ILM flap. Three months after surgery, fundus photography revealed complete removal

C.-M. Yang, *Surgery for Complications of Diabetic Retinopathy*,
https://doi.org/10.1007/978-981-96-2848-3_15

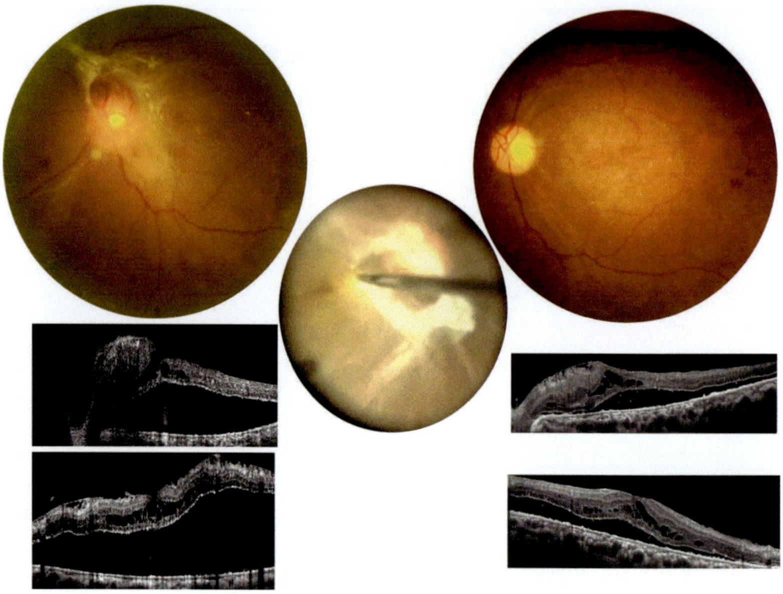

Fig. 15.1 Preoperative color and OCT images (left) showing fibrotic proliferative tissue around the disc and TRD with LMH and parafoveal schisis/cysts. Intraoperative video image shows that the MH was created during proliferative tissue removal (center). Three months after surgery with the inverted ILM flap, the MH was sealed; there was residual SRF and intraretinal cysts (right color photo and OCT images). (Courtesy of Dr. Chung-May Yang)

of the FVP; the MH was closed, and the retina was reattached. Her BCVA was 0.025 in the left eye (Fig. 15.1).

15.2 Macular Hole During Diabetic Vitrectomy

FTMHs created during surgery are assured when the surgeon has direct visualization of the underlying retinal pigment epithelium (RPE) or notices the out-flowing of the subretinal fluid from the central fovea. If available, intraoperative OCT is the most accurate diagnostic tool.

We investigated the clinical features, management, and prognosis of FTMHs inadvertently created during vitrectomy for eyes with PDR and FVP [1]. A total of 11 eyes of 11 patients (5 males and 6 females) were included in the study group. We used age- and sex-matched subjects with PDR and FVP of similar severity who did not have intraoperative FTMHs as the control group. In this study, we defined premacular fibrosis as the presence of a hyperreflective fibrotic membrane over the macula on OCT, while central condensed preretinal tissue was defined as a thickened fibrotic tissue plaque over and connecting with the central or paracentral foveal structure. Our study revealed that central condensed and adherent preretinal tissue is a major risk factor associated with this intraoperative complication. The mere presence of a sheet-like preretinal membrane, however, did not increase the risk of intraoperative FTMHs. We also found that all eyes in the study group had moderate to severe (grade 2 or 3) FVP. In addition, there was a greater proportion of eyes with induced FTMHs having SO tamponade during the primary operation, indicating a more complicated intraoperative condition in the study group, such as multiple large retinal breaks (preexisting or iatrogenic), more strong preexisting traction, and/or residual vitreoretinal traction, than in the control group.

Thickened and condensed preretinal tissue usually strongly adhered to foveal or parafoveal tissue. This abnormal structure may be part of a thickened preretinal fibrotic membrane or in continuation with a thin posterior hyaloid. During the removal of the proliferative tissue adjacent to the arcade, the traction force may transfer to the fovea through this condensed tissue; the removal of this condensed tissue itself could also exert strong traction forces directly on the fovea. In addition, some eyes had preexisting foveal abnormalities, such as LMH or foveal cysts. The complex traction of the FVP and the amount and direction of force used to grasp and remove the central condensed preretinal tissue from a structurally weakened fovea during the operation play important roles in inducing FTMHs. Specific care should be taken to remove the FVP close to the arcade when central condensed tissue is present, and scissors, instead of forceps or cutters, should be used to remove this central tissue, especially when preexisting foveal structural weakening occurs.

Once inadvertently created FTMHs occur, after complete release of all the traction forces, ILM peeling or the inverted ILM flap technique should be performed. The choice of ILM peeling or an inverted ILM flap for treating FTMH is based on the degree of tissue loss and the size of the MH. If the surgeon feels that the tissue loss is substantial and the MH size is large, an inverted ILM flap should be applied. One convenient way to estimate the MH size is to compare it with that of the 25G vitrector tip. A MH equal to or larger than the tip diameter was considered a large MH.

Our study showed that, compared with those in the control group, eyes in the study group had worse BCVA at 3 months, but there was no significant difference in the final BCVA between the two groups. In the study group, BCVA significantly improved 3 months after the operation, and anatomical closure of the MH was 100%, suggesting that the prognosis of intraoperatively created FTMHs treated with either ILM peeling or the inverted ILM flap technique was relatively favorable.

The foveal contour after surgery is quite different from the postoperative foveal contour in idiopathic MH or PDR patients with preexisting MH. In idiopathic MHs, U-shaped closures and/or V-shaped closures predominate, while U-shaped closures and/or W-shaped closures predominate in PDRs with preexisting MHs. No U-shaped closure was observed in the intraoperative MH group. We suspect that there is more trauma to the fovea and more tissue loss when iatrogenic FTMHs are created during surgery than when FTMHs are spontaneously formed in PDR, causing the absence of U-shaped closure in this study. In addition, foveal thinning, as well as LMH on OCT after surgery, was much more commonly observed in MHs with PDR than in idiopathic MHs. These configurations may be attributed to unwanted tissue loss during surgical manipulations.

Case examples of MH created during DV are shown in Figs. 15.2 and 15.3.

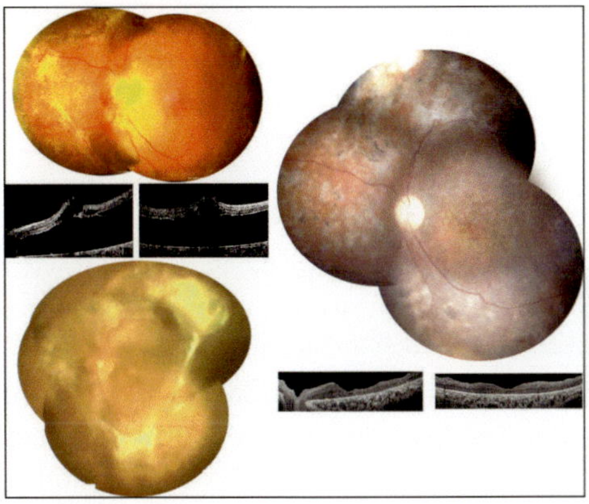

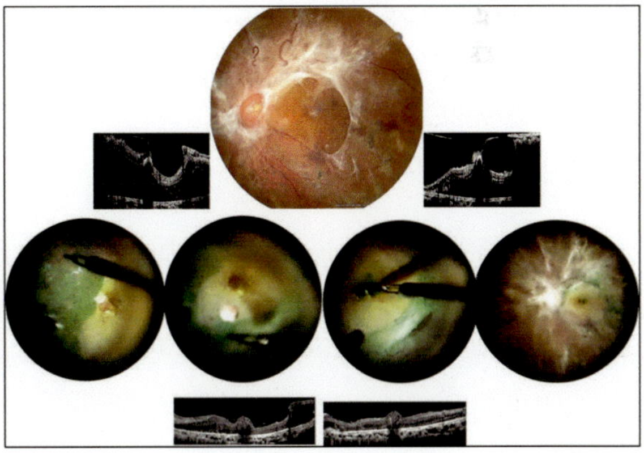

Fig. 15.2 Two examples of MHs created during operation. The right panel shows a case of TRD with an active FVP around the arcade and on the nasal side; LMH with cysts and a thin outer lining was noted on OCT (left upper composite color photo and OCT images and left lower composite color photo from intraoperative video images). During surgery, MH was created, and ILM peeling was performed (not shown here). After surgery, the retina was reattached, and the MH was sealed (right composite color photo and OCT images). The right panel shows a case of TRD with prominent fibrosis around the disc and arcade, with condensed tissue over the fovea (upper color photo and OCT images). A large MH was created during ILM peeling and condensed tissue removal; the inverted ILM flap technique was then performed (midoperative four video images). After surgery, the MH was sealed, and residual SRF was noted on the temporal side (lower horizontal and vertical OCT images). (Courtesy of Dr. Chung-May Yang)

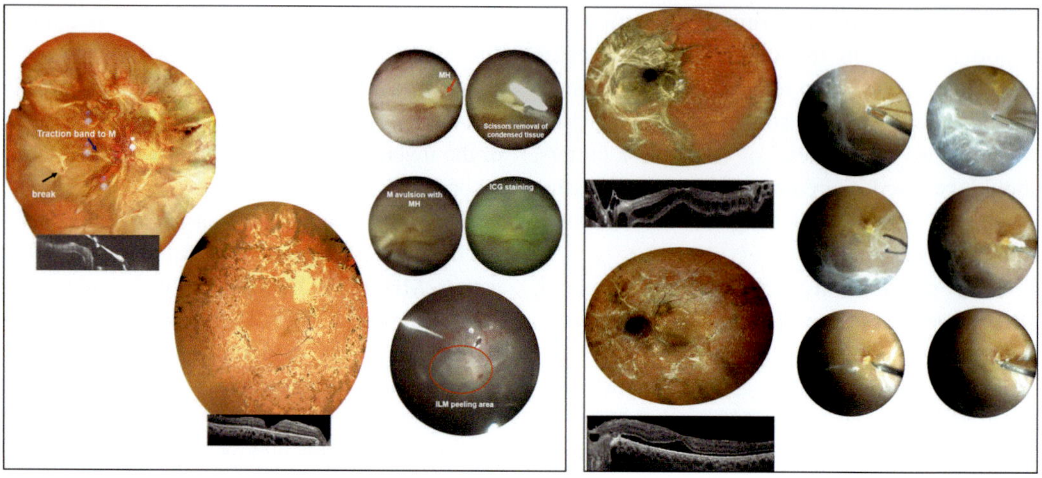

Fig. 15.3 Two examples of MH created during operation for PDR with severe FVP. The left panel shows a patient with combined RD in the right eye (upper left color and OCT). A break at the temporal midperiphery was identified (black arrow); there was a temporal horizontal traction band with condensed premacular tissue adjacent to the fovea (blue arrow). Intraoperative video images show MHs created during the removal of condensed premacular tissue. FVP removal and ILM peeling were performed (right side five intraoperative video images). After surgery, the retina was reattached, and the MH was sealed (lower). The right panel shows a patient with severe fibrotic proliferation and TRD (upper left wide angle color photo and OCT image). Intraoperative video images show MHs created during the removal of condensed premacular tissue with forceps. Scissors were used to leave the condensed tissue attached to the edge of the MH, and the tissue was inserted into the MH (right six images). One month after FVP removal and ILM peeling, the retina became reattached, and the MH was sealed (lower left wide angle color photo and OCT image). (Courtesy of Dr. Chung-May Yang)

Reference

1. Tsui MC, Yang CM, Wang LC. Characteristics and outcomes of full-thickness macular holes created during vitrectomy for proliferative diabetic retinopathy. Int Ophthalmol. 2023;43(10):3479–90. https://doi.org/10.1007/s10792-023-02753-8.

16 Recurrent Vitreous Hemorrhage After Diabetic Vitrectomy

Abstract

Recurrent VH after successful DV may lead to prolonged and severe visual loss and sometimes requires surgical intervention (Schachat et al., Ophthalmology 90:522–530, 1983). Previous studies have shown that after successful surgery, approximately one-third of these patients develop recurrent VH; among these patients, one-third ultimately require gas-fluid exchange or vitreous lavage to restore vision (Brown et al., Arch Ophthalmol 110(4):506–510, 1992; Yang, J Formos Med Assoc 97(7):477–484, 1998; Blankenship, Ophthalmology 93(1):39–44, 1986; Blumenkranz et al., Arch Ophthalmol 104(2):291–296, 1986; Han et al., Retina 11(3):309–314, 1991). With the use of modern microincision techniques, this complication is reduced but still affects a fair number of patients. This complication may slow visual recovery and jeopardize an otherwise successful operation with additional procedures. In this chapter, risk factors, bleeding sources, proper preventive management, and treatment of recurrent VH after surgery are discussed. It should be recognized that the optimal management method has not been well established.

16.1 Case Report

This 52-year-old woman had type 2 DM for 2 years. She also had hypertension (HT). Both diseases were under oral medication control. She did not take anticoagulants. She was diagnosed with proliferative diabetic retinopathy (PDR) and received panretinal photocoagulation (PRP) and anti-vascular endothelial growth factor (VEGF) treatment in both eyes at an outside hospital. She came to our clinic because of blurred vision in the right eye. On examination, best-corrected visual acuity (BCVA) was hand motion (HM) at 50 cm in the right eye and 0.7 in the left eye. The intraocular pressure (IOP) was normal in both eyes. The anterior segment in both eyes was unremarkable. Fundus examinations revealed dense VH in the right eye and mild nasal FVP in the left eye. She smoothly underwent vitrectomy, retinal ablation, and IVI of anti-VEGF in the right eye. Two weeks after surgery, she developed VH, hyphema, mild RI, and high IOP. After anterior chamber irrigation and IVI of anti-VEGF, the intraocular hemorrhage improved, but the IOP remained high because of lens swelling and angle narrowing. She underwent phacoemulsification with posterior chamber intraocular lens (PCIOL) implantation

C.-M. Yang, *Surgery for Complications of Diabetic Retinopathy*,
https://doi.org/10.1007/978-981-96-2848-3_16

3 weeks later. Her condition stabilized, and her BCVA improved to 0.3. She subsequently had progressive FVP on the nasal side and tractional retinal detachment (TRD) with VH in the left eye 8 months after cataract operation in the right eye. She underwent vitrectomy, retinal ablation, and IVI of anti-VEGF in the left eye. The early post-operative course was smooth, but recurrent VH developed 3.5 months after surgery in the left eye. After IVI of the anti-VEGF agent, the VH subsided within 2 weeks, and supplementary PRP was applied to the left eye. However, recurrent VH was noted 11 months later. VH subsided 2 weeks after IVI of anti-VEGF. Since then, there has been no episode of recurrent VH in either eye. She underwent a cataract operation in the left eye 3.5 years later. The BCVA (7 years after cataract surgery in the left eye) was 0.6 in the right eye and 0.8 in the left eye (Fig. 16.1).

16.2 Recurrent VH After Diabetic Vitrectomy

Persistent or recurrent VH after successful surgery is a major complication of DV [1]. Recognition of risk factors and bleeding sources and proper preventive management are very important for reducing the incidence and severity of recurrent VH.

Systemic risk factors are similar to risk factors for recurrent VH in a nonvitrectomized eye. Because major intraoperative vascular injury bleeding inevitably prolongs the postoperative vitreous clear-up time, known systemic risk factors should be specifically avoided to reduce both the possibility of uncontrolled intraoperative bleeding and recurrent postoperative bleeding. Accordingly, systemic intake of aspirin, NSAIDs, or other anticoagulants may be stopped for

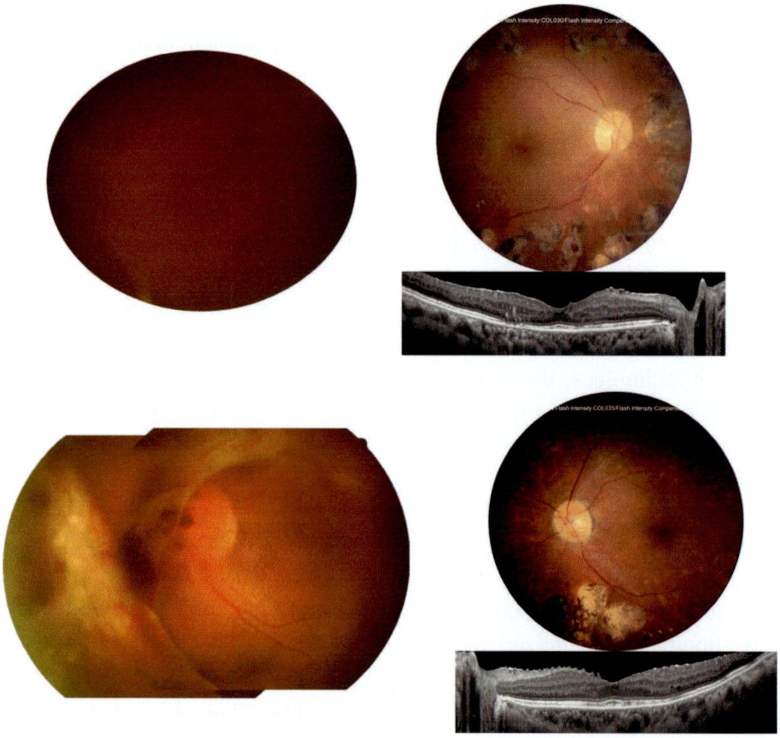

Fig. 16.1 Preoperative fundus color photograph showing dense VH in the right eye (upper left). After surgery, recurrent VH and hyphema were noted. After IVIA, anterior chamber irrigation and subsequent cataract surgery, the condition is improved, and no recurrent VH was noted (upper right color photo and OCT image). The left eye developed nasal and upper arcade FVP with preretinal hemorrhage and VH (lower left composite color photo). The postoperative course was complicated by two episodes of recurrent VH. After IVI of Avastin and supplementary PRP, the condition stabilized (lower right color photo and OCT image). (Courtesy of Dr. Chung-May Yang)

10–14 days if possible to ensure the complete elimination of their effects on hemostasis. No solid evidence has been established regarding the hemorrhagic complications of continuous use of aspirin or anticoagulants prior to vitreoretinal surgeries, and no consensus has been reached concerning the optimal duration of medication discontinuation before surgery [6–8]. Some authors have suggested that 1 week should be sufficient for reversing any bleeding side effects based on pharmacological studies [8]. Studies indicate that for aspirin, although 10 days are needed for complete loss of its effect, not using aspirin for only 2 days may be sufficient to significantly reduce its antiplatelet aggregation effect; NSAIDs act synergistically with aspirin and show a similar duration of action lasting for 1–2 weeks. Heparin has a short duration of action (less than 2 days), while Coumadin (warfarin) needs 4–5 days to reverse its effect. Sporadic case reports have shown that hemorrhagic complications may occur even after 1 week of discontinuation of all systemic anticoagulants. For these reasons, it is best to consult the patient's internal medicine doctors for the possibility of stopping the use of anticoagulants for 10–14 days. For similar reasons, anticoagulants should also be discontinued during hemodialysis for at least 1 week before surgery.

Locally within the eye, extensive active FVP is an important factor of intraoperative bleeding, prolonged vitreous clear-up, and recurrent VH. Blood retained in the vitreous base may be shed after surgery and cause recurrent VH. Residual FVP or unreleased vitreoretinal traction is another source of recurrent VH. Ischemia or inflammation induced by excessive manipulation during surgery may promote new vessel growth in the vitreous base or even the anterior segment, causing recurrent VH. Postoperative anterior hyaloidal fibrovascular proliferation (AHFVP), postoperative NV at the sclerotomy site, so-called entry site NV, or fibrovascular ingrowths are also important causes of recurrent VH [3, 9–13]. The source of early recurrent VH (within 2–3 weeks after DV) may differ from that of late VH, although overlap may be considerable. In the early postoperative period, the distinction between persistent hemorrhage and recurrent hemorrhage may not be obvious; VH occurring in this period is more closely related to unabsorbed blood within the peripheral vitreous skirt, NV stumps, or surgically injured retinal vessels [3, 14]. Sources of late bleeding include NV from residual fibrovascular tissue, postoperative NV that develops in the vitreous base, and NV that grows from surgical sclerotomy sites [9–11, 15, 16]. Many patients experience recurrent bleeding despite thorough removal of FVP tissue and blood clots in the peripheral vitreous skirt, suggesting that newly formed postoperative NV in the vitreous base or sclerotomy sites may be a significant source of recurrent bleeding.

Strictly defined, VH from lyses of residual retained blood clots at the end of surgery or from blood shedding from the vitreous base is not truly recurrent VH. However, these sources have similar effects as other factors on prolonged vitreous clear-up and are difficult to distinguish from early recurrent VH secondary to bleeding from injured retinal vessels or incompletely removed fibrovascular tissues. We thus include them as sources of early recurrent VH in our discussion.

16.3 Prevention of Early Postoperative VH

To counter the risk factors and reduce early postoperative VH, one should aim to do the following: (1) Minimizing intraoperative vascular injuries; (2) The amount of vitreous blood and blood clots were reduced at the end of surgery; (3) Promoting early recovery of injured retinal vessels; (4) Vitreoretinal traction and FVP tissue should be eliminated as thoroughly as possible; and (5) The development of NV at the vitreous base, anterior segment, and sclerotomy sites should be prevented. The last two items are also important for preventing late-onset recurrent VH. The above categories will be discussed sequentially:

1. **Avoidance of vascular injury**: Important points to avoid vessel injury are proper identification of the surgical plane and gentle trac-

tion on the hyaloid membrane or on the proliferative membrane. When performing scissor delamination, proliferative tissue should be slightly lifted and dissected closer to the FVP membrane than to the retinal tissue when the epicenter is adjacent to or on top of a retinal vessel. As small gauged vitrectomy has become popular, vitrectors are being used more frequently than before for the removal of FVP tissue. Care should be taken to circumvent large new vessels during tissue dissection.

2. **Reduction of vitreous blood and the amount of blood clots at the end of surgery**: Blood in the vitreous base should be removed as much as can be safely done. Scleral indentation with cutting and suction allows more complete removal of the peripheral blood. Blood adherent to the vitreous skirt that does not come off easily after suction, mostly in the inferior part, may be left in position; it usually remains within the vitreous base after surgery. Inadequate hemostasis during surgery not only increases the amount of blood clots but also jeopardizes the success of the surgery. For a discussion of proper hemostasis, please refer to Chap. 1.

Patients with active FVPs are more prone to bleeding complications than those with inactive fibrosis. As mentioned before, intravitreal bevacizumab is capable of inducing rapid regression of retinal and iris NV. Many studies have shown that presurgical administration of intravitreal bevacizumab may reduce intraoperative bleeding during membrane dissection in PDR patients with FVP or traction retinal detachment [17–23]. Our studies showed that in active FVP with mild to moderate severity, i.e., active FVP with vitreoretinal adhesions at three or more sites but not extending beyond the equator in more than one quadrant, intravitreal injection of bevacizumab 1.25 mg in 0.05 mL 1 week before primary vitrectomy induces significant regression of NV [20]. Active FVP is defined as visible new vessels within proliferative membranes with any degree of fresh vitreous or preretinal hemorrhage. In our study, we found that intraoperative bleeding and subsequent blood clot remaining at the end of the operation were significantly less common in the bevacizumab-pretreated group than in the group without bevacizumab pretreatment, ensuring a shortened reabsorption time after clot lysis. The temporal regression of active fibrovascular proliferation by bevacizumab decreases the extent of bleeding during tissue segmentation and delamination. This result, in turn, facilitates visualization of the surgical plane and a more precise separation of the proliferative tissue from the retina, avoiding accidental retinal vascular damage. One possible complication of bevacizumab pretreatment is the development or progression of traction retinal detachment [24]. When anti-VEGF is used, although proliferation may be inhibited, fibrosis may be enhanced, causing contraction of the fibrovascular tissue. The manifested result may be more vitreoretinal traction, frank traction retinal detachment, or even combined detachment. There may be a surgical window when the fibrovascular tissue activity has already been significantly reduced while the contraction of these tissues has not increased to a great extent. In our study with moderate fibrovascular proliferative tissue, no increased retinal elevation or enlarged area of traction detachment was noticed when bevacizumab was given 7–10 days before surgery [21]. Instead, the minor increase in contraction of the proliferative tissues may actually make identification of point adhesions between the proliferative tissue and the retina easier and may create more safe space for instrument manipulation during delamination, which may, in turn, decrease the possibility of accidental retinal injury or vessel avulsion. In more recent practices, we found that IVI of anti-VEGF agents 2–7 days before surgery may be a good window for treating PDR patients with moderate FVP. Because bevacizumab may reduce the likelihood of intraoperative bleeding, surgeons may have a false sense of safety in thinking that blood vessels are not disrupted to a great extent, while in reality, the severed vessels merely maintain temporary hemostasis. This may result in a paradoxical increase in postoperative hemorrhage. For this reason, any active bleeder should be checked carefully before air-fluid exchange. The retina was examined carefully after intentionally lowering the infusion bottle for a short period of time to ensure that no fresh blood was oozing from the injured blood vessels. For the use of anti-VEGF therapy in the treatment of severe active FVP when intraoperative bleeding is a major concern, please refer to Chap. 6.

3. **Promoting early recovery of injured retinal vessels**: To prevent recurrent vitreous hemorrhage, mechanical tamponade of the bleeding sites by air or a nonexpansile SF_6-air mixture has been attempted for hemorrhage prevention [25, 26]. We hypothesize that a long-acting gas bubble within the vitreous cavity may mechanically tamponade fragile retinal vessels and concentrate coagulation factors close to bleeding sites. This action would thus allow the gradual reestablishment of vascular integrity and reduce the occurrence of early postoperative recurrent vitreous hemorrhage. To investigate this hypothesis, a clinical prospective study was undertaken to examine the effect of long-acting gas infused into the vitreous cavity at the end of diabetic vitrectomy to prevent early (<4 weeks) recurrent vitreous hemorrhage [14]. C_3F_8 (10%) was used intravitreally as a way to achieve hemostasis. Prolonged (>5 weeks) vitreous clearance after surgery or recurrent VH lasting more than 2 weeks were considered to indicate significant recurrent VH. The frequency of significant recurrent hemorrhage in the gas-treated group was significantly lower than that in the non–gas-treated group. The combined number of patients who experienced significant recurrent hemorrhage plus prolonged vitreous clear-up was also significantly lower in the gas-treated group. The significance persisted in logistic regression analysis for risk factors among all study cases. These results suggested that the incidence of significant early recurrent vitreous hemorrhage was reduced in patients receiving the intravitreal long-acting gas 10% C_3F_8. The study also showed that patients with active FVP benefitted more than those without active FVP. We reasoned that short-acting intravitreal gas may not provide the long-lasting tamponade needed for vascular healing. In previous studies, either air or 20% SF_6 was used intravittruly, with the tamponade to the posterior retina lasting no more than 10 days. In contrast, at the proper head position, 10% C_3F_8 tamponade was applied to the posterior retina for at least 3 weeks. The posterior retina is the area that may have sustained the most surgical manipulations and may contain vessels susceptible to rebleeding. In another study, we further found that combined preoperative bevacizumab and intraoperative gas infusion may increase the vitreous clearance time for patients with mild to moderate FVP [20]. For a discussion of recurrent hemorrhage under SO, please refer to Chap. 6.
4. **Vitreoretinal traction and FVP tissue should be eliminated as thoroughly as possible**: The key point is to identify the surgical plane beneath the last layer of the vitreous schysis or under the ERM and ensure that the adjacent traction has been completely released. In doubt, a scleral buckle should be considered to counter residual traction. A residual FVP with persistent traction is an important cause of postvitrectomy recurrent VH. For the detailed surgical technique, please refer to Chap. 1.
5. **Preventing the development of NV at the vitreous base, anterior segment, and sclerotomy sites**: Retinal ischemia and excessive inflammation are the most important factors contributing to the development of fibrovascular tissue at the vitreous base, anterior segment, and sclerotomy sites. The growth of these abnormal tissues may be important because of late postvitrectomy recurrent VH. Through either direct observation during surgery or UBM examination, several studies have confirmed the strong correlation between fibrovascular ingrowth (FVIG) and recurrent vitreous hemorrhage after PPV for PDR [27–30]. Although prominent FVIGs at sclerotomy sites after PPV have been noted to be associated with

various conditions, the single most important factor related to FVIG is PPV after PDR [9, 10, 27–30]. The combination of surgical wounds, vitreous scaffolds, angiogenic factors produced by the ischemic retina, various growth factors contained in fresh or old blood, and cytokines induced by postoperative inflammation provides a suitable environment for the development of fibrovascular proliferation in the sclerotomy area. Standard PRP alone may not be intensive enough to fully inhibit the production of angiogenic factors. We hypothesize that anterior retinal ablation together with direct cryoapplication to sclerotomy sites may inhibit FVIG and hence decrease the incidence of postoperative recurrent vitreous hemorrhage. Our retrospective study showed that the presence of FVIG at sclerotomy sites was strongly correlated with the development of recurrent postoperative vitreous hemorrhage; furthermore, we found that sclerotomy site cryotherapy may decrease the incidence of sclerotomy NV and the rate of recurrent vitreous hemorrhage by rendering the ciliary body atrophic. However, cryotreatment may also induce inflammation and, in turn, increase the possibility of NV formation, which is definitely an unwanted effect. Considering that sclerotomy NVs may not play a role as important as before in microincision surgery, emphasis should be given to a more complete peripheral PRP; sclerotomy site cryo, if performed, should reduce treatment number and time, and anti-VEGF therapy at the end of surgery may be applied to counter the possible effect of NV stimulation by cryotreatment. At the time of this writing, we saved the cryotherapy for recurrent VH after DV and always simultaneously added IVI of anti-VEGF to gain the greatest advantage.

To conclude, the best preventive methods for persistent/recurrent hemorrhage after DV may include applying presurgical anti-VEGF, intraoperative adequate tissue removal and anterior retinal ablation, as well as gas infusion, anti-VEGF injection, and sclerotomy site cryotherapy at the end of surgery to treat active fibrovascular ingrowth (FVP) and omitting presurgical anti-VEGF for patients with inactive fibrosis. In this way, most facets of recurrent hemorrhage have been addressed, and the possibility and severity of recurrent VH may be reduced to a minimal extent.

Despite every precaution, recurrent VH may occur after vitrectomy surgery. One must ensure that recurrent VH (or hyphema) does not come from the AHFVP. The treatment of AHFVP is beyond the scope of this chapter. Treatment options for recurrent VH include observation, fluid-air exchange, vitreous lavage, and vitrectomy with dissection of entry-site fibrovascular proliferation [1, 2, 3–5]. For intractable cases, especially in patients with a single functioning eye, silicone oil has been infused after vitreous lavage to obtain long-term clear media [31].

Since most recurrent VHs clear spontaneously, observation is suggested if the IOP is within the normal limit, no echographic evidence of retinal detachment is noted, and the patient has relatively good vision. Prolonged VH may be managed by one-port or two-port air-fluid exchange [5, 32, 33]. The patient was instructed to lie on one side with the lesion eye in the dependent position. The operating table should be raised to ensure a slightly upward direction of the syringe during manipulation by the operator in a sitting position. A 27- or 30-gauge needle is connected with a 5 c.c. syringe containing prefiltered air. The needle was inserted through the pars plana into the vitreous cavity. A small volume of air is then injected, followed by gentle suction of the intravitreal blood. This "push-pull" maneuver should be continued until most of the vitreous blood has been replaced with air. Care should be taken not to induce great fluctuations in IOP, as a sudden increase in IOP may stretch the peripheral vitreous, causing retinal tear if residual VR adhesion exists, or increasing retinal ischemia, and too low pressure may cause the eye to become deformed and injured by the needle. Other methods include nasal upper insertion of a 30-gauge needle connected to an air pump and insertion of another 27- or 30-gauge needle into the temporal lower quadrant connected to a 5 c.c. syringe without a plunge. The air pump pressure was increased to 30 mmHg, and vitreous blood was allowed to drain spontaneously from the dependent temporal side syringe through gravity [5, 32, 33]. IOP fluctuations may be greatly reduced by this method, but it is not easy to perform smoothly with small lid fissures because lens damage is more likely.

Vitreous lavage may achieve a more complete wash out of the vitreous blood, and additional peripheral ablation and sclerotomy site cryotherapy may be performed in the same setting [15]. Any residual traction may be removed. The chance of future recurrence of VH may be reduced but cannot be eliminated. Steel DH et al. suggested that entry-site neovascularization was correlated with the need for vitreous lavage. Some authors have specifically performed dissection of entry-site fibrovascular proliferation if echographic evidence of FVIG existed or if peripheral indentation showed FVIG. This is followed by ciliary body laser or cryotherapy over sclerotomy sites. Good results have been reported [27, 34].

Since the most likely source of bleeding is NV, intravitreal injection of bevacizumab in eyes with late recurrent vitreous hemorrhage should be able to induce regression of new vessels and reduce the possibility of repeated bleeding, thus shortening the reabsorption time and reducing the need for surgery. We conducted a retrospective case-control study to investigate whether intravitreal bevacizumab facilitates vitreous clearance after late-onset recurrent vitreous hemorrhage [35]. Eighteen consecutive patients with postoperative recurrent VH $\geq$2 weeks after primary diabetic vitrectomy were treated with intravitreal bevacizumab. Repeated injections were performed after 2–3 weeks in the case of no obvious blood reabsorption. The criteria for reinjection were no improvement in best corrected visual acuity plus no improvement in vitreous opacity according to clinical examinations. Twenty consecutive patients with the same complication but without bevacizumab injection served as the historical control group. Vitreous surgeries in both groups were indicated if no clinical improvement was noted 10–12 weeks after the initial bleeding. In the study group, the vitreous clear-up time (VCT) after the first recurrent VH was 6.5 ± 1.5 weeks with 2.2 ± 0.8 injections. Nine patients had more than one episode of VH, but no surgery was needed. In the control group, 13 eyes exhibited spontaneous reabsorption (at 6.4 ± 1.3 weeks), 5 eyes underwent surgery, and 3 of the 13 eyes eventually underwent surgery after further recurrent VH. The rates of vitreous surgery in the two groups were 0/20 and 8/18 ($p = 0.01$). Our study suggested that intravitreal bevacizumab treatment may reduce the need for revitrectomy for recurrent vitreous hemorrhage after diabetic vitrectomy [36]. Repeated recurrent vitreous hemorrhage suggests the presence of protracted NV or sustained release of angiogenic factors. The addition of peripheral retinal cryotherapy and sclerotomy site cryotherapy under the cover of anti-VEGF therapy may be used [37]. Because bevacizumab has only temporal effects, the possibility of recurrent vitreous hemorrhage raises the question of whether bevacizumab should be used at regular intervals as a preventive method [38, 39]. In our study, prolonged vitreous clearance was achieved after blood reabsorption in most patients, and when recurrent bleeding occurred, further bevacizumab treatment was effective. The average hemorrhage-free period among patients in our study was 5.9 months. Thus, we believe that prophylactic injection on a nonselected base may not be necessary. However, if certain risk factors arise during follow-up, such as intraocular surgery, intraocular inflammation, hemodialysis, or anticoagulant use, one or two booster injections of bevacizumab may be a reasonable option. On the other hand, there is no evidence demonstrating that multiple injections induce permanent NV regression in severe cases; therefore, supplementary retinal ablation, especially to the anterior retina, should be performed as an adjunct treatment to decrease the likelihood of reactivation and bleeding during neovascularization. In general, vitreous clearance is 2 or 3 times faster in vitrectomized eyes than in nonvitrectomized eyes [40]. We thus chose 3 weeks as the interval between two bevacizumab injections when prolonged hemorrhage developed. The optimal interval for repeated injection requires further study. The available data in our study cannot be used to determine whether patients with entry-site neovascularization may need more frequent bevacizumab injections or are prone to having more episodes of recurrent bleeding.

Other investigators have shown that IVI of triamcinolone can effectively shorten the VH time after DV [41]. It reduces inflammation and possibly NV activity, and TA particles mixed with blood cells or components may facilitate blood reabsorption. Our standard regimen is combined IVI TA 0.02 mL and IVI anti-VEGF (Avastin 0.05 mL) for the first time for recurrent VH, followed by cryotreatment (one spot, 4 s for three sclerotomy sites) for persistent or recurrent VH. Cataract progression assessment, IOP measurement, and observation of the RI should be performed carefully.

Examples of post-DV VH cases are shown in Figs. 16.2 and 16.3.

Vitreous surgery, including vitreous lavage with fill-in PRP, IVI of anti-VEGF, and/or peripheral retinal cryotherapy, was performed if the above manipulations failed. For intractable cases, SO may be used as the last resort (Fig. 16.3, upper panel).

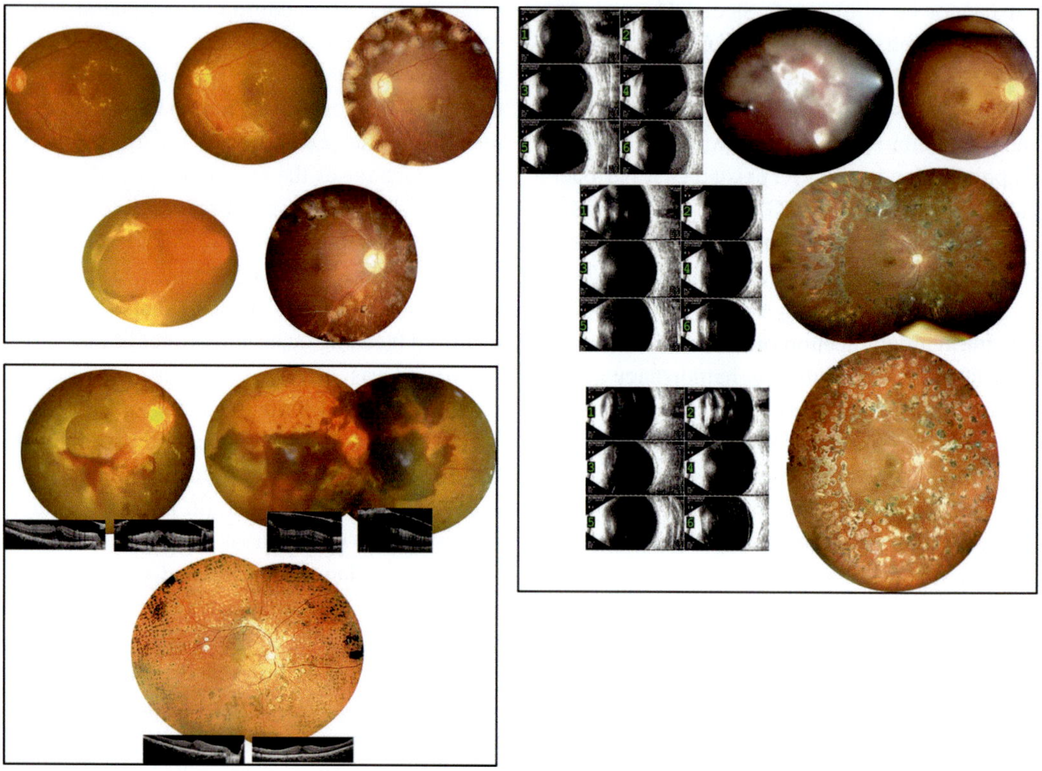

Fig. 16.2 Three examples of postoperative recurrent VH in patients who underwent bilateral DV. In the upper left panel, the left eye had DME (upper left color photo) and then developed FVP in the lower arcade (upper center color photo), followed by VH. She underwent smooth cataract surgery and vitrectomy in the left eye, and the retina was attached (upper right color photo). She also had FVP around the arcade and VH in the right eye (lower left color photo). After vitrectomy, recurrent VH was noted 2.5 months later. She received IVI of Avastin and the ARC with a good response. However, two more episodes of VH occurred within 1.5 years. IVIA and IVTA were given. She underwent cataract surgery 3 years after her last episode of VH. After surgery, she had one more VH in her right eye, which was reabsorbed after IVIA. No additional VHs were noted for 3 years (lower right color photo). In the lower left panel, active FVP with progression was noted in the right eye of a young man (upper color photos and OCT images). After surgery, recurrent VH was noted three times within 2 years; each time, it was controlled with IVI Avastin and the ARC. No additional VHs were noted for 3 years (lower wide angle photo and OCT images). The left eye with severe FVP and TRD had a smooth surgical course. In the right panel, FVP, dense VH and preretinal hemorrhage were noted by US and intraoperative imaging (upper left and center). The retina was attached after surgery (upper right). She experienced recurrent VH three times during a 10-month period with transient clear fundus (middle left ultrasonography, middle right wide angle color photo, and lower left US). IVTA was added after the third recurrent VH event. The fundus was clear, with the retina attached for 2 years (lower right wide angle color photo). The left eye underwent uneventful cataract surgery and vitrectomy. (Courtesy of Dr. Chung-May Yang)

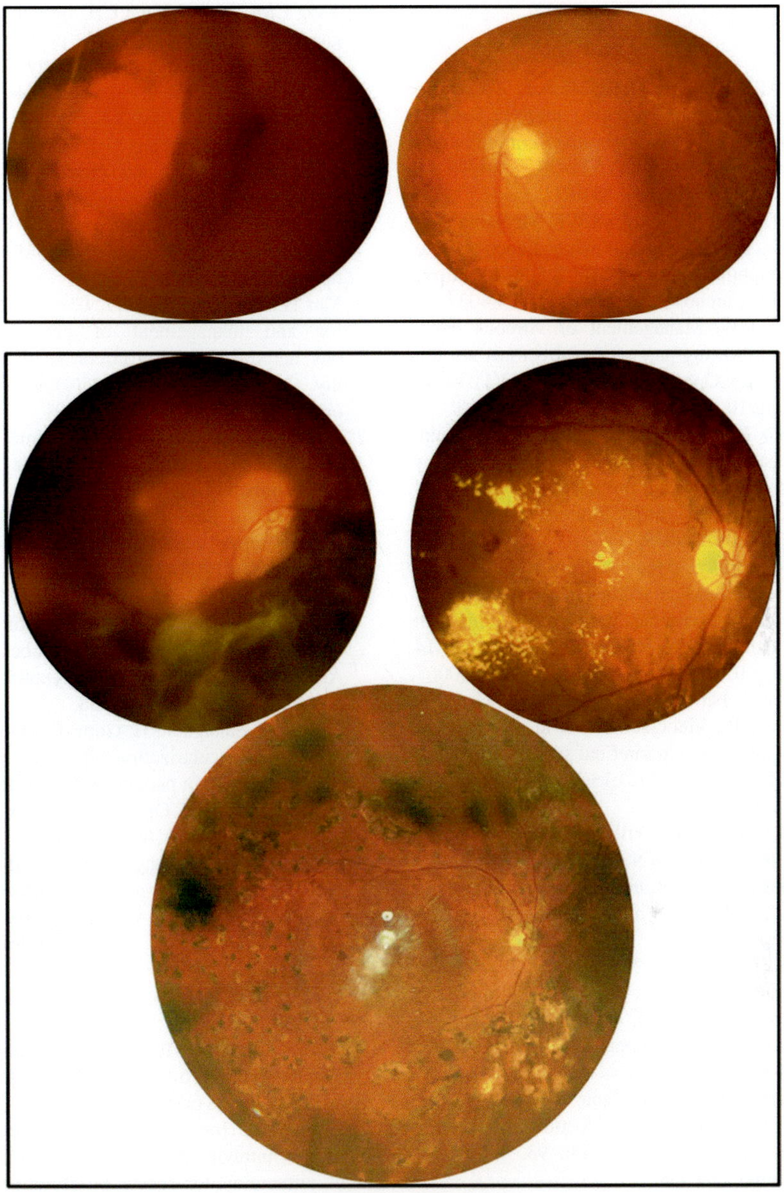

Fig. 16.3 Two examples of post-DV recurrent VH in the only functioning eye. In the upper panel, the preoperative color photo shows dense VH in the left eye (left). Postoperative color photo shows the attached retina (right). Recurrent VH was noted 16 months after surgery, and IVI Avastin and ARC were given. Cataract surgery was performed 2 months later. Five more IVIAs were given for repeated recurrent VH. He eventually received SO infusion to stop VH. The lower panel shows the preoperative FVP, preretinal hemorrhage, VH and FVP, mainly in the lower retina (upper left color photo). After surgery, the retina was attached to the parafoveal hard exudates (upper right color photo). She experienced recurrent VH 8 months later, and IVI of Avastin and the ARC were performed. Recurrent VH was noted again 14 months after the first episode. IVI Avastin and intravitreal TA were given. There was no additional VH for 2 years (lower wide angle color photo). (Courtesy of Dr. Chung-May Yang)

References

1. Schachat AP, Oyakawa RT, Michels RG, Rice TA. Complications of vitreous surgery for diabetic retinopathy. II. Postoperative complications. Ophthalmology. 1983;90(5):522–30. https://doi.org/10.1016/s0161-6420(83)34540-1.
2. Brown GC, Tasman WS, Benson WE, McNamara JA, Eagle RC Jr. Reoperation following diabetic vitrectomy. Arch Ophthalmol. 1992;110(4):506–10. https://doi.org/10.1001/archopht.1992.01080160084037.
3. Blankenship GW. Management of vitreous cavity hemorrhage following pars plana vitrectomy for diabetic retinopathy. Ophthalmology. 1986;93(1):39–44. https://doi.org/10.1016/s0161-6420(86)33791-6.
4. Blumenkranz M, Gardner T, Blankenship G. Fluid–gas exchange and photocoagulation after vitrectomy. Indications, technique, and results. Arch Ophthalmol. 1986;104(2):291–6. https://doi.org/10.1001/archopht.1986.01050140149039.
5. Han DP, Murphy ML, Mieler WF, Abrams GW. Outpatient fluid-air exchange for severe postvitrectomy diabetic vitreous hemorrhage. Long-term results and complications. Retina. 1991;11(3):309–14. https://doi.org/10.1097/00006982-199111030-00007.
6. Confalonieri F, Ferraro V, Di Maria A, Gaeta A, Vallejo-Garcia JL, Vinciguerra P, et al. Antiplatelets and anticoagulants in vitreoretinal surgery: a systematic review. Life (Basel). 2023;13(6):1362. https://doi.org/10.3390/life13061362.
7. Fu AD, McDonald HR, Williams DF, Cantrill HL, Ryan EH Jr, Johnson RN, et al. Anticoagulation with warfarin in vitreoretinal surgery. Retina. 2007;27(3):290–5. https://doi.org/10.1097/01.iae.0000243033.39301.10.
8. Dayani PN, Grand MG. Maintenance of warfarin anticoagulation for patients undergoing vitreoretinal surgery. Arch Ophthalmol. 2006;124(11):1558–65. https://doi.org/10.1001/archopht.124.11.1558.
9. Koch FH, Kreiger AE, Spitznas M, Glasgow B, Foos RY, Yoshizumi MO. Pars plana incisions of four patients: histopathology and electron microscopy. Br J Ophthalmol. 1995;79(5):486–93. https://doi.org/10.1136/bjo.79.5.486.
10. Kreiger AE. Wound complications in pars plana vitrectomy. Retina. 1993;13(4):335–44. https://doi.org/10.1097/00006982-199313040-00012.
11. Kreiger AE. Ultrasound biomicroscopy of sclerotomy sites. Ophthalmology. 2001;108(7):1175–6. https://doi.org/10.1016/s0161-6420(01)00616-9.
12. Novak MA, Rice TA, Michels RG, Auer C. Vitreous hemorrhage after vitrectomy for diabetic retinopathy. Ophthalmology. 1984;91(12):1485–9. https://doi.org/10.1016/s0161-6420(84)34099-4.
13. Tolentino FI, Cajita VN, Gancayco T, Skates S. Vitreous hemorrhage after closed vitrectomy for proliferative diabetic retinopathy. Ophthalmology. 1989;96(10):1495–500. https://doi.org/10.1016/s0161-6420(89)32700-x.
14. Yang CM, Yeh PT, Yang CH. Intravitreal long-acting gas in the prevention of early postoperative vitreous hemorrhage in diabetic vitrectomy. Ophthalmology. 2007;114(4):710–5. https://doi.org/10.1016/j.ophtha.2006.07.047.
15. Yeh PT, Yang CM, Yang CH, Huang JS. Cryotherapy of the anterior retina and sclerotomy sites in diabetic vitrectomy to prevent recurrent vitreous hemorrhage: an ultrasound biomicroscopy study. Ophthalmology. 2005;112(12):2095–102. https://doi.org/10.1016/j.ophtha.2005.07.010.
16. Yan H, Cui J, Lu Y, Yu J, Chen S, Xu Y. Reasons for and management of postvitrectomy vitreous hemorrhage in proliferative diabetic retinopathy. Curr Eye Res. 2010;35(4):308–13. https://doi.org/10.3109/02713680903572491.
17. Avery RL, Pearlman J, Pieramici DJ, Rabena MD, Castellarin AA, Nasir MA, et al. Intravitreal bevacizumab (Avastin) in the treatment of proliferative diabetic retinopathy. Ophthalmology. 2006;113(10):1695.e1–15. https://doi.org/10.1016/j.ophtha.2006.05.064.
18. Mason JO III, Nixon PA, White MF. Intravitreal injection of bevacizumab (Avastin) as adjunctive treatment of proliferative diabetic retinopathy. Am J Ophthalmol. 2006;142(4):685–8. https://doi.org/10.1016/j.ajo.2006.04.058.
19. Oshima Y, Sakaguchi H, Gomi F, Tano Y. Regression of iris neovascularization after intravitreal injection of bevacizumab in patients with proliferative diabetic retinopathy. Am J Ophthalmol. 2006;142(1):155–8. https://doi.org/10.1016/j.ajo.2006.02.015.
20. Yang CM, Yeh PT, Yang CH, Chen MS. Bevacizumab pretreatment and long-acting gas infusion on vitreous clear-up after diabetic vitrectomy. Am J Ophthalmol. 2008;146(2):211–7. https://doi.org/10.1016/j.ajo.2008.04.028.
21. Yeh PT, Yang CM, Lin YC, Chen MS, Yang CH. Bevacizumab pretreatment in vitrectomy with silicone oil for severe diabetic retinopathy. Retina. 2009;29(6):768–74. https://doi.org/10.1097/IAE.0b013e3181a3b7ef.
22. Ishikawa K, Honda S, Tsukahara Y, Negi A. Preferable use of intravitreal bevacizumab as a pretreatment of vitrectomy for severe proliferative diabetic retinopathy. Eye (Lond). 2009;23(1):108–11. https://doi.org/10.1038/sj.eye.6702983.
23. Chen E, Park CH. Use of intravitreal bevacizumab as a preoperative adjunct for tractional retinal detachment repair in severe proliferative diabetic retinopathy. Retina. 2006;26(6):699–700. https://doi.org/10.1097/01.iae.0000225351.87205.69.
24. Arevalo JF, Maia M, Flynn HW Jr, Saravia M, Avery RL, Wu L, et al. Tractional retinal detachment following intravitreal bevacizumab (Avastin) in patients with severe proliferative diabetic retinopathy. Br J Ophthalmol. 2008;92(2):213–6. https://doi.org/10.1136/bjo.2007.127142.
25. Joondeph BC, Blankenship GW. Hemostatic effects of air versus fluid in diabetic vitrectomy. Ophthalmology.

1989;96(12):1701–6; discussion 6–7. https://doi.org/10.1016/s0161-6420(89)32649-2.
26. Koutsandrea CN, Apostolopoulos MN, Chatzoulis DZ, Parikakis EA, Theodossiadis GP. Hemostatic effects of SF6 after diabetic vitrectomy for vitreous hemorrhage. Acta Ophthalmol Scand. 2001;79(1):34–8. https://doi.org/10.1034/j.1600-0420.2001.079001034.x.
27. West JF, Gregor ZJ. Fibrovascular ingrowth and recurrent hemorrhage following diabetic vitrectomy. Br J Ophthalmol. 2000;84(8):822–5. https://doi.org/10.1136/bjo.84.8.822.
28. Bhende M, Agraharam SG, Gopal L, Sumasri K, Sukumar B, George J, et al. Ultrasound biomicroscopy of sclerotomy sites after pars plana vitrectomy for diabetic vitreous hemorrhage. Ophthalmology. 2000;107(9):1729–36. https://doi.org/10.1016/s0161-6420(00)00213-x.
29. Hershberger VS, Augsburger JJ, Hutchins RK, Raymond LA, Krug S. Fibrovascular ingrowth at sclerotomy sites in vitrectomized diabetic eyes with recurrent vitreous hemorrhage: ultrasound biomicroscopy findings. Ophthalmology. 2004;111(6):1215–21. https://doi.org/10.1016/j.ophtha.2003.08.043.
30. Hotta K, Hirakata A, Ohi Y, Yamamoto R, Shinoda K, Oshitari K, et al. Ultrasound biomicroscopy for examination of the sclerotomy site in eyes with proliferative diabetic retinopathy after vitrectomy. Retina. 2000;20(1):52–8. https://doi.org/10.1097/00006982-200001000-00010.
31. Bodanowitz S, Kir N, Hesse L. Silicone oil for recurrent vitreous hemorrhage in previously vitrectomized diabetic eyes. Ophthalmologica. 1997;211(4):219–22. https://doi.org/10.1159/000310793.
32. Lambrou FH, Devenyi RG, Han DP. Fluid–gas exchange after vitrectomy using long-acting gases in an outpatient setting. Arch Ophthalmol. 1988;106(10):1344. https://doi.org/10.1001/archopht.1988.01060140508003.
33. Miller JA, Chandra SR, Stevens TS. A modified technique for performing outpatient fluid-air exchange following vitrectomy surgery. Am J Ophthalmol. 1986;101(1):116–7. https://doi.org/10.1016/0002-9394(86)90477-0.
34. Steel DH, Habib MS, Park S, Hildreth AJ, Owen RI. Entry site neovascularization and vitreous cavity hemorrhage after diabetic vitrectomy. The predictive value of inner sclerostomy site ultrasonography. Ophthalmology. 2008;115(3):525–32. https://doi.org/10.1016/j.ophtha.2007.08.034.
35. Yeh PT, Yang CH, Yang CM. Intravitreal bevacizumab injection for recurrent vitreous hemorrhage after diabetic vitrectomy. Acta Ophthalmol. 2011;89(7):634–40. https://doi.org/10.1111/j.1755-3768.2009.01821.x.
36. Huang YH, Yeh PT, Chen MS, Yang CH, Yang CM. Intravitreal bevacizumab and panretinal photocoagulation for proliferative diabetic retinopathy associated with vitreous hemorrhage. Retina. 2009;29(8):1134–40. https://doi.org/10.1097/IAE.0b013e3181b094b7.
37. Neely KA, Scroggs MW, McCuen BW II. Peripheral retinal cryotherapy for postvitrectomy diabetic vitreous hemorrhage in phakic eyes. Am J Ophthalmol. 1998;126(1):82–90. https://doi.org/10.1016/s0002-9394(98)00066-x.
38. Bakri SJ, Snyder MR, Reid JM, Pulido JS, Singh RJ. Pharmacokinetics of intravitreal bevacizumab (Avastin). Ophthalmology. 2007;114(5):855–9. https://doi.org/10.1016/j.ophtha.2007.01.017.
39. Heiduschka P, Fietz H, Hofmeister S, Schultheiss S, Mack AF, Peters S, et al. Penetration of bevacizumab through the retina after intravitreal injection in the monkey. Invest Ophthalmol Vis Sci. 2007;48(6):2814–23. https://doi.org/10.1167/iovs.06-1171.
40. Yanyali A, Aytug B, Horozoglu F, Nohutcu AF. Bevacizumab (Avastin) for diabetic macular edema in previously vitrectomized eyes. Am J Ophthalmol. 2007;144(1):124–6. https://doi.org/10.1016/j.ajo.2007.02.048.
41. Lee SY, Yoon YH, Lee HG, Chung H, Kim JG. Intravitreal triamcinolone acetonide in eyes with recurrent postvitrectomy diabetic vitreous hemorrhage. Am J Ophthalmol. 2006;142(3):501–3. https://doi.org/10.1016/j.ajo.2006.03.045.

17 Epiretinal Membrane After Diabetic Vitrectomy

Abstract

Epiretinal membrane (ERM) is a common complication after diabetic vitrectomy (Messmer et al., Klin Monbl Augenheilkd 200(4):267–272, 1992; Yang et al., Acta Ophthalmol 88(2):193–198, 2010). One of our studies analyzing post-DV complications showed that more than 60% of the various complications were related to ERM (Yang et al., Acta Ophthalmol 88(2):193–198, 2010). It may cause macular thickening, macular folds, a vertically sloped foveal pit, lamellar macular hole (LMH), macular hole (MH), cystic degeneration, subretinal fluid, etc. (Yang et al., Acta Ophthalmol 88(2):193–198, 2010). The clinical features, prevention, and management will be discussed in this chapter.

17.1 Case Report

Patient 1: This was a 29-year-old woman with a family history of DM and a history of DM for 10 years. She had good control of DM and no HT or renal disease. She first came to our clinic because of VH in the left eye. She lost to follow-up after complete panretinal photocoagulation (PRP) in the left eye. Two years later, she visited our clinic complaining of blurred vision in her left eye for 3 weeks. On examination, best-corrected visual acuity (BCVA) was 0.8 in the right eye, and hand motion was observed in the left eye. Tractional retinal detachment (TRD) and severe active fibrovascular proliferation (FVP) with broad adhesions on the upper and lower arcades were noted in the left eye. After vitrectomy with SO infusion, the retina reattached. However, the epiretinal membrane (ERM) gradually developed and worsened with time, and the BCVA was 0.05. The patient underwent SO removal and ERM peeling. After the operation, the BCVA improved to 0.2, but recurrent ERMs gradually developed. The BCVA was maintained at 0.2 (Fig. 17.1).

Patient 2: This was a 39-year-old woman. She had been diagnosed with DM and HT for 1 year, with good control. She had a history of VH and PRP in her left eye in Thailand 1 year before. Severe vision loss was recently noted in her left eye. On examination, BCVA was 0.5 in the right eye, and light perception in the left eye. Her intraocular pressure (IOP) was normal in both eyes; no rubeosis was noted in the left eye. Fundus examination revealed moderate FVP in the right eye with an attached retina but no FVP in the left eye from the dense VH. She underwent vitrectomy in the left eye. Broad adhesions at

C.-M. Yang, *Surgery for Complications of Diabetic Retinopathy*,
https://doi.org/10.1007/978-981-96-2848-3_17

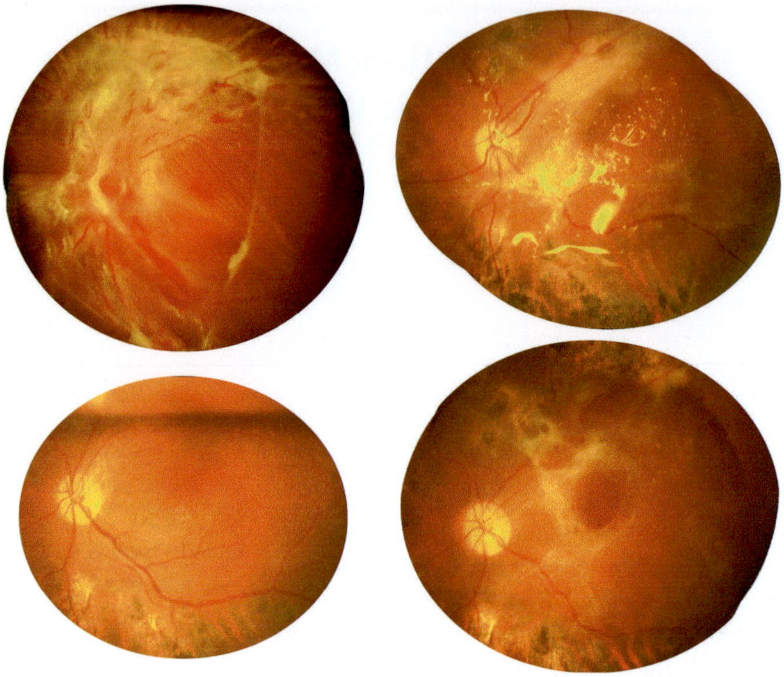

Fig. 17.1 This 29-year-old woman had severe TRD (upper left). After surgery with SO, severe ERMs developed (upper right). ERM peeling and SO removal were performed (lower left), but recurrent ERMs were noted (lower right). (Courtesy of Dr. Chung-May Yang)

two sites without macular detachment were noted during the operation. After surgery, BCVA improved to 0.05. Severe ERM with macular pucker was noted during follow-up visits (FU) with worsening of BCVA. ERM peeling was performed on the left eye 6 months later. However, recurrent ERMs with irregular macular thickening were noted again during FU. She underwent ERM and internal limiting membrane (ILM) peeling combined with cataract surgery 3.5 years later. Her BCVA improved to 0.4. Her right eye also underwent vitrectomy with FVP tissue removal and ERM and ILM peeling. No postoperative ERMs were noted. Her final BCVA in her right eye was 1.0 (Fig. 17.2).

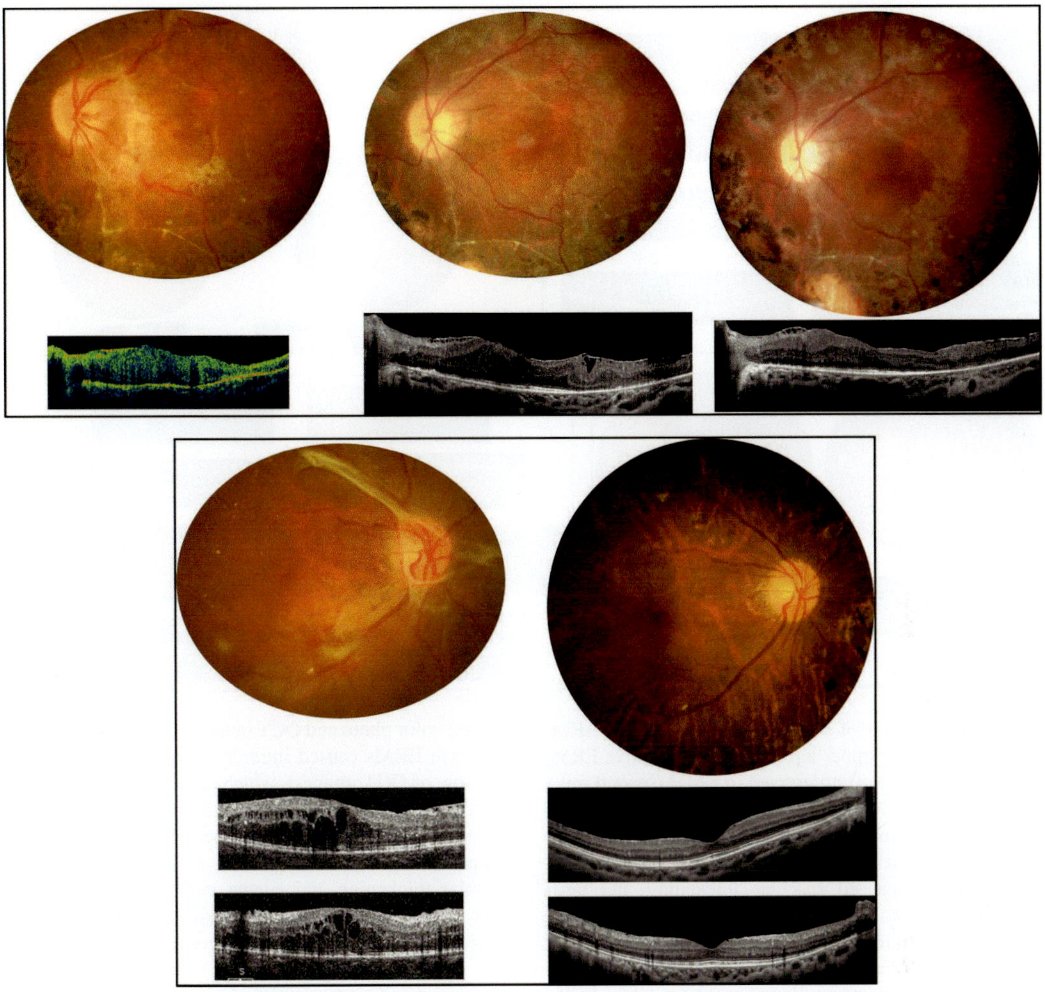

Fig. 17.2 Two sets of images showing pre- and postoperative retinal changes in a patient who underwent bilateral surgery for FVP and macular thickening. In the upper panel, severe ERMs with macular thickening and intraretinal cysts after DV were noted in the left eye (left color photo and OCT images). At 6 months after the initial surgery, recurrent ERMs with irregular macular contours were noted (middle images). ERM and ILM peeling combined with cataract surgery were performed 3.5 years later, and the macular contour improved (right images). In the lower panel, FVPs with traction thickening and cysts/schisis in the right eye were noted (left color photo and OCT images). After vitrectomy with ERM and ILM peeling, the macular contour normalized with an intact EZ (right color photo and OCT images). (Courtesy of Dr. Chung-May Yang)

17.2 ERM After Diabetic Vitrectomy

Because of the pro-proliferative microenvironment, ERMs frequently develop after successful surgery [1, 2]. The ischemic environment in eyes with PDR may persist or even worsen after DV, increasing the risk of cellular infiltration and epimacular membrane formation [3, 4]. Intraoperative bleeding or postoperative recurrent hemorrhage produces a proinflammatory environment and stimulates ERM formation [5–9], especially in patients with SO infusion, because of the high concentration of various growth factors between the retina and the SO [10]. Eyes with active and high-grade FVPs that were more difficult to remove were prone to significant ERM formation since FVP stumps and associated ERMs near the arcade may send an avascular membrane to the macula, creating

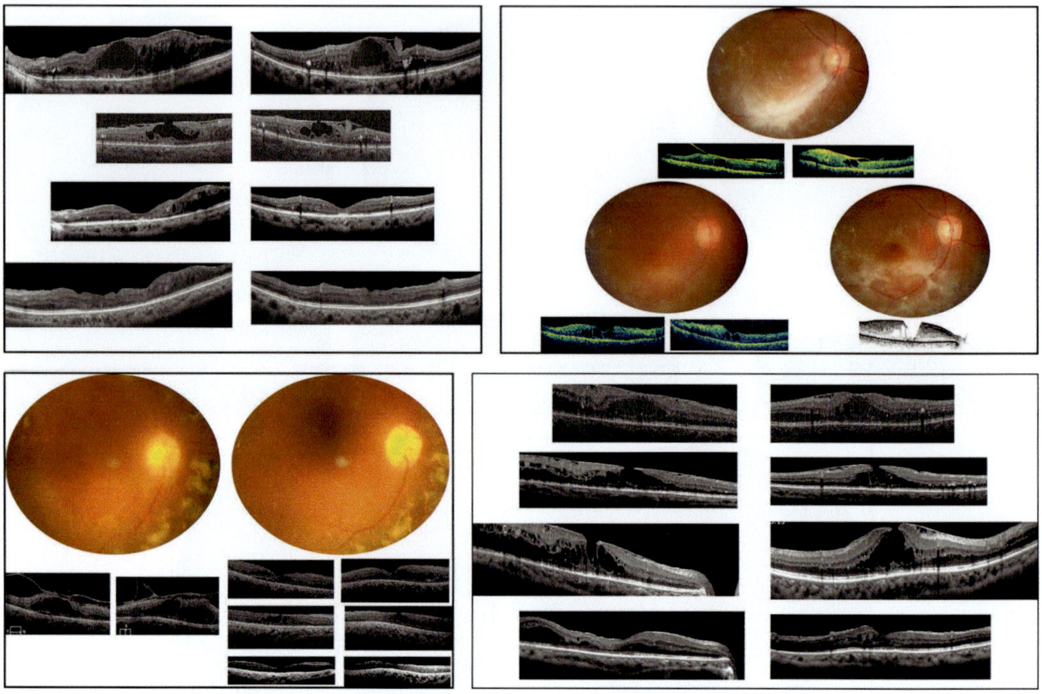

Fig. 17.3 Four sets of images showing post-DV ERMs with LMHs. In the upper left panel, postoperative ERMs and severe DME (top) progressed to LMH (second row). After ERM and ILM peeling, the foveal contour improved at 1 month (third row) and 5 years (bottom row) (Courtesy of Dr. Chang-Hao Yang). In the upper right panel, lower arcade fibrosis caused macular thickening and cysts (upper color photo and OCT images). After surgery, the ERMs and intraretinal cysts were noted (lower left images); parafoveal schisis and LMH developed later without further operation (lower right images). In the lower left panel, premacular traction caused macular schisis (left color photo and OCT images). After surgery, postoperative ERMs caused intraretinal cysts (right column, first row of OCT images), which progressed to LMH and outer schisis (right column, second row of OCT images). Spontaneous LMH closure developed later (right column, bottom row of OCT images). In the lower right panel, macular thickening and edema with ERM were noted after surgery for preretinal fibrosis (top row of OCT images). An ERM with LMH developed (second row), with gradual worsening (third row). After ERM and ILM peeling, the foveal contour improved (bottom row). (Courtesy of Dr. Chung-May Yang)

ERMs. Postoperative prolonged inflammation, a retained ERM, or posterior hyaloid fragments contribute to ERM formation [2] (Figs. 17.3, 17.4, and 17.5).

ERM severity varies among individual patients. ERMs may be localized, defined as thickened bands or sheets of membrane involving the macula and extending to either the upper or lower arcade, or more often widespread, consisting of bands or sheets involving the posterior pole and extending beyond both the upper and lower arcades [2]. The membrane itself may also have a wide range of thicknesses. Macular structural changes include thickening, cysts, schisis, folding, LMH, submacular fluid pockets, or even full-thickness macular hole (FTMH) or TRD [1]. ERM in the presence of diabetic macular edema (DME) may progress to LMH. If we defined a significant ERM as a visibly thickened membrane causing macular distortion or structural changes and a progressive decrease in vision, then our study showed that the preoperative severity of the FVP was positively correlated with a significant ERM [2] (Fig. 17.6). Postoperative hemorrhage and the presence of a residual fibrovascular stump were also significantly correlated. Our study revealed that the interval of ERM formation following primary DV was 9.69 ± 11.99 months (range, 1–45 months), and approximately 90% of the

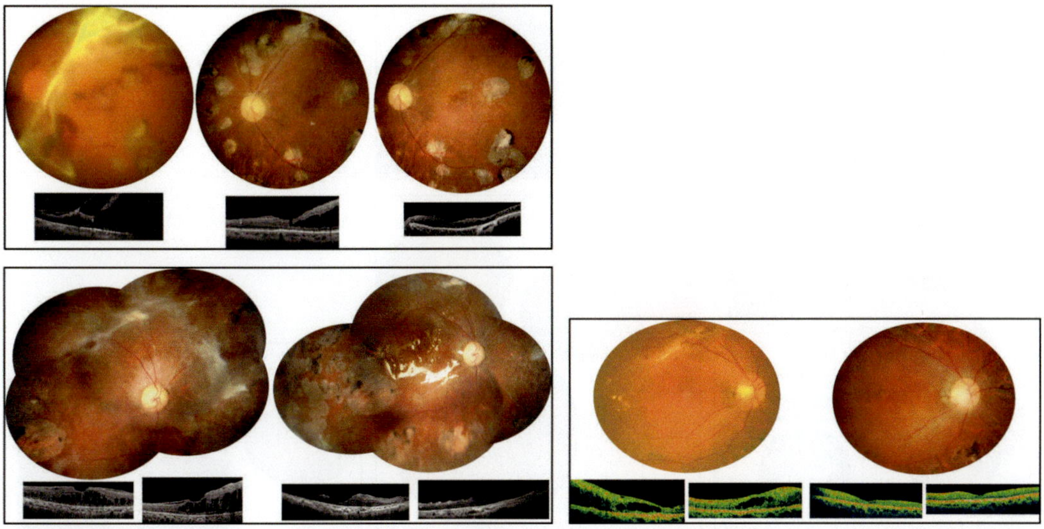

Fig. 17.4 Three sets of images showing ERM with schisis. In the upper panel, FVP tissue with traction macular schisis was noted preoperatively (left color photo and OCT images). After surgery, persistent schisis with LMH was present (center images). Further ERM and ILM peeling resulted in improved macular structure (right images). In the lower left panel, residual fibrosis outside the arcade with macular schisis was noted after DV (left composite color photo and OCT images). Further surgery to remove the FVP tissue and SO infusion was performed, and the macular structure improved (right composite color photo and OCT images). In the lower right panel, a residual fibrotic band at the upper arcade along with ERM-induced traction schisis is shown (left color photo and OCT images). After ERM and ILM peeling, the macular structure improved (right images). (Courtesy of Dr. Chung-May Yang)

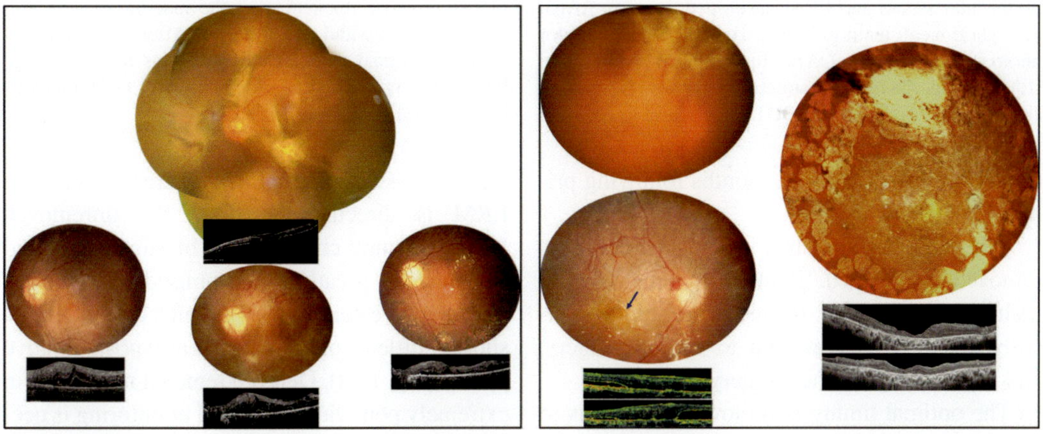

Fig. 17.5 Two sets of images showing ERM with submacular fluid. In the left panel, the FVP involving the macula and TRD were noted preoperatively (upper composite color photo and OCT image). After surgery, ERMs with SRF were noted (lower left color photo and OCT image). The ERM became more prominent during follow-up (lower middle color photo and OCT image). After further surgery to remove the ERM and ILM, the macula structure improved (lower right color photo and OCT image). In the right panel, active FVP with VH was noted before surgery (upper left color photo). After vitrectomy, an ERM with SRF developed (lower left color photo and OCT images). The blue arrow points to the ERM band. Further surgery improved the macular contour (right column wide angle color photo and OCT images). (Courtesy of Dr. Chung-May Yang)

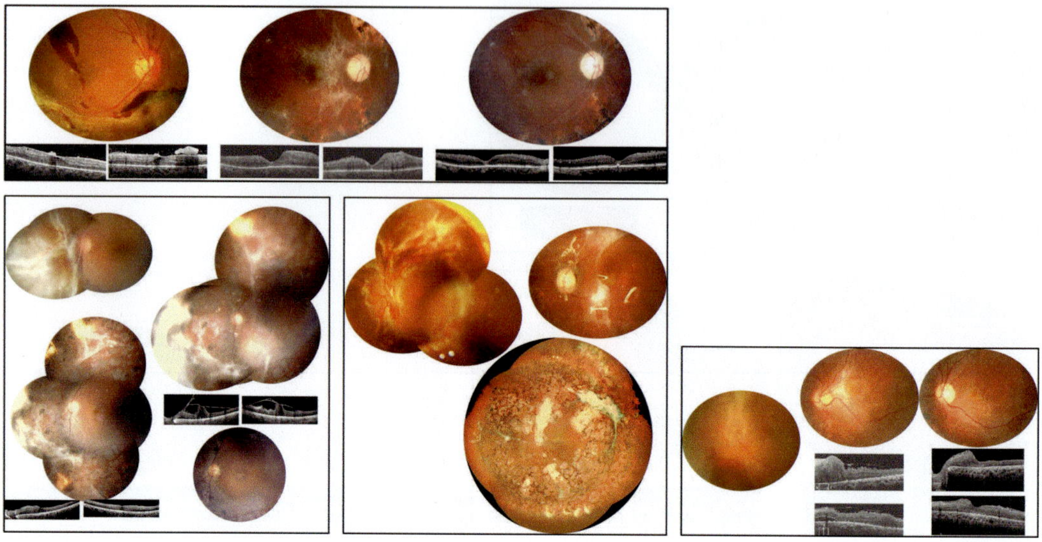

Fig. 17.6 Four sets of images showing various preoperative severities and postoperative ERM-induced macular changes. In the upper panel, an active FVP with an ERM was noted preoperatively (left). After surgery, a dense premacular membrane formed, causing parafoveal thickening (middle). After ERM and ILM peeling, the macular structure improved (right). In the left lower panel, nasal side fibrosis was noted preoperatively (upper left composite color photo). After surgery, the premacular strand and ERM developed, causing foveal and parafoveal tenting (upper right composite color photo and OCT images). After further ERM removal and ILM peeling, the macular structure improved (lower left composite color photo and OCT images and lower right color photo). In the lower middle panel, severe FVP was noted preoperatively (upper left). After surgery, dense vertically oriented premacular fibrosis under SO was noted (upper right color photo). ERM and SO removal were subsequently performed, and the macula was allowed to settle (lower wide angle color photo). In the lower right panel, active upper FVP with VH was noted preoperatively (left color photo). After surgery, dense premacular fibrosis developed nasal to the fovea, causing asymmetric thickening of the macula (middle column color photo and OCT images). After ERM and ILM peeling, residual macular elevation was noted nasal to the fovea (right column color photo and OCT images). (Courtesy of Dr. Chung-May Yang)

events occurred within 12 months following primary DV [2].

Whether postoperative ERMs should be removed is debated. Points for consideration include the following: degree of technique difficulty, complications related to further surgery, and functional gain after surgery (Fig. 17.7).

The optimal timing to remove the ERM is to balance between a worse functional outcome by prolonged traction and increased inflammation resulting from the short interval between the two operations. A second operation soon after primary DV may increase inflammation and ischemia and stimulate NV formation in the vitreous base or sclerotomy sites, causing recurrent VH or even RI and neovascular glaucoma (NVG). If possible, at least half a year should be allowed for gradual recovery from the first DV surgical trauma before the ERM operation. Two situations may necessitate early ERM operation: (1) The ERM is directly related to the unremoved FVP. Structural changes may be substantial, and VA may be greatly compromised in the early postoperative period. (2) The thick clot under SO showed little resolution in the early postoperative period (Fig. 17.8). Delayed removal may result in extremely poor vision. Careful monitoring is necessary, as RIs or NVGs may develop at any time after ERM surgery.

The functional prognosis is important when considering whether ERM removal is necessary. Optic atrophy, major vessel sheathing in all four quadrants, and optical coherence tomography (OCT) evidence of macular thinning are associated with poor functional recovery (please see Chap. 26). The ERM outside the macular area without disturbing the macular structure should be left undisturbed.

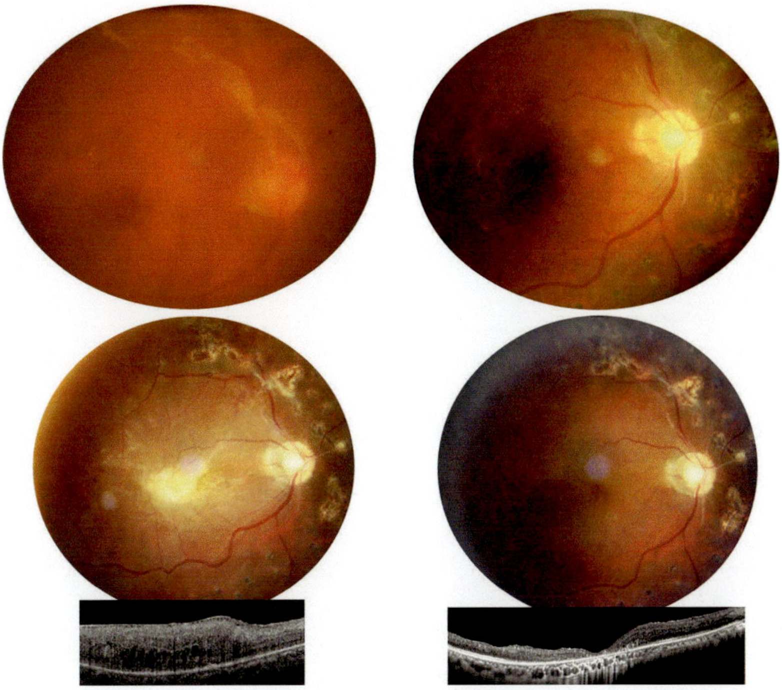

Fig. 17.7 This 49-year-old man had PDR with VH and FVP mainly in the upper arcade (upper left color photo), and BCVA was 0.05. After surgery, the retina was flat. There was a residual FVP band along the upper arcade (upper right color photo). However, a thick ERM soon developed and progressed within 3 months after surgery (lower left color photo and OCT images), and the BCVA was 0.02. After ERM and ILM peeling, the condition improved, but the fovea showed atrophy (lower right). The final BCVA was 0.05. (Courtesy of Dr. Chung-May Yang)

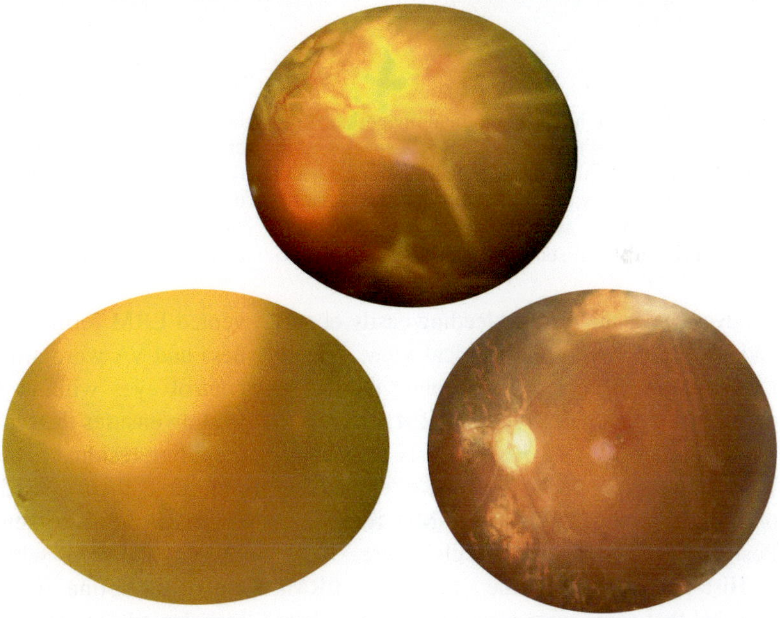

Fig. 17.8 This 56-year-old woman had CTRRD in the left eye (upper color photo). After surgery with SO, a fibrin clot extending from the macula to the upper arcade was noted (lower left color photo). The fibrin clot was trimmed to the upper arcade. Residual fibrosis was noted in the upper arcade (lower right color photo). Please see Fig. 6.6. (Courtesy of Dr. Chung-May Yang)

Operative procedures must be tailored to individual cases depending on the severity, adhesiveness, and distribution of the ERM. A thin and avascular membrane can be peeled as in idiopathic cases; thick and widespread membranes usually connect with retinal vessels. An attempt to completely remove such ERMs may result in excessive bleeding and retinal tears, greatly compromising the surgical results. Care should be taken not to disturb the retinal vascular structure attached to the ERM by trimming the ERM with a cutter or scissors. The ERM should not be

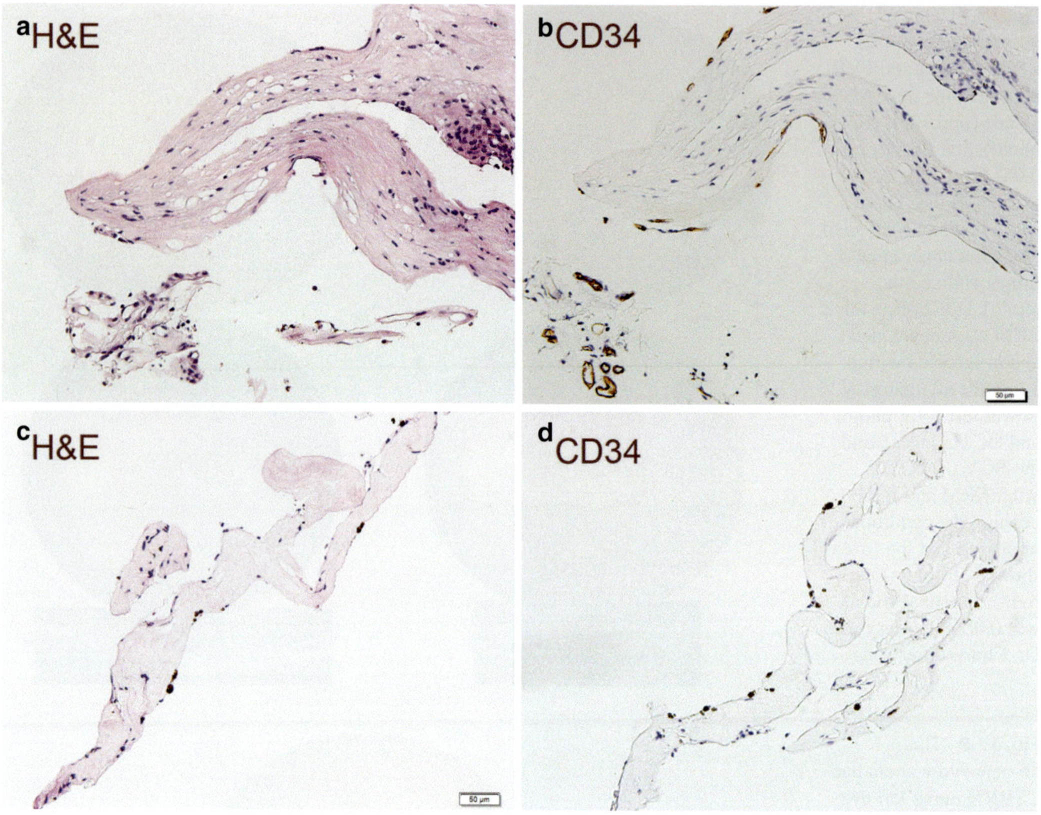

Fig. 17.9 One set of histopathological images showing the characteristics of the ERM. The ERM specimens in **a** and **b** were taken from one surgically removed ERM piece without vessels; the ERM specimens in **c** and **d** were taken from one surgically removed ERM piece with vessels. (**a**) H&E staining showing abundant collagen with epithelial cells. (**b**) CD34 immunohistochemical staining showing no vascular endothelium. (**c**) H&E staining showing abundant collagen with epithelial cells. (**d**) CD34 immunohistochemical staining showing the presence of vascular endothelium. (Courtesy of Dr. Po-Ting Yeh)

removed under the SO, as bleeding easily occurs and rapidly obstructs the surgical view. During ERM removal surgery, ILM peeling should be performed if possible to prevent ERM recurrence. When LMH or LMH with schisis is present, an ILM flap covering or the insertion or embedding of EP, if present, may prevent MH formation. Postoperative MH is discussed elsewhere.

Histopathology of the removed ERMs revealed that some were avascular, while others contained vascular structures, indicating different origins of the ERMs (Fig. 17.9).

Studies have shown that ILM peeling during primary surgery may prevent postoperative ERM formation [11]. Our study showed that in eyes with mild to moderate FVP, ILM peeling up to the arcade (5–6 DD) significantly prevented ERM formation, and the macular thickness and VA were greater in these eyes than in control eyes without ILM peeling [11]. ILM peeling ensures the removal of preretinal tissue, including residual hyaloid tissue and ERM [12, 13]. One theory holds that as ILM peeling removes the basement membrane of Muller cells, it alternates with the protoplasmic skeleton of the retina and aids in the resolution of macular edema. However, ILM peeling during primary surgery is sometimes difficult in severe cases, and the retained FVP stump may become the original site of newly developed ERMs, even after ILM peeling; thus, it is not clear whether postoperative ERMs can be completely prevented even when ILM peeling is performed during primary surgery.

References

1. Yang CM, Yeh PT, Cheng SF, Yang CH, Chen MS. Macular appearance after diabetic vitrectomy for fibrovascular proliferation: an optical coherence tomography study. Acta Ophthalmol. 2010;88(2):193–8. https://doi.org/10.1111/j.1755-3768.2008.01420.x.
2. Hsu YR, Yang CM, Yeh PT. Clinical and histological features of epiretinal membrane after diabetic vitrectomy. Graefes Arch Clin Exp Ophthalmol. 2014;252(3):401–10. https://doi.org/10.1007/s00417-013-2479-0.
3. Yagi T, Sakata K, Funatsu H, Hori S. Evaluation of perifoveal capillary blood flow velocity before and after vitreous surgery for epiretinal membrane. Graefes Arch Clin Exp Ophthalmol. 2012;250(3):459–60. https://doi.org/10.1007/s00417-011-1618-8.
4. Krepler K, Polska E, Wedrich A, Schmetterer L. Ocular blood flow parameters after pars plana vitrectomy in patients with diabetic retinopathy. Retina. 2003;23(2):192–6. https://doi.org/10.1097/00006982-200304000-00009.
5. Roldan-Pallares M, Rollin R, Mediero A, Martinez-Montero JC, Fernandez-Cruz A, Bravo-Llata C, et al. Immunoreactive ET-1 in the vitreous humor and epiretinal membranes of patients with proliferative vitreoretinopathy. Mol Vis. 2005;11:461–71.
6. Schoenberger SD, Kim SJ, Sheng J, Rezaei KA, Lalezary M, Cherney E. Increased prostaglandin E2 (PGE2) levels in proliferative diabetic retinopathy, and correlation with VEGF and inflammatory cytokines. Invest Ophthalmol Vis Sci. 2012;53(9):5906–11. https://doi.org/10.1167/iovs.12-10410.
7. Iannetti L, Accorinti M, Malagola R, Bozzoni-Pantaleoni F, Da Dalt S, Nicoletti F, et al. Role of the intravitreal growth factors in the pathogenesis of idiopathic epiretinal membrane. Invest Ophthalmol Vis Sci. 2011;52(8):5786–9. https://doi.org/10.1167/iovs.10-7116.
8. Abu El-Asrar AM, Struyf S, Opdenakker G, Van Damme J, Geboes K. Expression of stem cell factor/c-kit signaling pathway components in diabetic fibrovascular epiretinal membranes. Mol Vis. 2010;16:1098–107.
9. Abu El-Asrar AM, Missotten L, Geboes K. Expression of advanced glycation end products and related molecules in diabetic fibrovascular epiretinal membranes. Clin Experiment Ophthalmol. 2010;38(1):57–64; quiz 87. https://doi.org/10.1111/j.1442-9071.2010.02194.x.
10. Yeh PT, Yang CM, Lin YC, Chen MS, Yang CH. Bevacizumab pretreatment in vitrectomy with silicone oil for severe diabetic retinopathy. Retina. 2009;29(6):768–74. https://doi.org/10.1097/IAE.0b013e3181a3b7ef.
11. Chang PY, Yang CM, Yang CH, Chen MS, Wang JY. Pars plana vitrectomy for diabetic fibrovascular proliferation with and without internal limiting membrane peeling. Eye (Lond). 2009;23(4):960–5. https://doi.org/10.1038/eye.2008.334.
12. Michalewska Z, Bednarski M, Michalewski J, Jerzy N. The role of ILM peeling in vitreous surgery for proliferative diabetic retinopathy complications. Ophthalmic Surg Lasers Imaging Retina. 2013;44(3):238–42. https://doi.org/10.3928/23258160-20130503-05.
13. Rush RB, Del Valle Penella A, Reinauer RM, Rush SW, Bastar PG. INTERNAL LIMITING MEMBRANE PEELING DURING VITRECTOMY FOR DIABETIC VITREOUS HEMORRHAGE: a randomized clinical trial. Retina. 2021;41(5):1118–26. https://doi.org/10.1097/IAE.0000000000002976.

18 Secondary Macular Hole After Diabetic Vitrectomy

Abstract

Postvitrectomy macular hole (MH) has been reported after surgery for rhegmatogenous retinal detachment (RRD), epiretinal membrane (ERM), or myopic tractional maculopathy, with incidence rates ranging from 0.2% to 1.9% (Garcia-Arumi et al., Retina 31(9):1777–1782, 2011; Fabian et al., Retina 32(3):511–519, 2012; Medina et al., Retina 37(6):1065–1072, 2017; Rush et al., Retina 34(5):890–896, 2014; Kang et al., Sci Rep 9(1):19535, 2019; Gaucher et al., Am J Ophthalmol 143(3):455–462, 2007). The possible mechanisms include iatrogenic trauma or microhole formation during the induction of posterior vitreous detachment (PVD) or membrane peeling, cystoid macular edema (CME), tangential traction caused by residual posterior hyaloid (PH) or ERM, and underlying macular weakening. Secondary MHs may have distinct pathogenesis and clinical manifestations depending on the underlying disease. Few studies have been performed to specifically investigate postoperative MH after diabetic vitrectomy (DV). In this chapter, the various clinical manifestations, surgical choices, and outcomes are discussed.

18.1 Case Report

Patient 1: A 48-year-old woman with DM for more than 10 years underwent vitrectomy with SO tamponade in the right eye for tractional retinal detachment (TRD) at an outside hospital. She suffered from blurred vision in her left eye for 1 month. On examination, best-corrected visual acuity (BCVA) was 0.1 in the right eye and 0.05 in the left eye. Fundus examinations revealed vitreous hemorrhage, grade 3 fibrovascular proliferation (FVP) along the upper and lower arcades and at the nasal side, as well as a macula-involved the TRD. After surgery, the retina was attached under SO tamponade. Optical coherence tomography (OCT) revealed foveal thinning and an epiretinal membrane (ERM). Cataract operation and SO removal were performed after 14 months. Progressive foveal thinning and lamellar MH (LMH) formation were noted. Full-thickness MH and retinal detachment (RD) develop 3 weeks later. The retina was attached, and the MH was sealed after ERM removal, internal limiting membrane (ILM) peeling, and inverted ILM flap insertion. Her BCVA improved to 0.3 in the left eye (Fig. 18.1).

Patient 2: A 54-year-old man with DM and HT had previous PPV and SO for PDR with TRD and

C.-M. Yang, *Surgery for Complications of Diabetic Retinopathy*,
https://doi.org/10.1007/978-981-96-2848-3_18

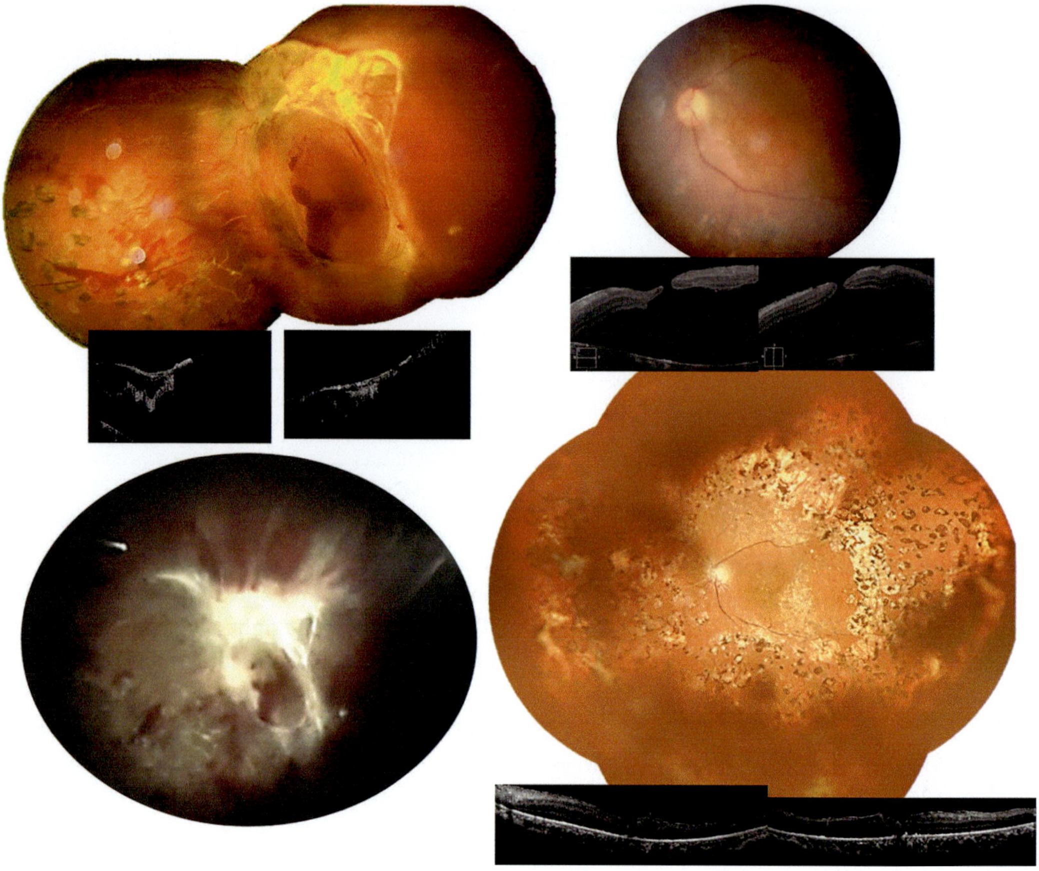

Fig. 18.1 Preoperative color photo, OCT images, and intraoperative image showing severe active FVP with TRD (left). Vitrectomy and SO infusion were performed. Three weeks after SO removal, MH with RD developed (upper right color photo and OCT images). After ERM removal and inverted ILM insertion, the retina was attached, and the MH was sealed. (Courtesy of Dr. Chung-May Yang)

VH in the left eye at an outside hospital. He complained of progressive blurred vision in the right eye. Ophthalmological examination revealed that BCVA was 0.3 in the right eye and 0.2 in the left eye. He underwent uneventful surgery to treat preretinal fibrosis and LMH with foveoschisis in the right eye in our hospital. Cataract surgery, SO removal, and ILM peeling were performed on the left eye 21 months after the right eye operation. Two weeks later, a full-thickness MH developed in the left eye. Lens posterior capsular tissue insertion and intravitreal infusion of C3F8 successfully sealed the MH. The BCVA was maintained at 0.1 (Fig. 18.2).

18.2 Secondary MH After Diabetic Vitrectomy

Postoperative MHs after DV are not common. The major predisposing factors for secondary MHs after DV include ERMs, residual FVP, anterior proliferative vitreoretinopathy (PVR), chronic CME, weakened foveal structure, and iatrogenic traction during surgery. The foveal structure is weakened in eyes with PDR due to longstanding CME and ischemia. Surgical manipulation during DV, induction of posterior vitreous detachment, ERM removal, and ILM

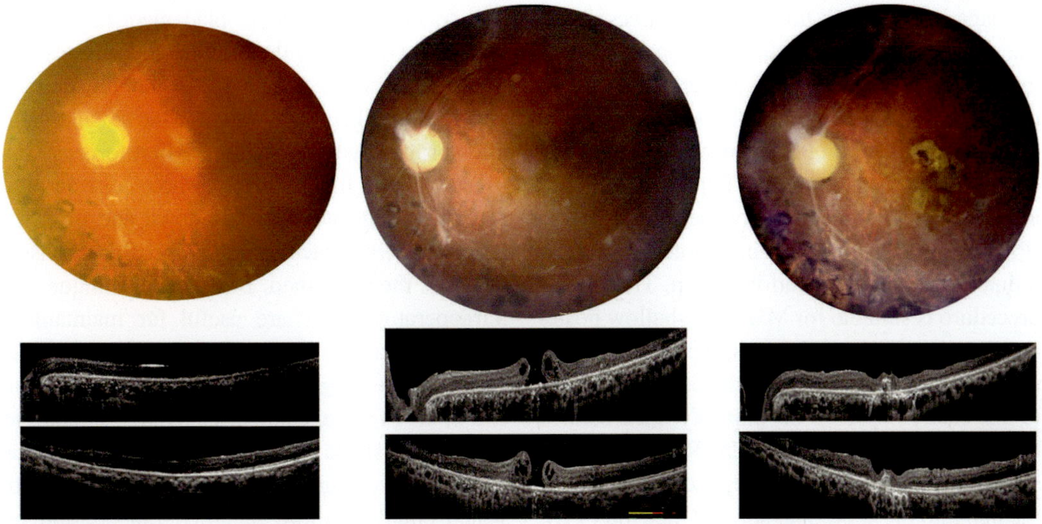

Fig. 18.2 Post-DV color photo and OCT images showing the attached retina under SO with macular thinning (left). After SO removal and ILM peeling, MH developed (center color photo and OCT). The MH was sealed after lens posterior capsular fragment insertion (right color photo and OCT images). (Courtesy of Dr. Chung-May Yang)

peeling may further damage fragile foveal structures. ERM was the most common predisposing factor for secondary MH after DV. LMH from ERM traction occurred in two-thirds of patients as a pre-MH condition. In general, ERM develops in more than half of post-DV eyes and has a multifactorial pathogenesis. (Please see Chap. 17 on post-DV ERM and related changes.)

In a retrospective, 10-year observational, and longitudinal study, we enrolled consecutive patients with PDR who developed MH after DV [1]. We found that three patients developed MH within 6 weeks, which was associated with foveal thinning, residual fibrovascular proliferation, or anterior proliferative vitreoretinopathy. Six patients developed MHs originating from the ERM with LMHs after a median interval of 16.5 months. Three of these patients had RD. The study showed that MH after surgery usually develops within a short period of time (within 6 weeks) when it is related to unreleased traction. On the other hand, MH caused by traction from the ERM takes longer to develop, usually through an intermediate stage of LMH, with subsequent progression to full-thickness MH (more than 12 months on average).

Depending on the complicated conditions of post-DV MHs, we applied different surgical techniques for MH repair. The indications for different surgical techniques were as follows. Standard ILM peeling was performed if no ILM peeling had been performed in the previous surgery and if the MH was <500 μm in diameter. A temporal inverted ILM flap or ILM flap insertion was performed if the MH was >500 μm in diameter or if RD was observed. Lens anterior capsular flap insertion was performed if cataract surgery was performed in the same setting, without available ILM tissue. Lens posterior capsular flap insertion was performed in pseudophakic eyes without available ILM tissue. A neurosensory retinal flap was created in eyes with complex RD lacking adequate ILM or lens capsular tissue. For the inverted ILM flap technique, meticulous ILM and ERM peeling and removal of residual FVP are pivotal for sealing MHs and preventing recurrence. In more complicated cases, the inverted ILM flap was the first choice. Inverted ILM insertion instead of an inverted ILM flap may be required when the size of the created ILM flap is inadequate and tends to flip back. In eyes without available ILM tissue, lens capsular fragments, neurosensory retinal tissues, or amniotic membranes can be used. Neurosensory retinal grafts (autologous retinal transplantation, ART) are useful for complicated RD, especially when peripheral retinectomy is needed. Peripheral retinectomy provides retinal tissue, facilitates subretinal fluid drainage, and releases traction. The harvested tissue may be placed in the subretinal space beneath the MH, inserted into the hole, or put on the preretinal surface covering the hole [2–4].

For flap insertion, two procedures may be adopted: neurosensory retinal flap harvesting and insertion followed by perfluorone carbon liquid (PFCL) injection; or PFCL injection followed by retinal flap harvesting and insertion. The former procedure is suitable for MH with shallow posterior detachment. In such cases, the elevated macular hole edge provides enough space for the flap to be easily inserted or partially incarcerated between the hole edge and the RPE, while the shallow detachment minimizes the risk of losing the flap into the subretinal space. Once the PFCL is injected to flatten the posterior retina, complete flap insertion may be accomplished with gentle manipulation. The size of the flap should be larger than the macular hole to prevent the flap from escaping into the subretinal space before or during PFCL injection. The second sequence of procedures has the following advantages: the PFCL reattachment of the posterior retina not only stabilizes the retina but also eliminates the possibility that the inserted tissue may be lost to the subretinal space.

There are some tips to be noted while using the PFCL to flatten the posterior pole before retinal flap harvesting. Because the retinal tissue fragment is lighter in density than the PFCL, it tends to flow up and drift to the PFCL bubble edge where the bubble is in contact with the retina. To avoid this tissue sticking to the far peripheral retina, one should not inject too much PFCL; rather, one should gently carry the retinal tissue fragment all the way to the posterior macular surface without loosening hold midway. Once it is in contact with the retina, it becomes stable and is subject to further fine manipulation and placement into the designated site. Another way is to first flatten the posterior pole with PFCL, then create the neurosensory retina (NSR) flap above the PFCL phase, but leave an attachment at the patch graft. Injection of the PFCL liquid to cover the donor is then carried out, followed by dragging the NSR patch graft to the MH. By doing this, the NSR flap may be kept from floating above the PFCL liquid. One way to facilitate a secure placement of the flap when it is covered by the heavy liquid is to remove a certain amount of the PFCL bubble until it becomes small enough to expose the macular hole after proper eyeball rotation. Microforceps was used to gently lift the macular hole edge and the NSR flap edge would settle down and properly covered by the macular hole edge. Secure insertion was then obtained. Bimanual technique and intraoperative OCT are useful for maintaining proper orientation during flap insertion. Another issue is preventing retinal flap dislodgement at the end of air-PFCL exchange. This may be achieved by reducing speed of exchange to minimize turbulence by inserting a larger piece of retinal flap, which could be more securely trapped, and by placing copious Viscoat® on top of the inserted tissue immediately after PFCL removal. With these manipulations, even if flap displacement should have occurred, it would have been minor, and repositioning of the flap could have been achieved. After the flap was in place with Viscoat® on top, SO infusion would not seem to cause flap dislodgement. Direct SO-PFCL exchange may be another option to decrease the likelihood of flap displacement.

For securing a preretinal flap on top of the MH, one may inject some viscoelastic substance within and around the MH before positioning the tissue flap. The sticky nature of the viscoelastic substance may help prevent flap from floating away by turbulence. After proper adjustment of the flap position, one may gently stroke and press the flap against the retina around the MH to maximize the surface contact area and strengthen the adherence between the free flap and the retina. Viscoelastic substance is then applied on top of the flap for flap stabilization during FAX. Another method is the SPOT technique described by Lai and associates (please see Chap. 4 MH treatment). It is particularly useful for this purpose. Tissue positioning can be performed under PFCL. PFCL may act as a compression tool to make the tissue flap firmly in contact with the macular surface. Viscoat is then injected onto the flap surface by passing the injection needle through the PFCL. When in contact with the flap, the Viscoat would form a smooth dome, making the flap very stable during FAX and after surgery. A large flap (>2DD) should be created. The advantage of a large flap is it may be better to counter the tendency of flap contraction and migration to ensure MH closure; it increases the contact area and adherence between the flap and the retinal surface to resist turbulence. After surgery, bending and curving of the flap toward RPE layer is expected, and the flap becomes integrated with normal retinal tissue. As the flap mainly serves as a barrier between the RPE and the vitreous, flap orientation is not a major concern for a successful surgery.

If the MH is too large and peripheral retinectomy is performed during the primary operation, an amniotic membrane graft may be a better option. Our study showed that although the MH closure rate may be high, the visual prognosis is poor in these patients due to complicated PDR and concomitant MH. The final visual acuity was poorer in these patients than in patients with other types of secondary MHs. However, all patients showed better visual acuity than that at the time of MH formation. The final visual acuity was noninferior to that of eyes with PDR complicated with MH before DV. Considering the complicated and challenging conditions in post-DV eyes, we suggest complete but meticulous ILM peeling during primary surgery to ensure total traction release and prevent MH formation.

Case examples of post-DV MH from different sources of traction are shown in Figs. 18.3 and 18.4.

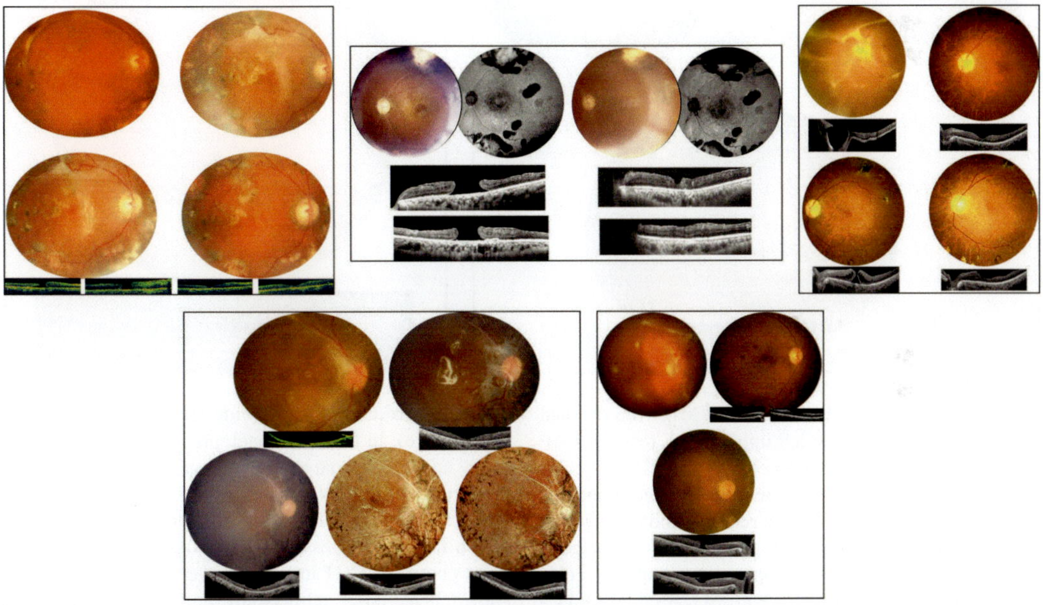

Fig. 18.3 Five cases of post-DV MH from the ERM. In the upper left panel, a preoperative color photo shows VH with the FVP band in the temporal arcade (upper left); after surgery, extensive ERM developed (upper right); MH developed 6 months or more after primary surgery (lower left); and after ERM/ILM peeling, the MH was sealed (lower right). In the upper middle panel, post-DV color photo and fundus autofluorescence image and OCT images show a large MH with ERM and epiretinal proliferation (left); after surgery with ERM peeling and EP embedding, the MH was sealed (right). In the upper right panel, a preoperative color photo and OCT images show the TRD (upper left); after surgery, the retina reattached (upper right); a tight ERM and MH developed later (lower left); and after ERM/ILM peeling, the MH was sealed (lower right). In the lower left panel, the upper two color photos and OCT images show pre- and postoperative changes. After cataract operation and SO removal, the ERM and foveal thinning developed gradually (lower left) and progressed to MH; the ERM was also apparent (lower middle). After ERM removal and ILM flap insertion, the MH was sealed (lower right). In the lower right panel, pre- and postoperative images are shown in the upper panel; the MH developed along with epiretinal proliferation (middle color photo and OCT images); the MH was sealed after the inverted ILM flap technique (lower OCT image). (Courtesy of Dr. Chung-May Yang)

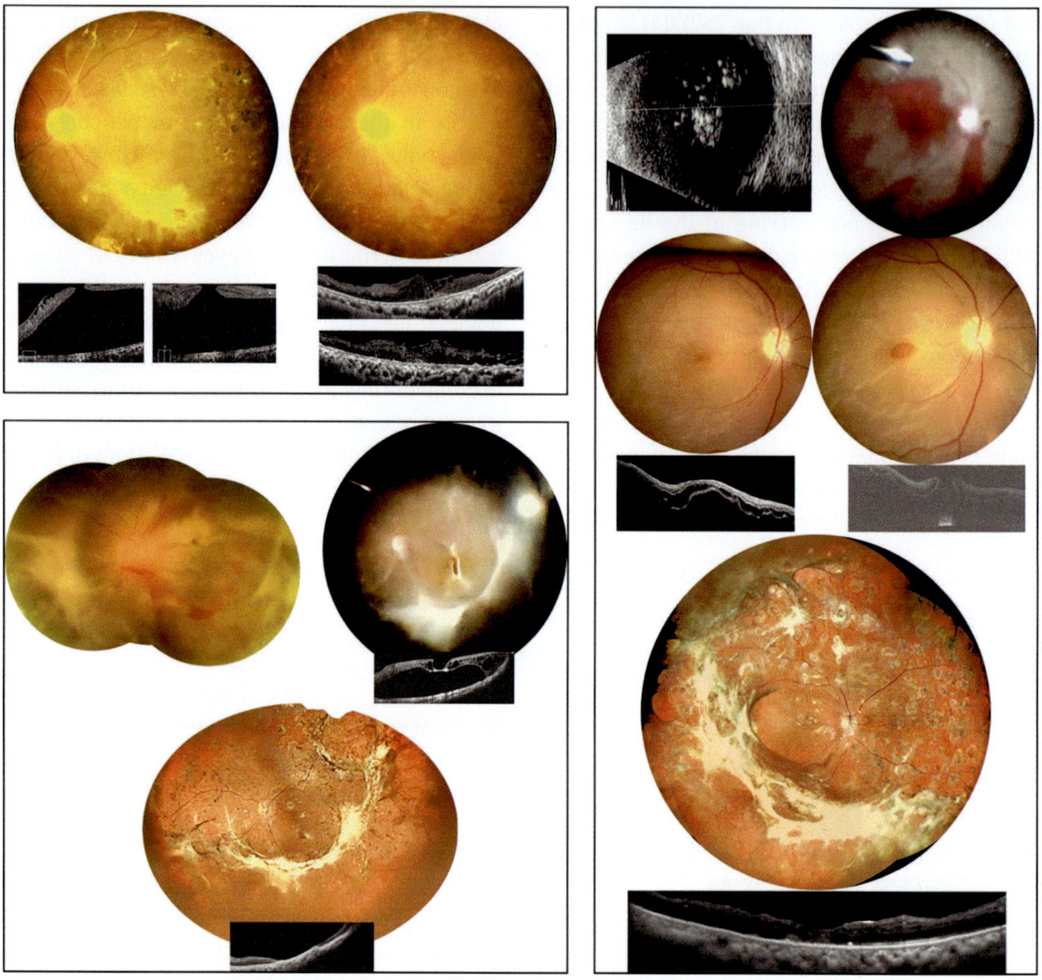

Fig. 18.4 Three examples of post-DV MH from residual FVP tissue traction. In the left upper panel, residual FVP tissue in the lower arcade induced MH and RD (left color photo and OCT images); the retina reattached, and the MH was sealed after FVP tissue removal and the inverted ILM flap technique (right color photo and OCT images). In the lower left panel, a preoperative composite color photo is shown. After surgery with SO, residual midperipheral fibrosis induced MH and RD, along with a submacular band (upper right intraoperative video image and OCT image). After retinectomy, ILM peeling and SO reinfusion, reattachment of the retina, and gap closure of the MH were noted (lower wide angle color photo and OCT image). In the right panel, preoperative ultrasonography and intraoperative video images show VH (upper); the midperipheral FVP is not shown here. After surgery, RD developed (middle left color photo and OCT image), which rapidly progressed to MH with RD (middle right color photo and OCT image); a lower anterior PVR is not shown here. After retinectomy and autologous retinal transplantation into the MH and SO infusion, the retina reattached, and the MH was sealed (lower wide angle color photo and OCT image). (Courtesy of Dr. Chung-May Yang)

References

1. Hsia Y, Yang CM, Hsieh YT, Wang LC. Secondary full-thickness macular holes after diabetic vitrectomy: clinical manifestations and rational approaches to the treatment. J Ophthalmol. 2022;2022:3156642. https://doi.org/10.1155/2022/3156642.
2. Thomas AS, Mahmoud TH. Subretinal transplantation of an autologous retinal free flap for chronic retinal detachment with proliferative vitreoretinopathy with and without macular hole. Retina. 2018;38(Suppl 1):S121–4.
3. Chen SN, Yang CM. Perfluorocarbon liquid-assisted neurosensory retinal free flap for complicated macular hole coexisting with retinal detachment. Ophthalmologica. 2019;242(4):222–33. https://doi.org/10.1159/000502443.
4. Chang Y, Liu P, Kao T, et al. Management of refractory large macular hole with autologous neurosensory retinal free flap transplantation. Retina. 2020;40:2134–9.

Retinal Detachment After Diabetic Vitrectomy

19

Abstract

Post-DV RD is a major complication after surgery. Approximately 1–20% of patients develop RD after DV for FVP (Schachat et al., Ophthalmology 90(5):522–530, 1983; Smiddy and Flynn, Surv Ophthalmol 43(6):491–507, 1999; La Heij et al., Graefes Arch Clin Exp Ophthalmol 242(3):210–217, 2004; Jackson et al., JAMA Ophthalmol 134(1):79–85, quiz 120, 2016; Yau et al., Semin Ophthalmol 33(1):126–133, 2018; Schrey et al., Retina 26(2):149–152, 2006). The risk of severe proliferation is high because of surgical difficulties and the excessive manipulations needed. New breaks, missed breaks, or proliferation from residual fibrovascular tissue or newly developed preretinal tissue may be the underlying causes (Smiddy and Flynn, Surv Ophthalmol 43(6):491–507, 1999; Yau et al., Semin Ophthalmol 33(1):126–133, 2018; Sternfeld et al., Clin Ophthalmol 9:1989–1994, 2015). Because of the preproliferative microenvironment and compromised choroidal and retinal circulation, recurrent RD after vitrectomy for PDR usually has poor anatomical and functional prognoses (Castellarin et al., Br J Ophthalmol 87:318–321, 2003). The detachment can have various manifestations and severities. There are few studies specifically focusing on this topic (Schrey et al., Retina 26(2):149–152, 2006; Brown et al., Arch Ophthalmol 110(4):506–510, 1992; Abdelhadi et al., Clin Ophthalmol 14:53–60, 2020). Different presentations and treatment options, as well as prognoses, will be discussed in this chapter.

19.1 Case Report

Patient 1: This was a 54-year-old woman who had a history of DM for more than 10 years. She underwent a successful vitrectomy for combined tractional and rhegmatogenous retinal detachment (CTRRD) in the right eye. She complained of rapid vision worsening in her left eye within 3 weeks. On examination, best-corrected visaul acuity (BCVA) was 0.3 in the right eye and 0.025 in the left eye. Fundus examination revealed an active fibrovascular proliferation (FVP) with macular involvement in the tractional retinal detachment (TRD). Vitrectomy with SO infusion was performed. However, VA did not improve. She visited our clinic, and fundus examination revealed widespread residual FVP tissue in the temporal midperiphery with macular thickening and paramacular subretinal fluid (SRF). Repeated surgeries, including cataract removal and posterior chamber intraocular lens (PCIOL) implantation, SO removal followed by membrane removal, endolaser, and SO reinjection, were performed.

C.-M. Yang, *Surgery for Complications of Diabetic Retinopathy*,
https://doi.org/10.1007/978-981-96-2848-3_19

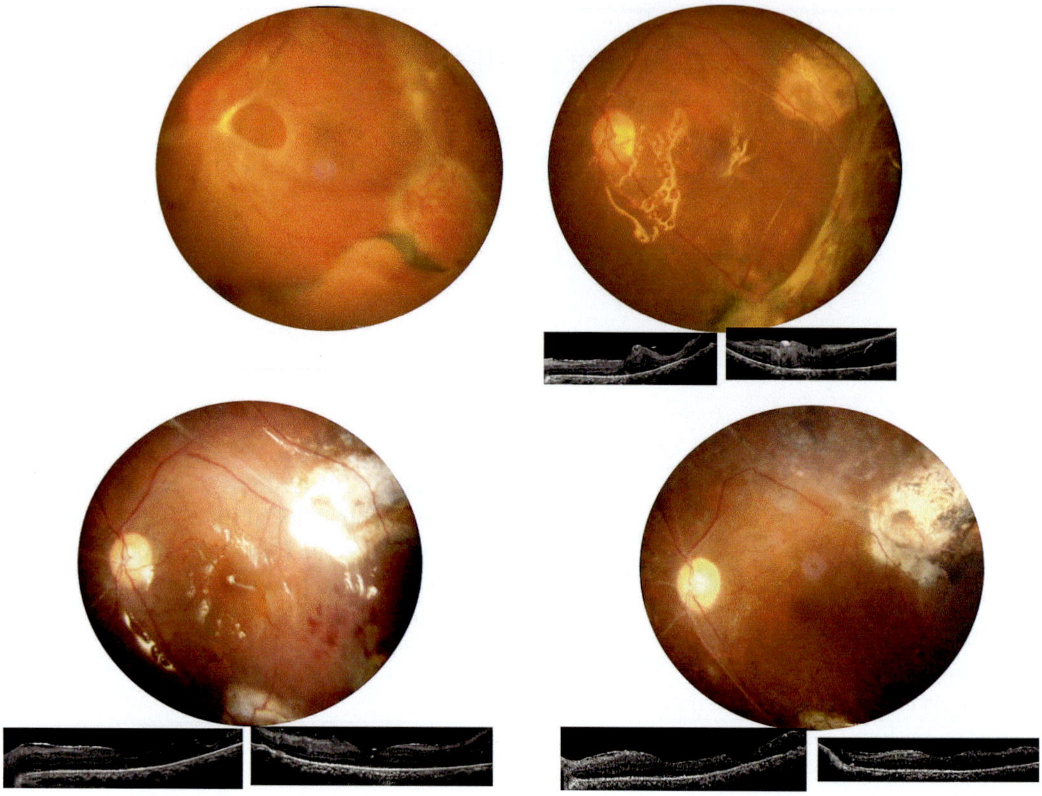

Fig. 19.1 Sequential images of the left fundus in a 54-year-old woman showing recurrent RD and treatment after primary DV. An active FVP with macular-involved TRD was noted preoperatively (upper left color photo). After surgery with SO infusion, widespread residual FVP tissue in the temporal midperiphery with macular thickening and paramacular SRF was noted (upper right color photo and OCT images). After cataract surgery, membrane removal, endolaser, and SO replacement, the retina was reattached (lower left color photo and OCT images). Further ERM and ILM peeling with SO removal was performed 4 years later (lower right color photo and OCT images). The BCVA improved to and stabilized at 0.15. (Courtesy of Dr. Chung-May Yang)

After surgery, the retina was reattached. Epiretinal membrane (ERM) and internal limiting membrane (ILM) peeling with SO removal were performed 4 years later. The BCVA improved to and stabilized at 0.15 (Fig. 19.1).

Patient 2: This was a 36-year-old woman with a history of DM for more than 10 years. She complained of blurred vision in the right eye for several months. She had panretinal photocoagulation (PRP) in both eyes at another hospital. On examination, BCVA was measured with a finger count of 50 cm in the right eye and 0.8 cm in the left eye. Fundus examinations revealed severe, broadly active FVP around the optic disc and macular subhyaloid hemorrhage in the right eye. Moderate active NV with scattered preretinal hemorrhage and a PRP scar were noted in the left eye. Optical coherence tomography (OCT) revealed TRD in the right eye. Vitrectomy with long-acting gas infusion was performed in the right eye 2 days after IVI of Avastin. During FU, RRD was noted 1 month after surgery. The BCVA was 0.05. No obvious changes in proliferation were noted. One break was noticed during the reoperation. She underwent SB 360°, vitrectomy, ERM removal, endolaser removal, and SO infu-

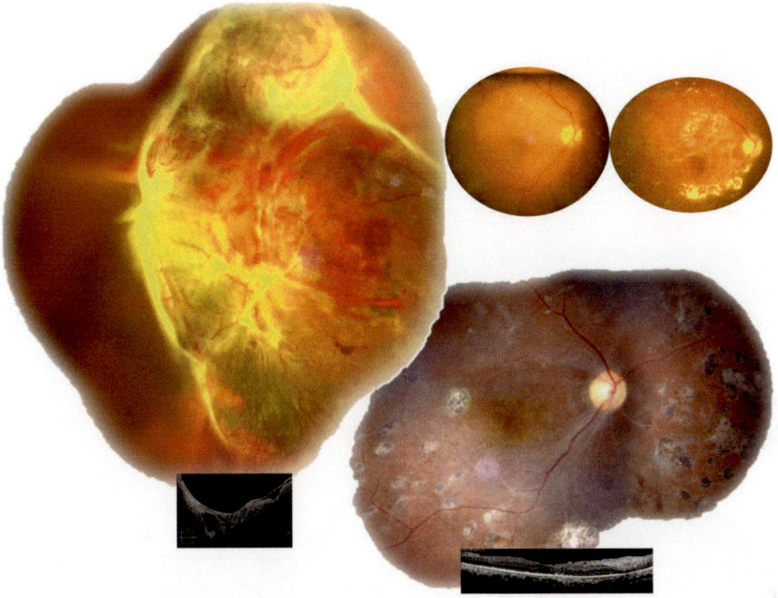

Fig. 19.2 One set of images showing recurrent RD after DV in a 36-year-old woman. Severe broadly active FVP around the optic disc with TRD and macular subhyaloid hemorrhage was noted in the right eye before surgery (left composite color photo and OCT image). After surgery, RD without PVR was noted (upper second right color photo). During repeated surgery, a single peripheral break was noticed. Postoperatively, the retina became reattached (upper right color photo and lower right composite color photo and OCT image). (Courtesy of Dr. Chung-May Yang)

sion. Phacoemulsification and SO removal were performed 7 months later. Her BCVA was 0.15. Her left eye had an uneventful vitrectomy, and her BCVA was 1.0 (Fig. 19.2).

Patient 3: This was a 62-year-old man who had underlying DM, HT, coronary artery disease, and hepatitis B. He was diagnosed with proliferative diabetic retinopathy (PDR) with VH, TRD, and RRD in the left eye and underwent PPV with SO injection at another hospital. Phacoemulsification with PCIOL was subsequently performed in the left eye. However, recurrent RD was noted, and repeated surgeries, including vitrectomy, buckle encircling, and SO reinjection, were performed. With persistent SRF in the inferior region, he was referred to our clinic. On examination, BCVA was 0.4 in the right eye, and ND was 60 cm in the left eye. The inferior RD of the macula with a fixed fold in the inferior macular area was noted in the left eye. Surgical procedures, including SO removal, residual FVP tissue removal, ERM and ILM peeling, lower peripheral retinectomy to release the anterior PVR, and SO injection, were performed. The retina was reattached after surgery, and the BCVA improved to 0.1. The patient subsequently underwent uneventful surgery in the right eye. Her BCVA was 0.5 in the right eye (Fig. 19.3).

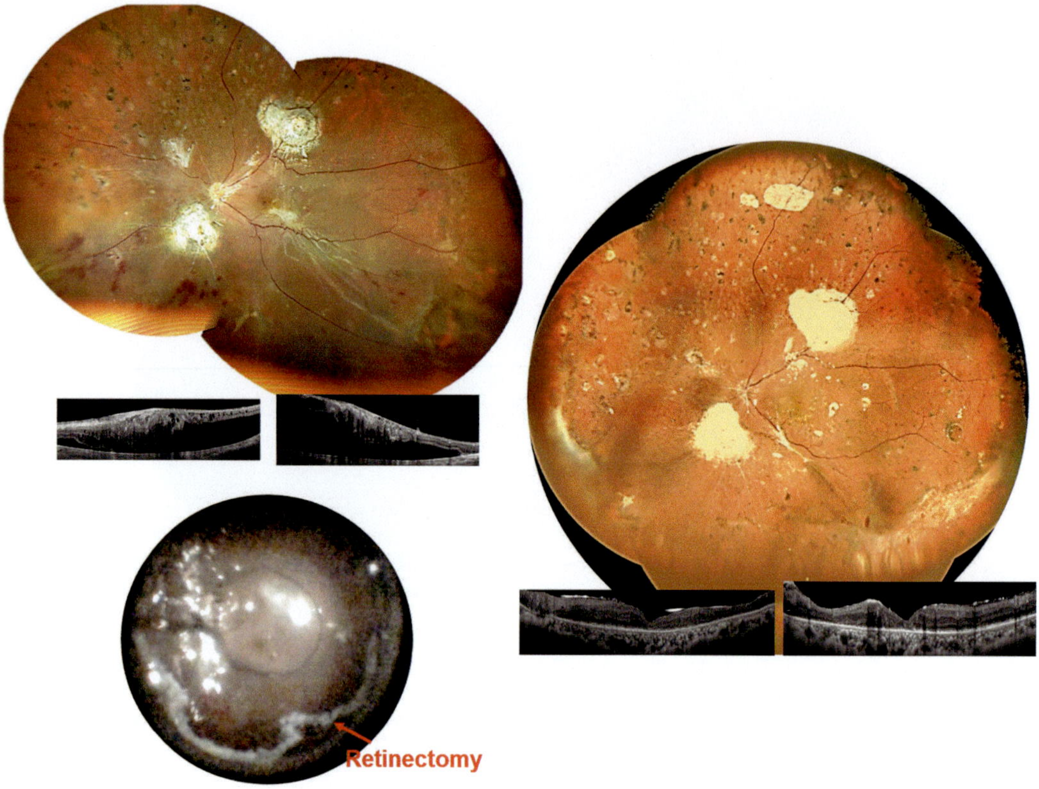

Fig. 19.3 One set of images showing treatment for recurrent RD after DV in the right eye in a 62-year-old man. After repeated surgery at an outside hospital, recurrent RD with persistent SRF in the inferior region with macular involvement was noted (upper left wide angle color photo and OCT images). ERM peeling and lower peripheral retinectomy were performed (lower left intraoperative video image). The retina became reattached under SO after surgery (right wide angle color photo and OCT images). (Courtesy of Dr. Chung-May Yang)

19.2 RD After Diabetic Vitrectomy

Despite advancements in surgical instruments and techniques, post-DV retinal detachment remains a major complication leading to total blindness [1–3]. Post-DV SRF may be caused by delayed reabsorption of SRF in TRD or exudative RD from surgical manipulation and inflammation [4–7]. These two benign conditions do not require surgery and are not discussed in this chapter.

We conducted a study to describe the clinical characteristics and surgical prognosis of patients treated for recurrent RD after DV [8]. We excluded patients who had multiple large retinal breaks with retinal tissue shortening and insufficiency resulting from severe traction. Patients with an opacified cornea, severe neovascular glaucoma (NVG), or without light perception vision were also excluded. Our results on those operable patients showed that recurrent RD had complex manifestations. It can be generally classified into two major categories: the pure RRD rhegmatogenous retinal detachment (RRD) group and the proliferative tissue-related group (proliferative group). The proliferative subgroup might include pure TRD (proliferative subgroup 1), combined RD with PVR and minor FVP (proliferative subgroup 2), or combined RD with PVR and severe FVP (proliferative subgroup 3). Here, PVR was defined as the presence of an avascular preretinal membrane in the posterior or anterior retina, causing fixed retinal folds or anterior retinal contraction. A minor FVP indicates that the FVP was distributed within the equator, and a severe FVP indicates that the proliferative tissue extended beyond the equator. Different sub-

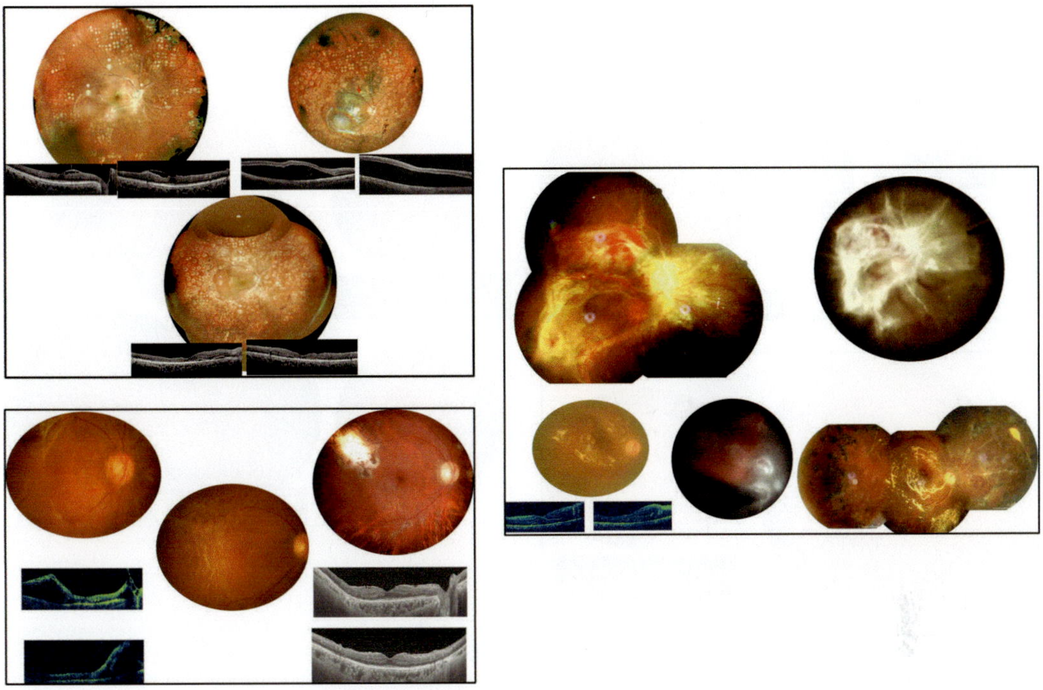

Fig. 19.4 Three sets of recurrent RDs with a pure RRD configuration. In the upper left panel, vitrectomy was performed for preretinal fibrosis and macular elevation (upper left color photo and OCT images). After surgery, a small break adjacent to the FVP stump in the upper arcade (red arrow) and macular RD were observed (upper right). After further surgery, the retina became attached (lower wide angle color photo and OCT images). In the lower left panel, TRD with moderate FVP was noted (left column). After vitrectomy, a small break within the temporal upper arcade and RD was noted (center color photo). After further surgery, the retina was reattached (right column). In the right panel, severe FVP with TRD was noted (upper left). The wide-angle surgical view is shown on the upper right. Shortly after vitrectomy with SO tamponade, RD was noted (lower left color photo and OCT images), and a break within lattice degeneration was found during surgery (picture not shown). SRF drainage under the SO through two iatrogenic holes was performed (lower center intraoperative image). The retina became reattached (lower composite color photo). (Courtesy of Dr. Chung-May Yang)

groups might be associated with different surgical outcomes. The overall reattachment rate of the 41 patients enrolled was 73.2%.

In the pure RRD group, there was no preretinal membrane or FVP tissue, as in Patient 2. The detachment came mainly from missed breaks created during intraoperative manipulation or breaks formed by vitreous traction after surgery. Iatrogenic breaks most commonly occurred within lattice degeneration, adjacent to prior FVP stumps, from one or more heavy laser scars, or close to the ora serrata corresponding to the instrument insertion sites. This type of RD recurred rapidly after the first operation. An increase in the RD area combined with a decrease in IOP are signs of RRD. All patients had reattached retinas in our study. If the surgeon intervened early and found and sealed the breaks, there would have been a better visual outcome without NVG complications (Fig. 19.4).

The majority of recurrent detachments were associated with proliferative tissue. The proliferative tissue came from DR-related residual or newly formed fibrovascular proliferation and PVR-related avascular tissue. An organized blood clot under SO is a unique and important source of thick preretinal tissue. Please see Chap. 6 for details. In subgroup 1, thick fibrotic bands or membranes caused retinal traction (Fig. 19.5). Traction macular thickening, schisis, lamellar macular hole (LMH), full-thickness macular hole (FTMH), or frank traction macular detachment

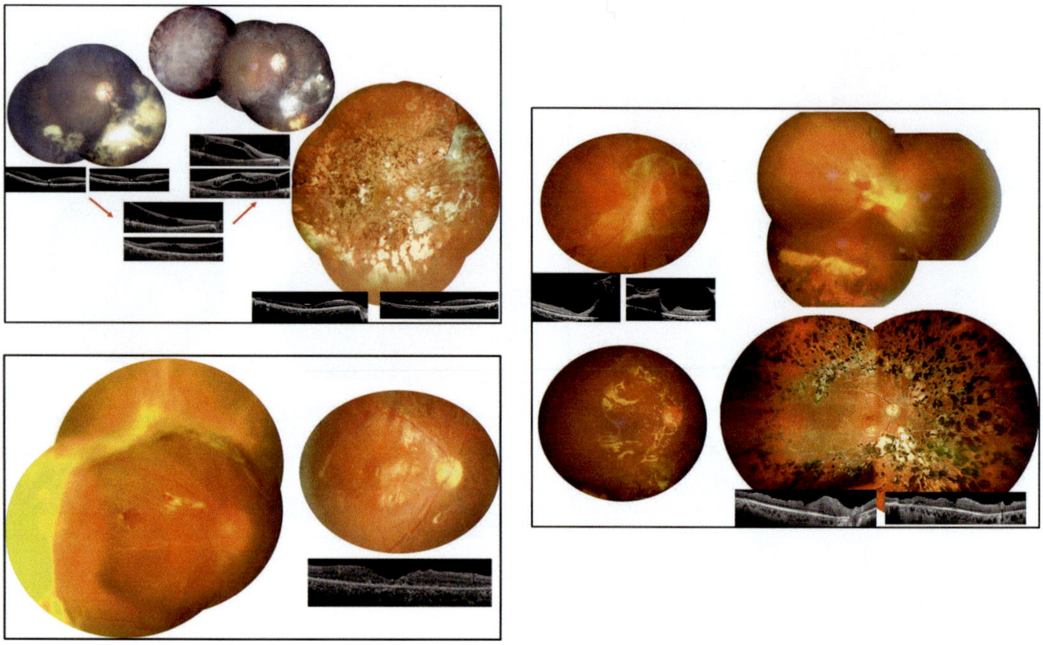

Fig. 19.5 Three sets of recurrent RD associated with postoperative fibrosis and TRD. In the upper left panel, postoperative images after vitrectomy for VH and preretinal fibrosis show residual lower arcade preretinal membrane and nasal lower massive hard exudates (upper left composite color photo and OCT images). Despite improved HE (upper center composite color photo), residual fibrosis caused schisis, which progressed to schisis and RD (sequential OCT images in the center). After further surgery to remove the fibrotic membrane, the retina was reattached (right wide angle color and OCT images). In the lower left panel, postoperative fibrosis along the upper arcade and in the temporal area caused TRD (left composite color photo). After further surgery and SO, the retina was reattached (right color photo and OCT image). In the right panel, preoperative color and OCT images showed fibrosis around the disc and traction macular schisis (upper left). Postoperative images showed residual fibrosis, causing TRD (upper right composite color photo). After surgery with SO, the fibrotic membrane was removed (lower left). The SO was removed later, and the foveal contour improved (lower right wide angle color photo and OCT images). (Courtesy of Dr. Chung-May Yang)

might develop. Extensive surgery is required because the tractional membrane is likely to be widespread; some patients require peripheral retinectomy. In subgroup 2, combined rhegmatogenous and tractional retinal detachment was induced by retinal breaks and some minor fibrotic membranes localized within the equator (Fig. 19.6). Both the avascular membrane from the PVR and the vascular membrane from the FVP were present. The removal of this minor FVP was usually attainable. However, peripheral retinectomy was still needed in most patients because of the presence of PVR. Subgroup 3 was the most frequently encountered and most challenging group. Anterior PVR was universally present in these eyes, and subretinal gas or subretinal SO was not uncommon. Some might also have extensive subretinal proliferative sheets or bands. The extensive proliferative tissue beyond the equator made complete removal more difficult, and the surgery was often complicated by bleeding and breaks even when using bimanual techniques (Fig. 19.7). In our study, less than 60% of patients in this subgroup had final reattachment. After reattachment, some patients gradually develop fibrosis around the PCIOL or rubeosis, causing vision deterioration. This evolution indicates persistent low-grade inflammation long after surgery. Despite these difficulties, significant VA improvement could be achieved on average because visual acuity markedly decreased at the time of recurrent detachment, and any anatomical or functional improvement may contribute to visual gain. In the proliferative

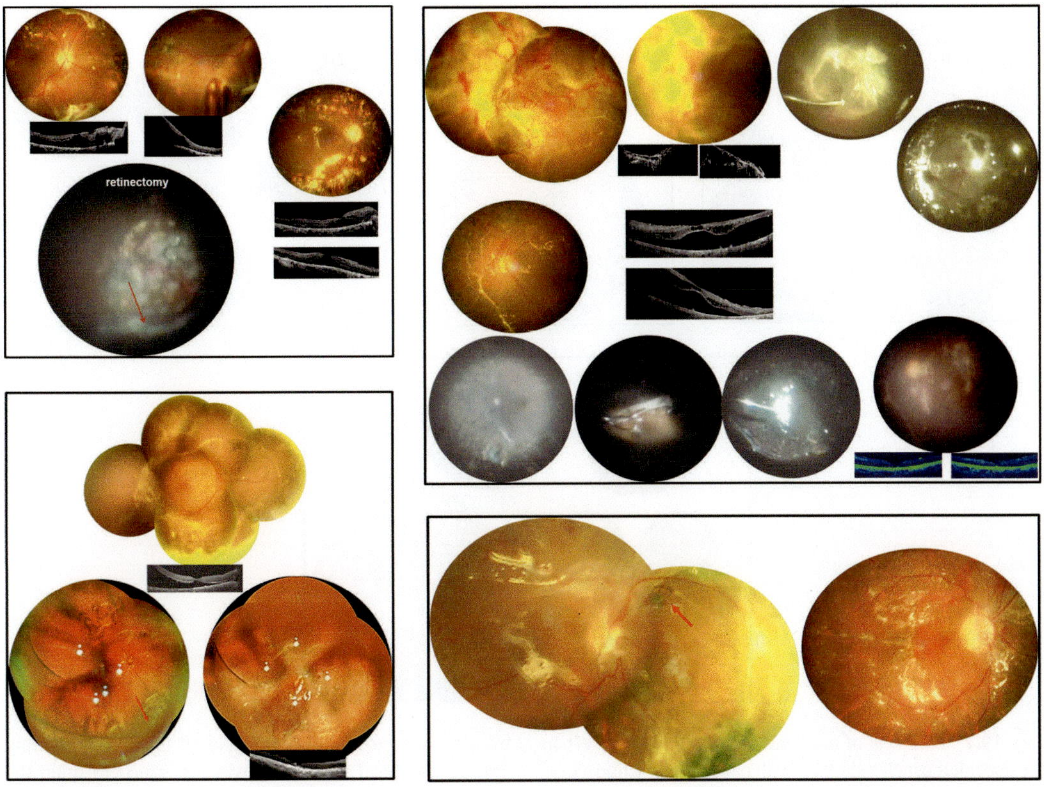

Fig. 19.6 Four sets of combined RDs with minor FVPs. In the upper left panel, post-DV retinal examinations show mild FVP in the lower retina and a large break (upper left color photos and OCT images). Surgery, including lower retinectomy, was performed (lower left intraoperative image). The retina reattached after surgery (right color photo and OCT images). In the upper right panel, severe active FVP with TRD was noted (upper left color photos and OCT images). FVP removal and localized retinectomy were performed (upper right two intraoperative images). After surgery, residual subretinal bands and RD under SO were noted (middle row color photo and OCT images). During reoperation, lower FVP tissue with anterior PVR was removed, and retinectomy was performed (lower left and middle two intraoperative images). The retina reattached under SO after surgery (lower right color photo and OCT images). In the lower left panel, preoperative composite color images and OCT images show the TRD and FVP mainly in the temporal upper, temporal, and temporal lower areas (upper). After surgery, a fibrotic membrane with a lower RD was noted (lower left wide angle color photo; red arrow points to the RD area). After surgery with lower retinectomy and SO, the retina was reattached (lower right wide angle color photo and OCT image). In the lower right set, post-DV color photo showed RD with minor FVP and a break under SO (left composite color photo; red arrow points to the break). After proliferative tissue removal, the retina was reattached under SO (right color photo). (Courtesy of Dr. Chung-May Yang)

subgroup, the bimanual technique and peripheral retinectomy are frequently applied for releasing preretinal and subretinal traction. SO tamponade, which has the advantages of early visual rehabilitation and a better opportunity to prevent recurrent detachment, is widely used in this situation (Fig. 19.8).

This classification can be used to assess the degree of surgical difficulty and predict anatomical and short-term functional outcomes. A comparison among the three proliferative subgroups revealed better preoperative vision in subgroup 1; in addition, subgroup 1 tended to have a reduced chance of having a BCVA of less than 20/400. Subgroup 3 had the least reattachment achieved. The relatively better prognosis in subgroup 1 (the TRD group) may have resulted from better vision before the second operation, which in turn was due to the limited area of retinal detachment or less macular elevation and ischemia. Despite the

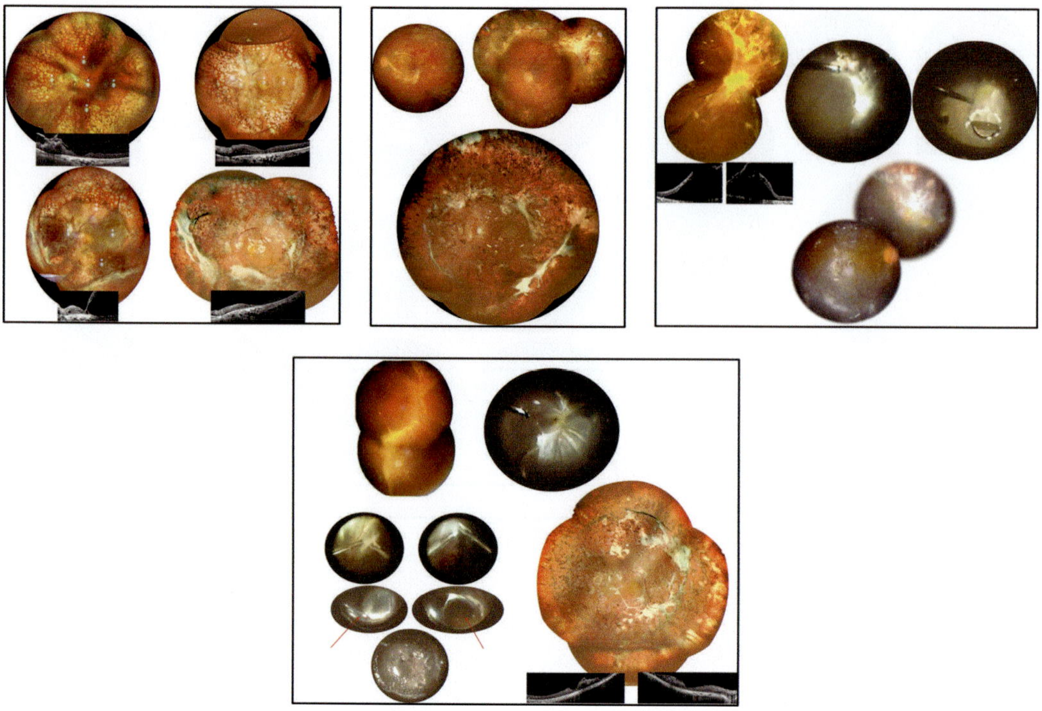

Fig. 19.7 Four sets of combined RD with severe FVP. In the upper left panel, mild FVP with parafoveal traction elevation and foveal thinning were noted before primary surgery (upper left). Early post-DV fundus showed an attached retina (upper right). However, FVPs with severe anterior PVR and RD were noted within 2 months (lower left). The retina reattached after reoperation, including extended lower retinectomy and SO (lower right). In the upper middle panel, severe active FVP with RD was noted under SO after primary surgery (upper color photos). The retina reattached after FVP removal and temporal retinectomy (lower wide angle color photo). In the upper right panel, post-DV composite color images and OCT images show RD with the FVP extending from the disc to the upper periphery (upper left). During reoperation, focal retinotomy was performed to drain the subretinal SO (upper middle and right two intraoperative video images). After surgery, the retina was reattached (lower composite color photo). In the lower panel, post-DV color photo and OCT images show RD with severe FVP extending to the lower periphery (upper left). During surgery, bimanual proliferative tissue removal, lower retinectomy for traction release, and subretinal SO removal were performed (upper right and lower left intraoperative video images; arrows point to the retinectomy site and subretinal SO). After surgery, the retina was reattached under the SO (lower right wide angle color and OCT images). (Courtesy of Dr. Chung-May Yang)

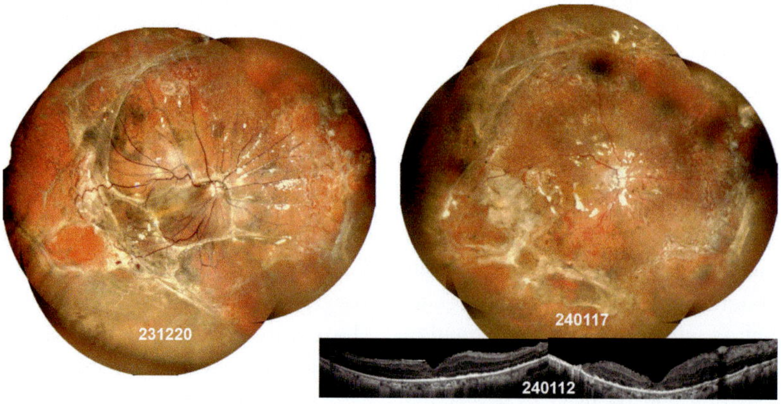

Fig. 19.8 One set of pre- and postoperative images showing retinal changes in a 75-year-old woman who had combined RD with extensive subretinal bands after diabetic vitrectomy (left wide-angle color photo). Lower retinectomy was performed to expose the undersurface of the retina for subretinal band removal. The retina was reattached under silicone oil (right wide-angle color and OCT images). (Courtesy of Dr. Chung-May Yang)

aforementioned differences, our study showed that the three subgroups were similar in many aspects. Visual improvement was achieved in approximately 50% of patients in each subgroup. The rates of NVG and long-term visual prognosis were similar. These unsatisfactory results indicate severe retinal pathological changes once recurrent RD develops.

It should be noted that not all recurrent RD cases are operable. Many patients with severe anterior or posterior pathological changes, as mentioned above, are not indicated for further surgery. Thus, the degree of anatomical/functional improvement in all patients with RD after primary surgery was much lower than that in our above study.

For operable cases, a standard 3-port pars plana vitrectomy with a 23-gauge system is used for more efficient suction if SO removal has been planned at the beginning of the surgery. Otherwise, a 25-gauge system is set up. After removing the preexisting SO, the retina was carefully inspected to determine the location and extent of the traction membrane. Any bizarre-shaped detachment should alert the surgeon to the possibility of subretinal SO, especially if there is a large retinal break with or without visible surrounding tissue under stretch. After removing the vitreous strands and the residual peripheral vitreous, the avascular epiretinal membrane is peeled directly with microforceps. Alternatively, microscissors and forceps are used for the delamination of thick fibrotic or fibrovascular tissue that is adherent to retinal vessels. Bimanual techniques are frequently adopted for the removal of extensive proliferation on the detached retina. Retinectomy of a limited area is performed posterior to the equator to remove the highly adherent, contracted thick membrane difficult to separate from the retina or isolated subretinal bands or to facilitate removal of a small subretinal SO bubble; circumferential peripheral retinectomy should be performed for significant vitreous base traction unreleasable by other manipulations, for a large subretinal SO bubble, or for extensive subretinal fibrotic bands. Direct fluid-air exchange or perfluorocarbon liquid injection followed by fluid-air exchange is performed to reattach the retina. Laser photocoagulation around the breaks and the peripheral retina is subsequently performed. SO infusion is then performed after an intravitreal injection of a small amount of anti-VEGF. For recurrent RD associated with FVP, SO may be a better option than gas for tamponade. Recurrent detachment, recurrent VH, and rubeosis may occur less often under SO.

To prevent recurrent RD, one should avoid or vigorously check for missed breaks or vitreous traction-induced breaks and remove the FVP tissue likely to cause traction as completely as possible. If there is unresolved extensive and thick preretinal blood under SO, prompt removal of the thick clot is suggested.

References

1. Cruz-Inigo YJ, Acaba LA, Berrocal MH. Surgical management of retinal diseases: proliferative diabetic retinopathy and traction retinal detachment. Dev Ophthalmol. 2014;54:196–203. https://doi.org/10.1159/000360467.
2. Issa SA, Connor A, Habib M, Steel DH. Comparison of retinal breaks observed during 23 gauge transconjunctival vitrectomy versus conventional 20 gauge surgery for proliferative diabetic retinopathy. Clin Ophthalmol. 2011;5:109–14. https://doi.org/10.2147/OPTH.S16414.
3. Newman DK. Surgical management of the late complications of proliferative diabetic retinopathy. Eye (Lond). 2010;24(3):441–9. https://doi.org/10.1038/eye.2009.325.
4. Barzideh N, Johnson TM. Subfoveal fluid resolves slowly after pars plana vitrectomy for tractional retinal detachment secondary to proliferative diabetic retinopathy. Retina. 2007;27(6):740–3. https://doi.org/10.1097/IAE.0b013e318030c663.
5. Algethami A, Talea M, Alsakran WA, Mura M, Alsulaiman SM. Persistent subretinal fluid following diabetic tractional retinal detachment repair: risk factors, natural history, and management outcomes. Int Ophthalmol. 2021;41(2):453–64. https://doi.org/10.1007/s10792-020-01595-y.
6. Tang J, Kern TS. Inflammation in diabetic retinopathy. Prog Retin Eye Res. 2011;30(5):343–58. https://doi.org/10.1016/j.preteyeres.2011.05.002.
7. Sun DF, Wang YL, Wang B, Xu CL, Zhang G, Li J, et al. Predictive risk factors for exudative retinal detachment after vitrectomy for proliferative diabetic retinopathy. Medicine (Baltimore). 2019;98(8):e14603. https://doi.org/10.1097/MD.0000000000014603.
8. Huang CH, Yang CM. Recurrent retinal detachment after diabetic vitrectomy. Int Ophthalmol. 2020;40(8):1931–9. https://doi.org/10.1007/s10792-020-01366-9.

20 Macular Atrophy in Diabetic Retinopathy

Abstract

Changes in the macular retinal pigment peithelium (RPE) are commonly observed in individuals with DR; in fact, hyperglycemia-induced changes in the RPE may contribute to the development of DR (Li et al., Mol Med Rep 28(4):185, 2023; Tonade and Kern, Prog Retin Eye Res 83:100919, 2021). Macular RPE atrophy can be observed in chronic or burn-out PDR retinas after the resolution of diabetic macular edema or after DV. Although it is an important cause of visual function disturbance in individuals with DR, few studies have investigated this topic. This will be briefly discussed in this chapter.

20.1 Case Report

Patient 1: This 66-year-old woman had DM for more than 20 years and was taking oral hypoglycemic agents. She denied having other systemic diseases. She had undergone cataract surgery with posterior chamber intraocular lens (PCIOL) implantation in both eyes 6 ~ 7 years prior. She was diagnosed with proliferative diabetic retinopathy (PDR) and received panretinal photocoagulation (PRP) in both eyes. As persistent blurred vision was noted, especially in the left eye, she was referred to our clinic for further evaluation. On examination, BCVA was 0.2 in the right eye, and ND was 50 cm in the left eye. Fundus examination revealed a whitish fibrotic membrane between the disc and the fovea and along the lower arcade, with mild VH and preretinal hemorrhage in the inferior part and an attached retina in the right eye; the left eye showed a dense whitish fibrotic membrane from the disc extending to the upper arcade and a fibrotic membrane nasal to the disc. Optical coherence tomography (OCT) revealed a thick premacular membrane with irregular macular thickening in the right eye and traction macular schisis in the left eye. She underwent vitrectomy with membrane removal in the left eye. After surgery, the retina became flat, and visual acuity improved. However, visual acuity in the right eye gradually deteriorated to 0.05. She underwent vitrectomy with epireitnal membrane (ERM) and internal limiting membrane (ILM) peeling in the right eye 18 months after left eye surgery. The macula contour was gradually removed after surgery. FU fundus examination and OCT revealed bilateral focal MA, which was enlarged and presented with progressive outer retina thinning over time. The BCVA was 0.3 and 0.025, respectively, 9 years later (Fig. 20.1).

Patient 2: A 59-year-old woman who had DM for more than 20 years and HT who was under oral medication control. She also had an atrial septal defect (ASD) and underwent ASD occluder placement. The patient complained of progressive blurred vision in both eyes, and fundus examina-

C.-M. Yang, *Surgery for Complications of Diabetic Retinopathy*,
https://doi.org/10.1007/978-981-96-2848-3_20

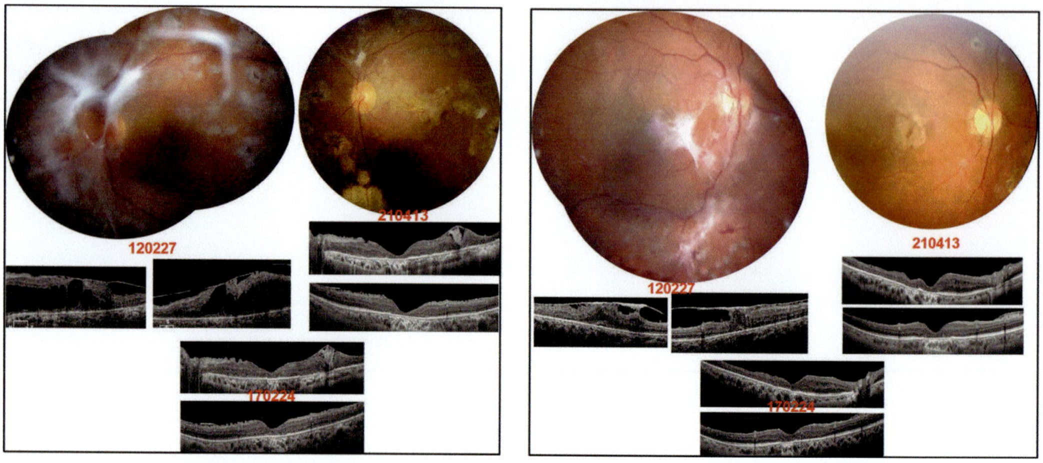

Fig. 20.1 Two sets of images showing post-DV MA in the two eyes of a patient. The numbers represent the date the images were obtained. In the left panel, a dense whitish fibrotic membrane from the disc extending to the upper arcade and a fibrotic membrane nasal to the disc are noted (upper left composite color photo). OCT images showing traction macular schisis in the left eye (upper left). After surgery, focal MA with loss of outer retinal tissue was noted (lower OCT images; upper right color photo and OCT images). In the right panel, whitish fibrotic membranes between the disc and the fovea and along the lower arcade are noted (upper left composite color photo). OCT images showing a thick premacular membrane with irregular macular thickening in the right eye (upper left). After surgery, focal MA with loss of outer retinal tissue, as in the left eye, was also noted (lower OCT images; upper right color photo and OCT images). Please also see Chap. 10, Fig. 10.4, the upper right panel. (Courtesy of Dr. Chung-May Yang)

tion revealed PDR in both eyes with tractional retinal detachment (TRD) in the left eye. PRP was applied to each eye. She was then referred to our clinic. On examination, BCVA was 0.16 in the right eye and 0.1 in the left eye. Fundus examination revealed an attached retina with mild VH and a visible PRP scar in the right eye. The left eye showed extensive fibrovascular proliferation (FVP) along the temporal upper and lower arcades and RD from 7 to 5:00 involving the upper macula. She underwent vitrectomy in the left eye. During surgery, combined tractional and rhegmatogenous retinal detachment (CTRRD) was confirmed. After surgery, the retina became reattached. She subsequently underwent phacoemulsification and PCIOL implantation in the left eye. Repeated vitreous hemorrhage in the right eye was noted during FU. Vitrectomy was performed smoothly 1.5 years after the left eye surgery. Postoperative follow-up fundus examination and OCT revealed focal macular atrophy with foveal thinning and outer retinal degeneration in the left eye but an intact outer retina in the macula in the right eye. The BCVA was 0.5 in the right eye and 0.2–0.3 in the left eye 12 M after the operation (Fig. 20.2).

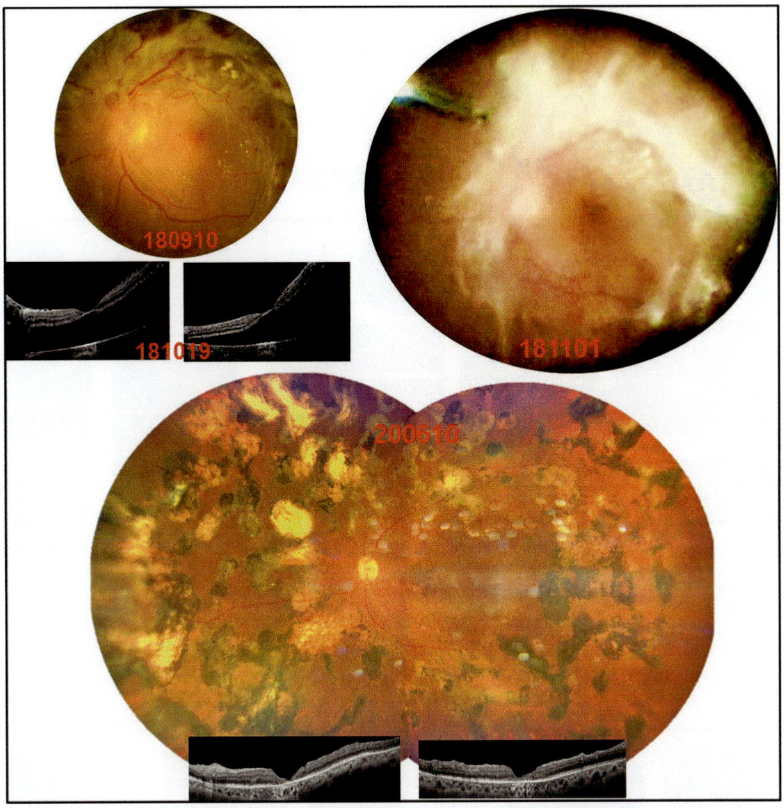

Fig. 20.2 The images show the pre- and postoperative retinal changes in a patient with CTRRD who developed post-DV MA in the left eye. Extensive FVP along the temporal upper and lower arcades and RD from 7 to 5:00 involving the upper macula are shown (upper left color photo and OCT images; upper right intraoperative video image). After surgery, the retina was reattached, but focal foveal thinning with MA was noted (lower wide angle color photo and OCT images). Please see Chap. 5 for further discussion on CTRRD. (Courtesy of Dr. Chung-May Yang)

20.2 Macular Atrophy in DR

Changes in the post-DV RPE may be an important cause of unsatisfactory vision recovery after surgery. We retrospectively collected 190 patients with postoperative macular atrophy. We found that this abnormality may exist before surgery or gradually develop after surgery. It usually became more prominent over time. Vision may be affected to various extents (as low as ND to a better level of 0.5). The severity of atrophy varied. We defined focal atrophy as an atrophic area of ≤3 DDs and broad atrophy as an atrophic area of >3 DDs. We found that the majority of the lesions exhibited focal atrophy (80%), but widespread or broad atrophy involving the arcade and/or beyond may be observed (20%). Fundus changes included irregular patches of pigmentary changes or irregularly shaped geographic-like atrophy. OCT may show incomplete outer retinal atrophy or complete outer retinal atrophy. When only the parafoveal area is involved, vision may be less affected than when central involvement is involved. Lesions in both eyes of the same patients were not uncommon and were usually of similar severity to MA. Many patients also had vessel sheathing.

Possible predisposing factors might include ME, hard exudates, subretinal blood, pigment dispersion, macular traction-related lamellar macular hole (LMH), macular thickening, TRD, TMS, retinal ischemia, and inflammation. It is possible that diabetic choroidopathy may play a role. To date, there is no known treatment or prevention for this condition.

It should be noted that MA may develop as a natural course of DR without surgery. Again, visual acuity may be affected to various extents. It is unknown whether but possibly whether surgery accelerates the MA process.

Examples of patients with macular or parafoveal atrophy are shown in Figs. 20.3, 20.4, 20.5, 20.6, 20.7, 20.8, and 20.9.

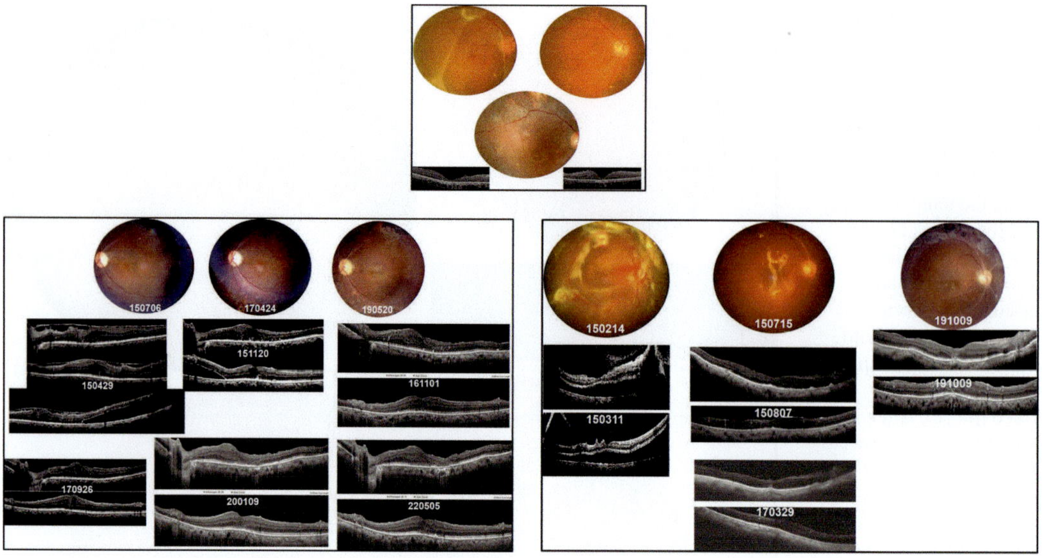

Fig. 20.3 Three sets of images showing pre- and postoperative retinal changes in patients with post-DV focal incomplete ORA. Preoperative retinal color images or OCT images show differences in the severity of proliferation. The numbers in the lower two panels indicate the dates of the images obtained. All OCT images at each time point are shown as horizontal and vertical scans. (Courtesy of Dr. Chung-May Yang)

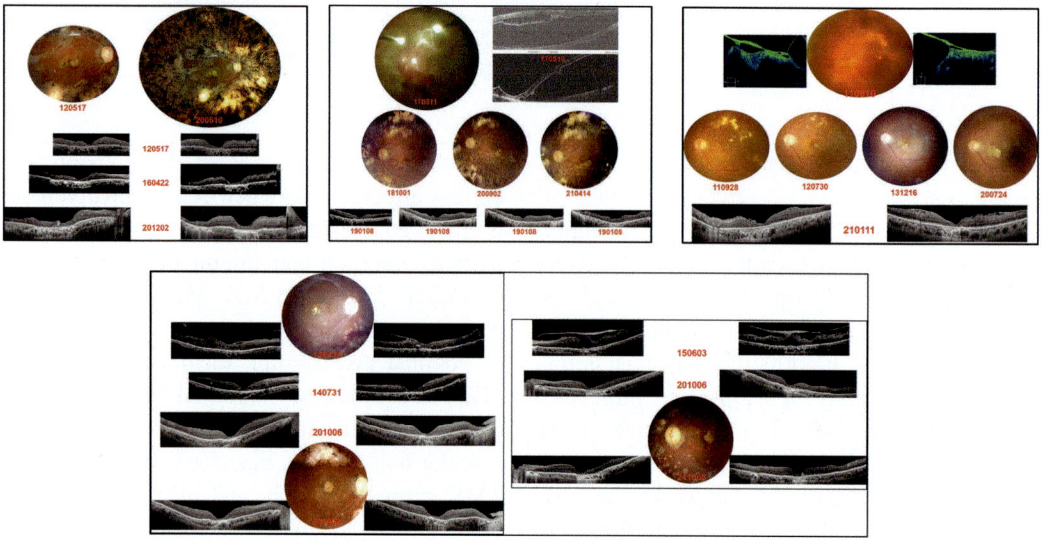

Fig. 20.4 Five sets of images showing pre- and postoperative retinal changes in patients with post-DV focal complete outer retinal atrophy. The lower large panel contains two sets (small panels) of images from the same patient. Preoperative retinal color images or OCT images also revealed differences in the severity of proliferation. Except for the upper center panel, all other patients had a FU time of more than 5 years. The numbers in all panels indicate the dates at which the images were obtained. (Courtesy of Dr. Chung-May Yang)

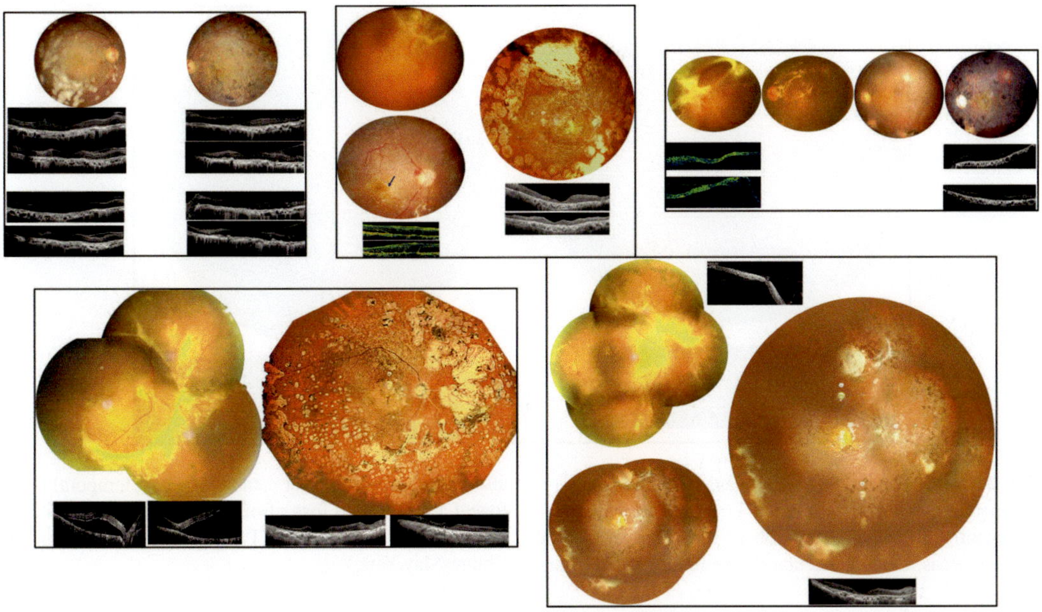

Fig. 20.5 Five sets of images showing pre- and postoperative retinal changes in patients with broad MA. Preoperative retinal color or composite color photos and OCT images revealed various degrees of proliferation. In the upper center panel, ERM-induced macular thickening and localized RD under SO were noted after the initial surgery (lower left color photo and OCT images; blue arrow points to the ERM location); after ERM peeling and SO removal, the macular contour improved, but a broad MA was noted (right wide angle color photo and OCT images). In the lower right panel, the CTRRD was noted before surgery (upper left composite color photo); the SO was not removed after the initial surgery (lower left and right wide angle color photos). (Courtesy of Dr. Chung-May Yang)

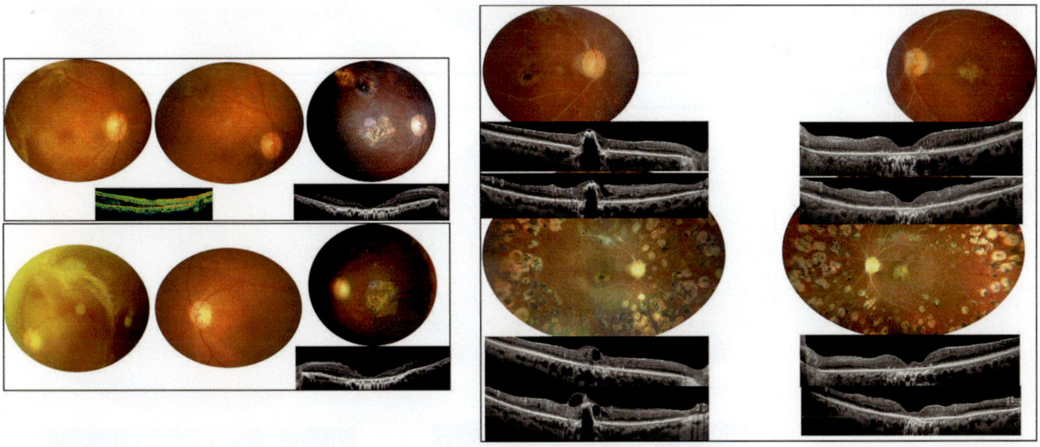

Fig. 20.6 Two sets of images showing post-DV MA in both eyes. In the left panel, the right eye developed combined rhegmatogenous and traction retinal detachment (upper left color photo), while the left eye had active FVP (lower left color photo). Distinct focal geographic atrophy developed after surgery (upper and lower right color photos and OCT images). In the left panel, all images were taken after vitrectomy for dense VH and a thick preretinal membrane in both eyes (right eye in the left column; left eye in the right column). A decrease in vision over time was associated with the gradual appearance of more focal MA in both eyes. The right eye also showed pigment proliferation and migration (left column). (Courtesy of Dr. Chung-May Yang)

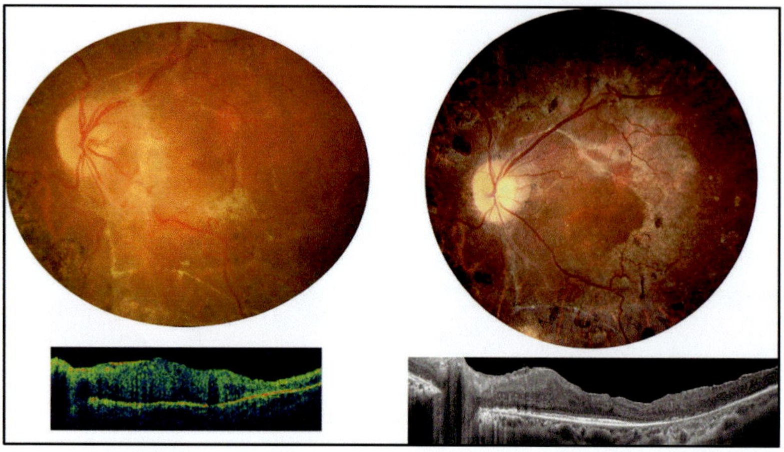

Fig. 20.7 An example of parafoveal MA after surgery. Preoperative color photo and OCT images showing predominantly fibrotic proliferation in the nasal and lower macular areas, causing macular thickening (left); 10 years after vitrectomy and after cataract surgery, temporal parafoveal atrophy with loss of outer retinal tissue was noted (right color photo and OCT images). (Courtesy of Dr. Chung-May Yang)

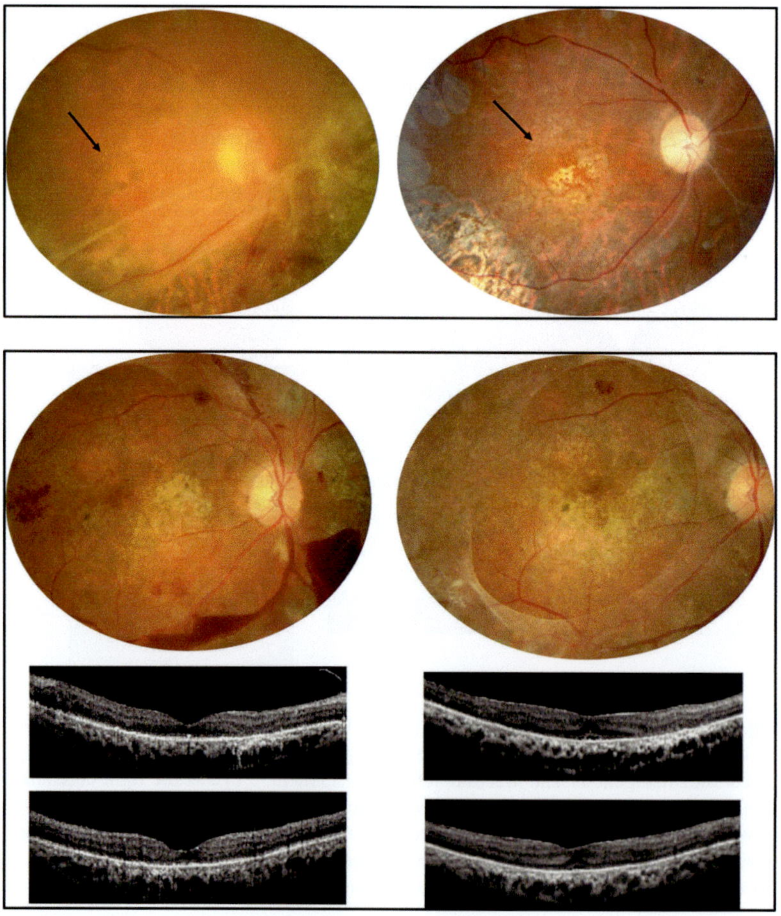

Fig. 20.8 Two sets of images showing MA in the early course of PDR. In the upper panel, MA became more pronounced after surgery, as indicated by the black arrows. In the lower panel, broad MA was noted in the early (left color photo and OCT images) and late (right color photo and OCT images) course of the disease without surgical intervention. (Courtesy of Dr. Chung-May Yang)

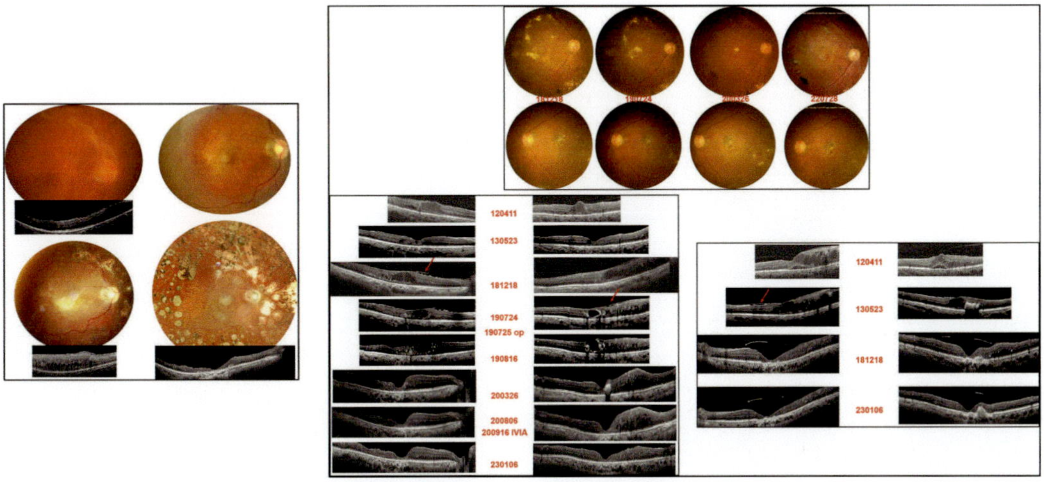

Fig. 20.9 Two sets of images showing possible predisposing factors for MA in PDR patients. In the right panel, preoperative images showing the FVP band along the upper arcade and mild VH; the macula was attached to an intact EZ (upper left color photo and OCT images). After surgery, the media was clear, and the retina was attached, but the ERM began to develop (upper right color photo). The ERM became a dense contractile membrane, causing macular thickening (lower left color photo and OCT image). After surgery, an attached macula with focal thinning was noted (lower right wide angle color photo and OCT image). In the right panel, macular edema and MA were noted in both eyes (upper sequential color photos). The sequential horizontal OCT images in the lower left and right show the macular structural changes before and after surgery in the right eye (lower left) and the natural course without surgery in the left eye (lower right). Red arrows point to the ERMs that developed during FU in both eyes. The numbers indicate the dates the images were obtained (please see the case report in Chap. 8 for a detailed history). (Courtesy of Dr. Chung-May Yang)

21 Retinal Vessel Occlusion After Diabetic Vitrectomy

Abstract

Retinal vascular occlusions may rarely occur following intraocular procedures (Fischer et al., J Ophthalmol 2017:9120892, 2017). Eyes that undergo diabetic vitrectomy (DV) usually have compromised blood circulation. It is not surprising that vascular occlusion may occur after successful DV. Post-DV paracentral acute middle maculopathy has been reported (Nakashima et al., Ophthalmology 125(12):1929–36, 2018). Because of retinal structural alterations and decreased visual function in patients with PDR, the typical presentations of retinal vessel occlusion become less obvious. The clinical features of vessel occlusion following DV are discussed in this chapter.

21.1 Case Report

A 55-year-old woman who was under insulin control had DM but no HT for more than 10 years. Panretinal photocoagulation (PRP) was performed in both eyes. She suffered from persistent VH after cataract surgery in her left eye at an outside hospital. She was referred to our clinic. Under the impression of proliferative diabetic reitnopathy (PDR) with vitreous hemorrhage (VH), she received intravitreal bevacizumab and retinal cryotherapy 3 times in the left eye. Although her VH improved, TRD developed 1 week after the last intravitreal bevacizumab treatment. On examination, best-corrected visual acuity (BCVA) was 0.4 in the right eye and 0.15 in the left eye. Fundus examinations revealed PDR and PRP laser scars in the right eye and nasal fibrovascular proliferation (FVP) and tractional retinal detachment (TRD) in the nasal and lower retina in the left eye. She underwent vitrectomy, FVP tissue removal, and buckle encircling in the left eye. The postoperative course was smooth. However, 4 months later, she developed bilateral VH, and BCVA was HM at 1 month in the right eye and 0.3 in the left eye. She received intravitreal bevacizumab treatment in both eyes. Sudden onset of VA loss was noted in the left eye 2 weeks later. Fundus examinations revealed cherry red spots in the macula in the left eye. Central retinal artery occlusion (CRAO) was diagnosed. Her BCVA was 0.4 in the right eye and 0.02 in the left eye. Retinal ischemia (RI) and high intraocular pressure (IOP) up to 40 mmHg were noted shortly thereafter. She underwent transscleral cyclophotocoagulation (TSCPC). Her IOP was approximately 30 mmHg under antiglaucoma medication. Her BCVA decreased to HM/10 cm in the left eye. One year later, she underwent uneventful vitrectomy for persistent VH in the right eye (Fig. 21.1).

C.-M. Yang, *Surgery for Complications of Diabetic Retinopathy*,
https://doi.org/10.1007/978-981-96-2848-3_21

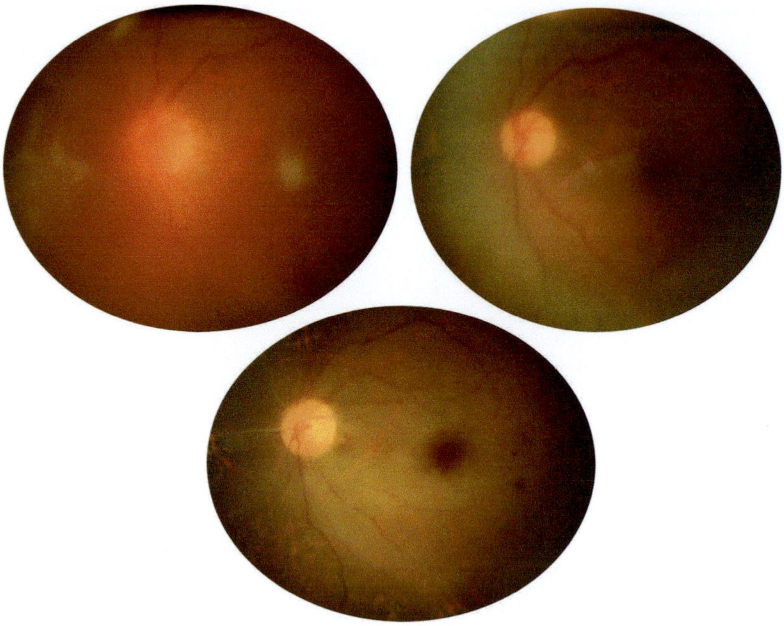

Fig. 21.1 Color photos of the pre- and postoperative fundus of the left eye are shown. Combined rhegmatogenous and tractional RD with VH was noted after repeated IVI of Avastin and anterior retinal cryo-treatment (upper left). After surgery, the retina was reattached (upper right). However, CRAO with cherry red spots developed later (lower color photo). (Courtesy of Dr. Chung-May Yang)

21.2 Retinal Vessel Occlusion After Diabetic Vitrectomy

Patients who undergo vitrectomy for complications of PDR often have a more severe degree of retinopathy and vasculopathy, which may render them more susceptible to vasoocclusive disease. Because DR, especially PDR, may cause significant retinal structural abnormalities, the clinical picture of retinal vessel occlusion may be modified after surgery. We retrospectively reviewed patients who were diagnosed with CRAO after successful DV and investigated the clinical presentations, risk factors, and prognoses [2]. CRAO was diagnosed when the patient had a sudden onset of visual loss in the operated eye, along with the typical CRVO fundus picture or delayed arterial filling for more than 30 s by fluorescein angiography (FA). Patients with previous neovascular glaucoma (NVG) and clinical follow-up for less than 4 months were excluded.

Twelve eyes from 12 patients (4 women and 8 men) with a mean age of 55.3 ± 6.2 years were included in this study.

We found some distinct and unique features of CRVO after DV. First, prominent cherry-red spots were not a hallmark of CRVO in these patients, and arterial constriction and emboli were usually not found. Second, increased reflectivity in the inner retinal layer on optical coherence tomography (OCT) was observed in the majority of patients. Third, RIs were more frequently observed in eyes with CRAO than in eyes with CRAO under other conditions. Other features, including systemic diseases such as HT, were common, and carotid artery Doppler showed various degrees of stenosis. The interval between the onset of CRAO and DV may be as short as 1 month to as long as 1.5 years.

We postulated that in this particular group of patients, there was preexisting atrophic inner retina induced by chronic ischemic changes, long-term macular edema, or macular grid laser use before the onset of CRAO, as well as a fluctuating IOP during and after surgery. The loss of inner retinal tissue prevents the development of cherry-red spots, which are caused by the swelling of ganglion cells and nerve fibers around the fovea.

Although arterial attenuation is an important sign of CRAO, this abnormality has already been widely present in many patients with PDR before surgery. This preoperative change can be attributed to the PRP, which causes retinal vessel constriction, and the diffuse silver wire appearance of arteries, which is not uncommon in end-stage

PDR with a burned-out retina. This preexisting alteration makes CRAO-associated arterial attenuation difficult to observe.

There may be several reasons why arterial emboli, which are present in 20% to 40% of eyes with CRAO, were not observed in the present study. First, the lumen of the central retinal artery in this group of patients may be narrow, preventing the emboli from reaching the optic nerve head to be visible. Second, the sheathing of vessels may mask the emboli. Third, some patients may have thrombosis, which is enhanced by the narrow lumen of arteries, instead of by emboli as the primary cause. Finally, many eyes in these patients may have underlying ocular ischemic syndrome with very low central arterial perfusion pressure; the vessel lumen may easily be closed by a transient high IOP without emboli.

Increased macular thickness compared with that of the fellow eye is a common phenomenon in patients at the acute stage of CRAO. In post-DV patients, however, because of the preexisting atrophic inner retina before the CRAO episode in the lesion eye and the frequent presence of macular edema or epiretinal membrane in the fellow eye, the comparison of macular thickness between the two eyes may not provide a good diagnostic clue for CRAO.

Finally, RI is more frequently observed despite previous complete PRP. Given that the RI is the hallmark of ocular ischemia syndrome and that DM is a major risk factor for ocular ischemic syndrome, this observation indicates that CRAO may be superimposed on preexisting ocular ischemia in lesioned eyes. It is possible that ocular ischemia was already present in most of the patients, which, on the one hand, contributed to the onset of CRAO in some of our patients and, on the other hand, caused the development of RI.

In summary, signs of CRAO may not be obvious in eyes with PDR with previous vitrectomy. Fewer typical cherry-red spots and a greater possibility of RI despite previous complete PRP are the characteristic features in this group of patients. To confirm the diagnosis, FA should be performed to look for delayed retinal major arterial filling time. Surgeons should keep the possibility of CRAO in mind when patients complain of sudden visual loss. If the diagnosis is confirmed, close FU is necessary for timely intervention because RIs and NVGs are more frequently noted in this group of patients.

In addition to CRAO, BRAO or cilioretinal artery occlusion may also occur after DV. The key point is to remain alert to this vessel occlusion complication.

It has been reported that paracentral acute middle maculopathy develops after pars plana vitrectomy for PDR, especially in younger and female patients. The incidence of PAMM was approximately 3.5%. No emboli were found in any of the 18 affected eyes; however, multiple segmental arterial constrictions were confirmed during vitrectomy in 1 eye. The BCVA decreased by more than two lines in two eyes (5%) [1].

Examples of RAO after DV are shown in Fig. 21.2.

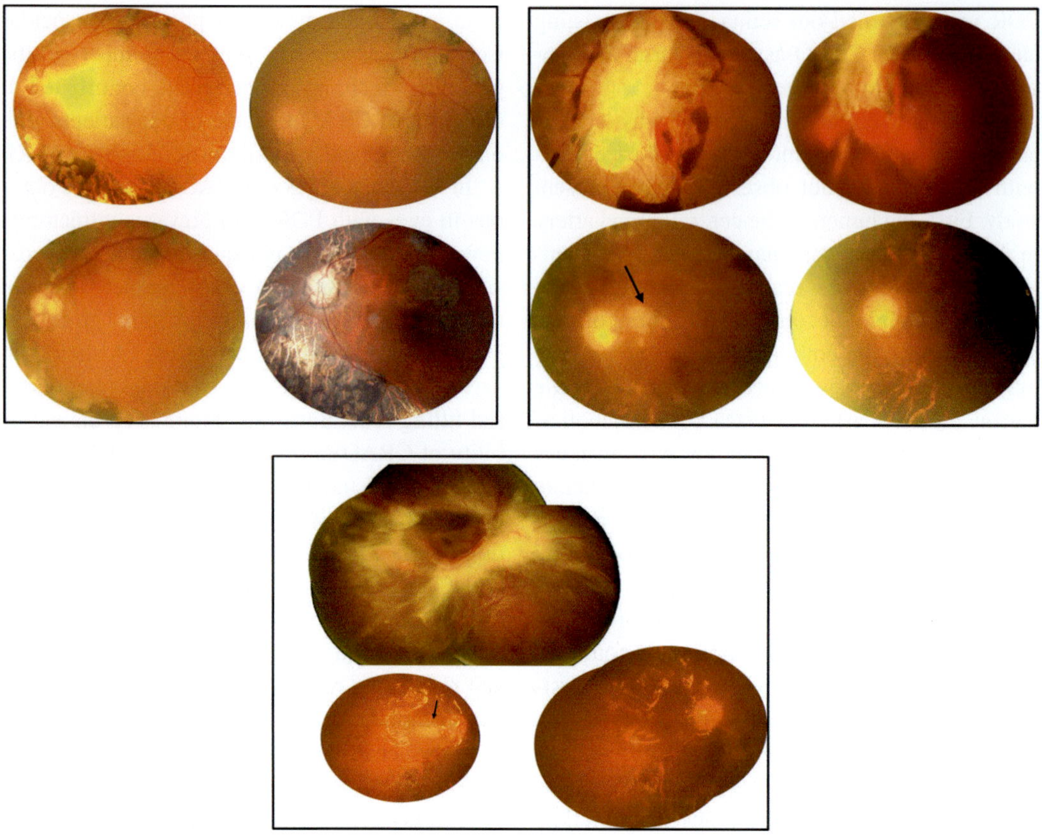

Fig. 21.2 Three sets of images showing post-DV retinal vessel occlusion. In the upper left panel, dense premacular fibrosis was noted in the left eye (upper left color photo). After surgery, temporal upper BRVO with retinal whitening in the upper macula was noted (upper right color photo). FU examinations revealed that the normal retinal color was restored (lower left color photo). After the cataract operation, the BCVA was 0.5 (lower right color photo). Please also see Chap. 4, Fig. 4.3, upper panel. In the upper right and lower panels, preoperative color photos of both patients show active FVP (upper 2 color photos in the upper right panel and composite color photo in the lower panel). Cilioretinal artery occlusion was noted in both patients after surgery (lower left color photo in the upper right and lower panels). The black arrows point to the retinal whitening area. Visual recovery was good in both patients. SO was used in the case in the lower panel. (Courtesy of Dr. Chung-May Yang)

Acknowledgement Most cases analyzed in this chapter were from Dr. San-Ni Chen; the author would like to thank Dr. San-Ni Chen for data sharing and text writing.

References

1. Nakashima H, Iwama Y, Tanioka K, Emi K. Paracentral acute middle maculopathy following vitrectomy for proliferative diabetic retinopathy: incidence, risk factors, and clinical characteristics. Ophthalmology. 2018;125(12):1929–36. https://doi.org/10.1016/j.ophtha.2018.07.006.
2. Chen SN, Chao CC, Hwang JF, Yang CM. Clinical manifestations of central retinal artery occlusion in eyes of proliferative diabetic retinopathy with previous vitrectomy and panretinal photocoagulation. Retina. 2014;34(9):1861–6. https://doi.org/10.1097/IAE.0000000000000158.

22 Submacular Hemorrhage After Diabetic Vitrectomy

Abstract

Subretinal blood may be observed in various conditions, including age-related macular degeneration (AMD), polypoidal choroidal vasculopathy (PCV), high myopia, arterial macroaneurysms, choroiditis, trauma, and Valsalva's retinopathy (Berrocal et al., Am J Ophthalmol 122(4):486–93, 1996). Subretinal blood may occur in proliferative diabetic retinopathy (PDR) (Morse et al., Retina 17(2):87–93, 1997). It is usually associated with tractional retinal detachment (TRD) or combined RD. It is located in the dependent part and is often unsuspected; it only shifts to the posterior pole to manifest during surgery. If not removed, it may be toxic to photoreceptors and adversely affect visual function (Glatt and Machemer, Am J Ophthalmol 94(6):762–73, 1982; Toth et al., Arch Ophthalmol 109(5):723–9, 1991). Few reports have focused on postoperative submacular blood in PDR patients (Morse et al., Retina 17(2):87–93, 1997). The significance and management of this complication will be discussed in this chapter.

22.1 Case Report

A 40-year-old man had PDR and panretinal photocoagulation (PRP) in both eyes. Sudden onset of blurred vision in the left eye was noted 2 months after treatment for left calf cellulitis. Vitreous hemorrhage (VH) in the left eye was diagnosed at another hospital. The blurred vision gradually recovered. However, massive darkness with multiple black lines over the lower visual field in the right eye was noted. He visited our clinic 3 weeks later. On examination, best-corrected visual acuity (BCVA) was 0.2 in both eyes. Fibrovascular proliferation (FVP) mainly in the upper arcade and localized macula-on upper TRD with VH were noted in the right eye. Within 3 weeks, the TRD area advanced to involve the macula area. Subretinal blood at the lower margin of the TRD was also noted. The BCVA decreased to 0.05. He received 0.05 ml of intravitreal Avastin and underwent surgery 3 days later. FVP tissue removal and subretinal blood drainage were performed. After surgery, the retina was reattached, and there was a thin layer of submacular blood in the early postoperative days. The blood reabsorbed rapidly, and BCVA improved to 0.5 with a moderate cat in the right eye 14 years later (Fig. 22.1).

C.-M. Yang, *Surgery for Complications of Diabetic Retinopathy*,
https://doi.org/10.1007/978-981-96-2848-3_22

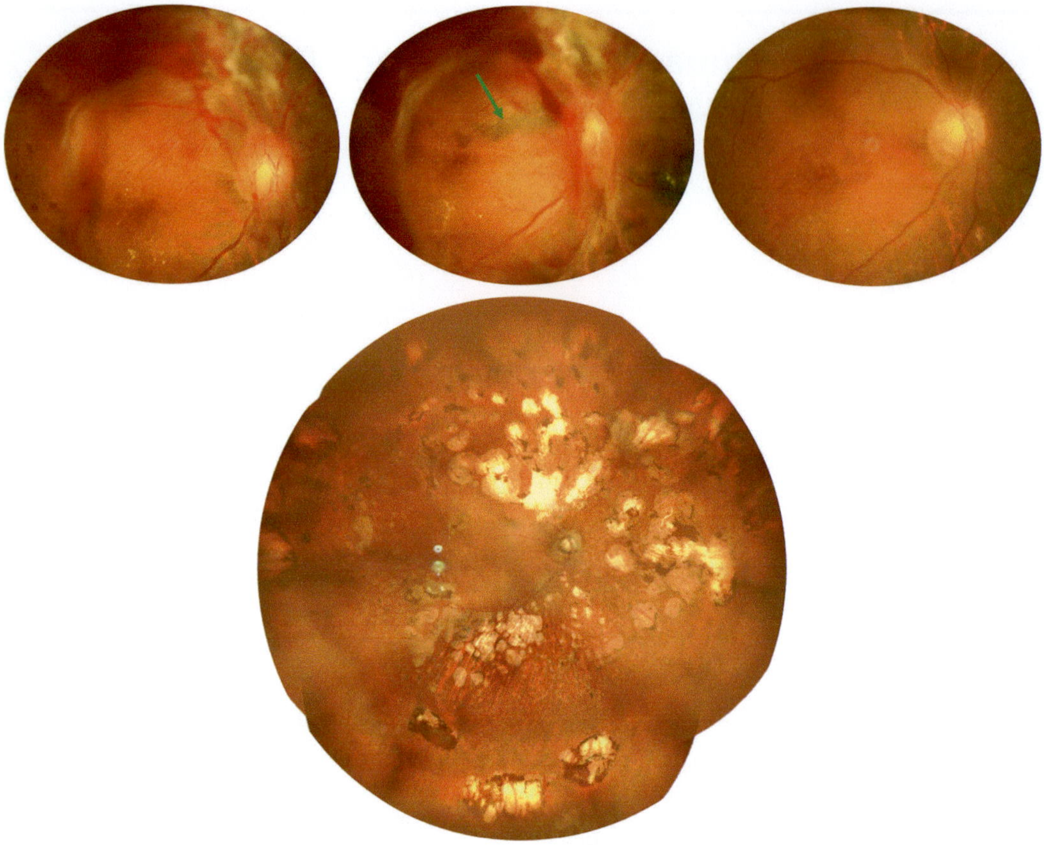

Fig. 22.1 The upper three color photos show the sequential fundus changes before and after surgery. The fundus change at presentation is shown on the left. There was an active FVP above the disc, and the lower margin of the TRD was indicated by the faint horizontally oblique line at the upper paramacular area. VH was evident. After 3 weeks, the TRD extended to the fovea. Subretinal blood (green arrow) was present (upper center). One month after surgery, faint submacular blood was observed. A lower wide angle color photo was taken 14 years after surgery, showing a reattached retina and a normal macula. (Courtesy of Dr. Chung-May Yang)

22.2 Submacular Hemorrhage After Diabetic Vitrectomy

A scattered area of subretinal blood may sometimes be observed in a reattached retina after successful surgery. Blood is usually reabsorbed without significantly affecting visual prognosis. However, on rare occasions, the subretinal blood involves the macula or is at the subfoveal area, and visual function may be greatly affected.

The major source of post-DV subretinal blood is residual preexisting subretinal blood before surgery that is incompletely removed during surgery or blood from ruptured vessels during or after surgery that passes through an unsealed break into the subretinal space.

Preoperative subretinal blood leakage usually occurs in TRD or combined RD with active FVP. The location, size, and clearance of subretinal hemorrhages vary widely. In one study by Morse and associates, 49 patients with subretinal hemorrhage who underwent DV were analyzed. Forty-two patients had focal subretinal hemorrhages, and 14 patients within this group had submacular hemorrhages. Retinal breaks were observed in 15 patients (31%) [1]. It is intriguing why subretinal blood may be present in TRD since there is no break to allow the preretinal or vitreous blood to enter the subretinal space. A possible explanation is that there is a microbreak, or traction may induce schisis with lamellar breaks; when the outer break develops at another location within the schisis area, the preretinal or vitreous blood may enter the schisis cavity and pass through the outer break. From this convoluted channel, the subretinal blood gradually builds up. Alternatively, similar to the breakthrough VH from subretinal hemorrhage without visible retinal defects in AMD or PCV, although in a reverse direction, blood may pass through the retina directly into the subretinal space. Nonetheless, one should always suspect the presence of retinal breaks when subretinal blood is noted, and a careful search for breaks is necessary in such cases. Subretinal blood signifies strong VR traction, with a more severe active FVP and greater retinal elevation. We have found that preoperative injection of anti-VEGF may increase the amount of subretinal blood in eyes with severe FVP [2].

Because of its medium opacity, VH, and dense FVP membrane, subretinal blood may not be readily detectable. The blood is noncoagulant, settles in the dependent part, and is easily obstructed by the lower VH. In the TRD, the detached margin may appear dark red. During surgery, the blood may shift to the posterior pole, giving a red hue to the posterior detached retina.

Because blood components damage photoreceptor cells, they should be removed as completely as possible. Blood can be drained through preexisting breaks or iatrogenic breaks. More complete drainage may be achieved through breaks close to the subretinal blood area. Repeated drainage under air at 1- to 2-min intervals is necessary to more thoroughly remove residual blood. The remaining submacular blood may be displaced to outside the macula by gas or SO through proper face-own positioning after surgery. In some cases, after traction has been released, the submacular blood can be displaced to the midperiphery by the injection of heavy liquid to facilitate complete drainage through an iatrogenic break. In severe cases, especially in those complicated by severe intraoperative bleeding with open retinal break(s), subretinal blood may accumulate rapidly; peripheral circumferential retinectomy should be carried out to invert the retina and expose the subretinal space for direct backflush needle drainage or blood clot removal.

Submacular blood that develops after surgery is more difficult to displace because the blood clots rapidly in the subretinal space.

The presence of significant amounts of submacular blood after surgery is a poor prognostic sign. The process may involve two pathways: gradual reabsorption and reabsorption with a fibrotic scar. As in other conditions, the blood first turns to yellow fibrin-like material, then decreases and is reabsorbed. In both pathways, OCT showed various degrees of damage to the outer retina. In some cases, the cause of subretinal blood after surgery is not clear.

Measures should be taken to reduce post-DV hemorrhage, so fresh blood may not be able to reach the subretinal space through poorly sealed retinal breaks. (Please see Chap. 18.)

Examples of para-surgery subretinal blood are shown in Fig. 22.2.

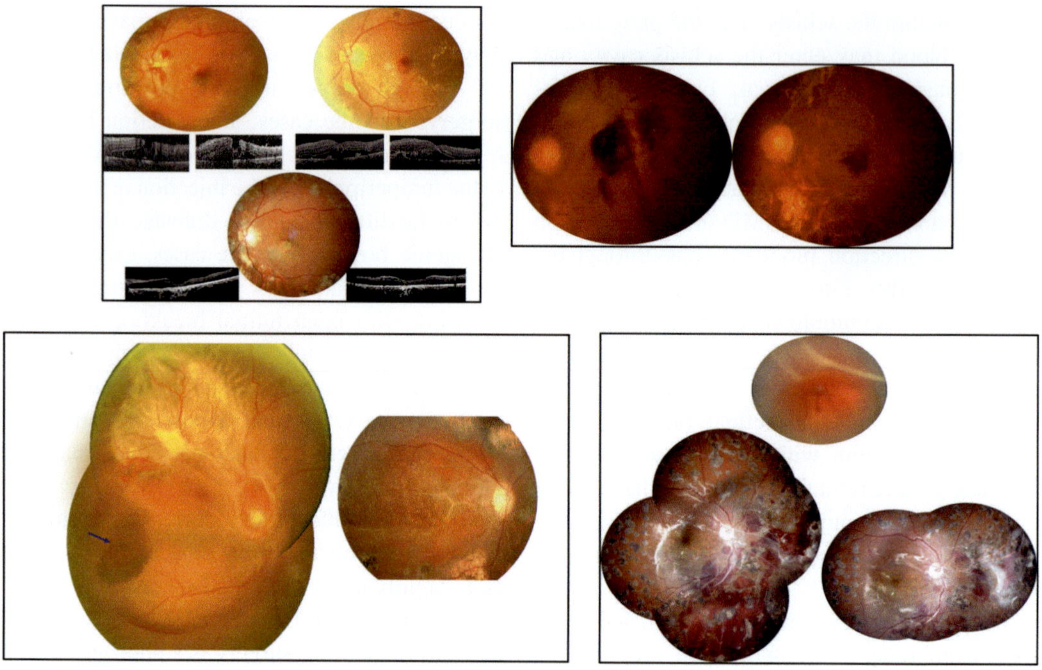

Fig. 22.2 Four sets of images showing different presentations of post-DV subretinal blood. In the upper left panel, preoperative images show MHs with submacular blood (upper left color photo and OCT images); early postoperative color photo and OCT images revealed MH closure with persistent submacular blood (upper right). The macula eventually reattached with reabsorption of submacular blood; however, macular atrophy was noted (lower color photo and OCT images). In the upper right panel, partial reabsorption of the subretinal blood was noted within 2 months after surgery. In the lower left panel, a preoperative composite color photo shows a broadly adherent FVP at the upper arcade, patchy subretinal blood (blue arrow) and boat-shaped subretinal blood at the lower margin of the TRD (left composite color photo). The retina was reattached with submacular bands after surgery (right color photo). The lower right panel shows a case of scattered subretinal hemorrhagic patches at different times after surgery. (lower two composite color photos); a preoperative color photo is shown on the upper image. (Courtesy of Dr. Chung-May Yang)

References

1. Morse LS, Chapman CB, Eliott D, Benner JD, Blumenkranz MS, McCuen BW 2nd. Subretinal hemorrhages in proliferative diabetic retinopathy. Retina. 1997;17(2):87–93. https://doi.org/10.1097/00006982-199703000-00001.
2. Yeh PT, Yang CM, Lin YC, Chen MS, Yang CH. Bevacizumab pretreatment in vitrectomy with silicone oil for severe diabetic retinopathy. Retina. 2009;29(6):768–74. https://doi.org/10.1097/IAE.0b013e3181a3b7ef.

23 Glaucoma After Diabetic Vitrectomy

Abstract

An increase in intraocular pressure (IOP) is an important complication after diabetic vitrectomy (DV). Persistent high IOP is a significant cause of visual loss after initial successful surgery. Different factors may contribute to high IOP during different postoperative periods.

23.1 Glaucoma After Diabetic Vitrectomy

In the early postoperative period, high IOP may be related to the surgical procedure or the patient's eye condition. A prolonged surgical time and a high volume of intraoperative panretinal photocoagulation (PRP) may increase inflammation and induce choroidal thickening or CD. In a gas- or SO-filled eye, the IOP may increase due to a decreased volume of the vitreous cavity. The angle is open most of the time. Severe CD may cause anterior rotation of the ciliary body and anterior lens displacement, creating angle narrowing or closure and inducing high IOP. Gas or SO overfill is another cause of high IOP and may last more than 1 week. Timely vitreous tapping to partially remove the vitreous substitute may be necessary. A large amount of blood clot left at the end of surgery creates a greater opportunity for the postoperative lysed blood to enter the anterior chamber and obstruct the trabecular meshwork, especially when the facedown position is adopted. A high SB may increase inflammation, impede blood flow to the anterior segment, or cause anterior lens displacement; all these factors may increase IOP. If the patient has a preexisting rubeosis iridis (RI) or severe ischemia, the RI may become more prominent shortly after surgery, causing an increase in IOP.

After 1–2 weeks of the postoperative period, increased IOP may be related to ghost cell glaucoma, lens swelling, anterior hyaloidal fibrovascular proliferation (AHFVP), early RI or neovascular glaucoma (NVG), and posterior synechia-induced pupillary block. Steroid-induced glaucoma may also play a role in some patients. The possibility of ghost cell glaucoma should be considered in patients with persistent or recurrent postoperative VH. It usually develops 3 or more weeks after VH. Khaki-colored RBCs should be specifically looked for in the anterior chamber. Medication to suppress aqueous production may be attempted first; however, surgical intervention, including AC paracentesis, vitreous lavage, or even trabeculectomy, is often necessary because of persistently elevated intraocular pressure under full antiglaucomatous medications [1–6]. Rapid cataracts may sometimes develop after surgery. The resultant lens swelling may cause an increase in IOP. RI may occur any time after surgery. An RI that appears within a few weeks after surgery should be considered for AHFVP

C.-M. Yang, *Surgery for Complications of Diabetic Retinopathy*,
https://doi.org/10.1007/978-981-96-2848-3_23

or recurrent RD. VH is common at this point, and ultrasonography is indispensable for making a correct diagnosis. In recurrent RD, IOP is usually low despite the presence of an RI. Reoperation may be needed for recurrent RD or AHFVP. If the retina is attached, anti-VEGF and antiglaucomatous treatment should be considered. For intractable cases, filtering surgery with shunt or transscleral cyclophotocoagulation (TSCPC) plus anti-VEGF therapy may eventually lower IOP, but the functional prognosis is poor. Persistent low-grade inflammation may cause posterior synechia and pupillary block. This situation is particularly likely to occur in a pseudophakic eye. Laser iridotomy is prone to occlusion even after repeated procedures. Surgical peripheral iridectomy is thus advised during combined phacoemulsification with IOL implantation and vitrectomy. Any factor that may increase intraocular inflammation, such as persistent corneal epithelium defects, should be treated aggressively to prevent the development of RIs and NVG. AHFVP is a severe complication with an extremely poor prognosis. It usually develops in young adults with active FVP and poorly controlled DM. FVP tissue grows from the vitreous base along the anterior hyaloid, forming a thick vascularized membrane. It is usually associated with hyphema, VH, TRD, RI, and high IOP. Fortunately, the incidence of AHFVP has decreased significantly in the modern micro-incision vitrectomy surgery (MIVS) era. Aggressive treatment, including crystalline lens removal, anterior proliferative membrane dissection, ciliary body photocoagulation, extensive peripheral PRP, and repeated IVI of anti-VEGF, may be necessary to preserve some visual function. (Please see Chap. 1, Fig. 1.22.)

The common cause of late-onset glaucoma is NVG, and less often, it gradually forms posterior synechia. In some cases, specific underlying factors cannot be identified. Perhaps these patients have undiagnosed primary open-angle glaucoma. The underlying causes of postoperative NVG include (1) persistent rubeosis or NVG from pre-existing changes before surgery; (2) postop inflammation induced; (3) postoperative retinal ischemia, possibly from retinal vessel occlusion or insufficient carotid artery perfusion; (4) the development of AHFVP.

NVG may be observed even after obvious improvement of postoperative inflammation and after complete retinal reattachment has been achieved. Possible causes may be progressive retinal ischemia from local partial or complete vessel occlusion or systemic circulation compromise. Several studies have shown that the incidence of NVG after DV in the modern micro-invasive surgery era is approximately 10%. Younger age, poor diabetes control, lack of preoperative PRP, and postoperative VH are risk factors for the development of NVG after vitrectomy [3, 4, 7–9].

Treatment of high IOP should be tailored to the underlying cause. In many cases, glaucoma surgery must be performed to control IOP. Retinal specialists should work closely with glaucoma specialists to provide timely and optimal care for patients.

Acknowledgement The authors would like to thank Dr. Jehn-Yu Huang for the critical review of this chapter.

References

1. Huang CH, Hsieh YT, Yang CM. Vitrectomy for complications of proliferative diabetic retinopathy in young adults: clinical features and surgical outcomes. Graefes Arch Clin Exp Ophthalmol. 2017;255(5):863–71. https://doi.org/10.1007/s00417-016-3579-4.
2. Miele A, Govetto A, Fumagalli C, Donati S, Biagini I, Azzolini C, et al. OCULAR HYPERTENSION AND GLAUCOMA FOLLOWING VITRECTOMY: a systematic review. Retina. 2018;38(5):883–90. https://doi.org/10.1097/IAE.0000000000001651.
3. Liang X, Zhang Y, Li YP, Huang WR, Wang JX, Li X. Frequency and risk factors for neovascular glaucoma after vitrectomy in eyes with diabetic retinopathy: an observational study. Diabetes Ther. 2019;10(5):1801–9. https://doi.org/10.1007/s13300-019-0644-0.
4. Sun D, Lin Y, Zeng R, Yang Z, Deng X, Lan Y. The incidence and risk factors for neovascular glaucoma secondary to proliferative diabetic retinopathy after vitrectomy. Eur J Ophthalmol. 2021;31(6):3057–67. https://doi.org/10.1177/1120672120980686.
5. Mansour AM, Chess J, Starita R. Nontraumatic ghost cell glaucoma—a case report. Ophthalmic Surg. 1986;17(1):34–6.

6. Honavar SG, Goyal M, Majji AB, Sen PK, Naduvilath T, Dandona L. Glaucoma after pars plana vitrectomy and silicone oil injection for complicated retinal detachments. Ophthalmology. 1999;106(1):169–76; discussion 77. https://doi.org/10.1016/S0161-6420(99)90017-9.
7. Sakamoto M, Hashimoto R, Yoshida I, Ubuka M, Maeno T. Risk factors for neovascular glaucoma after vitrectomy in eyes with proliferative diabetic retinopathy. Clin Ophthalmol. 2018;12:2323–9. https://doi.org/10.2147/OPTH.S184959.
8. Goto A, Inatani M, Inoue T, Awai-Kasaoka N, Takihara Y, Ito Y, et al. Frequency and risk factors for neovascular glaucoma after vitrectomy in eyes with proliferative diabetic retinopathy. J Glaucoma. 2013;22(7):572–6. https://doi.org/10.1097/IJG.0b013e31824d514a.
9. Kwon JW, Jee D, La TY. Neovascular glaucoma after vitrectomy in patients with proliferative diabetic retinopathy. Medicine (Baltimore). 2017;96(10):e6263. https://doi.org/10.1097/MD.0000000000006263.

24 Diabetic Vitrectomy in Young Patients

Abstract

The age of onset of DM is considered an important factor in the development and progression of DR (Yokoyama et al., Diabetes Care, 20(5): 844–7, https://doi.org/10.2337/diacare.20.5.844, 1997; Wong et al., Diabetes Care, 31(10): 1985–90, https://doi.org/10.2337/dc08-0580, 2008). A literature review showed that the prevalence of proliferative diabetic retinopathy (PDR) reached 30% in insulin-dependent DM (IDDM) patients, and the 10-year incidence of vitrectomy for complications by PDR in these patients was 6.4% (Giusti, Pediatr Diabetes, 2(2): 83–93, https://doi.org/10.1034/j.1399-5448.2001.002002083.x, 2001; Ostri et al., Acta Ophthalmol, 92(5): 439–43, https://doi.org/10.1111/aos.12249, 2014). In young adults, a greater risk of blindness was noted in patients with PDR than in older patients. The risk of retinopathy and vision-threatening retinopathy persisted even after stratification by HbA1c level. Recently, several epidemiologic studies have recognized the growing prevalence of young-onset NIDDM worldwide; this trend is even greater in Asian countries than in the United States (Yoon et al., Lancet, 368(9548): 1681–8, https://doi.org/10.1016/S0140-6736(06)69703-1, 2006; Fagot-Campagna et al., J Pediatr, 136(5): 664–72, https://doi.org/10.1067/mpd.2000.105141, 2000). Despite extensive studies on the epidemiology of young-onset DM and its relationship with DR, few reported studies have specifically investigated the prognosis of surgical outcomes and risk factors in young-onset DM patients (Liao et al., BMC Ophthalmol, 20(1): 416, https://doi.org/10.1186/s12886-020-01688-3, 2020; Kumar et al., Indian J Ophthalmol, 69(11): 3289–95, https://doi.org/10.4103/ijo.IJO_1293_21, 2021). Important questions are whether young adults who undergo vitrectomy for complications of PDR have different clinical presentations and prognoses than older patients do and whether surgically treated IDDM patients have different clinical features from young-onset NIDDM patients within the same young age group. These issues are discussed through our study in this chapter.

24.1 Case Report

A 29-year-old woman had insulin-dependent DM secondary to peritonitis-induced pancreatic damage in her childhood. She also had a history of pregnancy-induced HT, but her BP returned to normal after delivery. She underwent bilateral PRP for treating PDR at an outside hospital and was referred to our hospital for further treatment. On examination, her best-corrected visual acuity (BCVA) was 0.05 in the right eye and 0.3 in the left eye. The anterior segment was normal with-

C.-M. Yang, *Surgery for Complications of Diabetic Retinopathy*,
https://doi.org/10.1007/978-981-96-2848-3_24

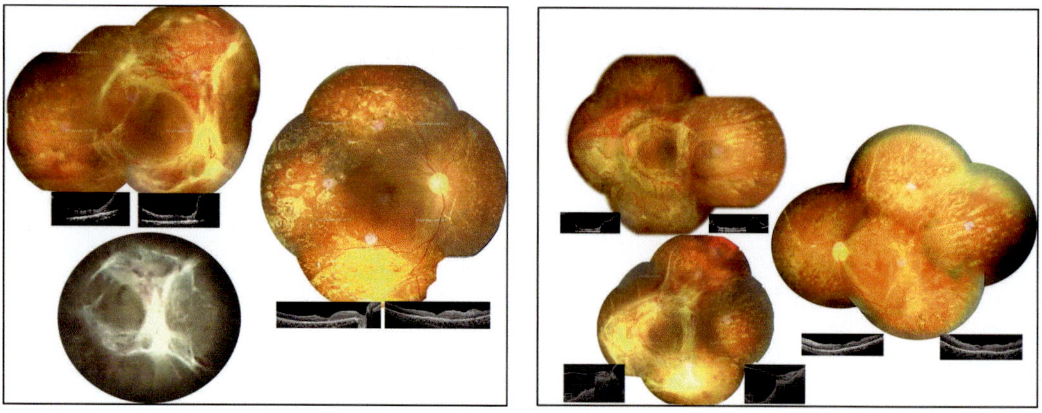

Fig. 24.1 Two sets of images showing pre- and postoperative fundus changes in the two eyes of the same patient. Both eyes had severe FVP. In the left panel, the preoperative composite color photo and OCT images as well as the intraoperative video images are shown on the left; after surgery, the composite color photo and OCT image show the attached retina. In the right panel, composite photos and OCT images on the left side show the advancement of the FVP before surgery. The retina was reattached after surgery (right composite color photo and OCT images)

out an RI in both eyes. Fundus examination revealed severe fibrovascular proliferation (FVP) and impending macula-off tractional retinal detachment (TRD) in the right eye and extramacular TRD in the left eye. She then received pars plana vitrectomy (PPV) and gas infusion. The retina reattached after surgery. Four months later, the left eye developed impending macula-off TRD, with BCVA decreasing to 0.05. The FVP turned into fibrotic tissue. She underwent similar surgery in the left eye. The retina reattached after surgery. The BCVA improved to 0.2 and 0.3, respectively, 6 months after surgery in the left eye (Fig. 24.1).

24.2 Diabetic Vitrectomy in Young Patients

Young DM patients have a steadily growing population. The increase in the number of patients with young NIDDM greatly contributed to this trend. While one study in the United States reported that approximately one-third of newly diagnosed children with DM had NIDDM, another study from Japan reported that 80% of patients in the same age group had NIDDM [1, 2]. Many studies have shown that there are similarities between IDDM and young-onset NIDDM with respect to the progression of DR and the prevalence of PDR [3–5]. Are there unique features in young adults who undergo vitrectomy for complications of PDR? We conducted a study attempting to answer this question [6].

We retrospectively reviewed the medical records of consecutive patients who received PPV secondary to PDR complications at 18–40 years of age by a single surgeon at National Taiwan University Hospital (NTUH); consecutive DR patients who received PPV after 40 years of age by the same surgeon in the same hospital were enrolled as the control group.

We chose 40 years of age as the cutoff point because in several previous studies, young-onset DM has been conventionally defined as DM onset before 30 years of age, and there may be a 5- to 10-year lag between disease onset and surgical intervention.

The analysis of various indications for vitrectomy revealed that VH was less likely, and TRD or combined tractional and rhegmatogenous retinal detachment (CTRRD) was more likely to be present in the young study group than in the older control group, implying rapid progression of proliferative vitreoretinopathy in youth with diabetes once retinal NV with VH occurred. In our study, we found that the younger onset group demonstrated a greater FVP grade and more extensive TRD than did the older onset group at the time of vitrectomy for complications of PDR. In addition, the possibility of having active FVP in the study group was also greater, despite a similar rate of IVI of anti-vascular endothelial growth factor (VEGF) and PRP in the two groups. These differences partly explain why a greater percentage of eyes in the study group required SO tamponade. With modern surgical techniques, although the overall anatomical success rates were high in both groups (91.2% and 100%, $p = 0.009$), the study group had a significantly greater rate of recurrent detachment requiring further surgeries.

Although young patients showed more severe VR changes, functional results measured by BCVA, on the other hand, showed similar improvements on average in both the study and the control groups.

Various manifestations and surgical results in young adults are shown in Figs. 24.2 and 24.3.

More closely, we found that most of the patients in either group could maintain ambulatory vision (79.1% in the study group vs. 76.9% in the control group). However, 11.9% and 1.5% of the patients in the younger-onset group had VA of the HM or less, respectively, compared with those in the control group. These results may be caused by a greater recurrent detachment rate and more severe vitreoretinal proliferation in younger patients, which are associated with severe retinal ischemia, longer operation times, increased postoperative inflammation, and IOP fluctuations. The accumulation of these factors contributes to poor BCVA despite eventual anatomical success. This issue is important because bilateral involvement of similar severity is common in young patients. On the other hand, the proportion of patients with vision better than 20/40 significantly increased with time within the 1-year follow-up in the younger onset group, from 5.1% at 2 months to 20.9% at 12 months, which was not found in the control group. This result may be partly due to a better retinal reserve in younger patients; once the retina becomes stable, functional improvement occurs more rapidly in younger patients than in older patients.

In the study group, the risk factors for inferior visual outcome included HTN and ESRD; poor preoperative VA; TRD; combined RD; and the use of SB during surgery.

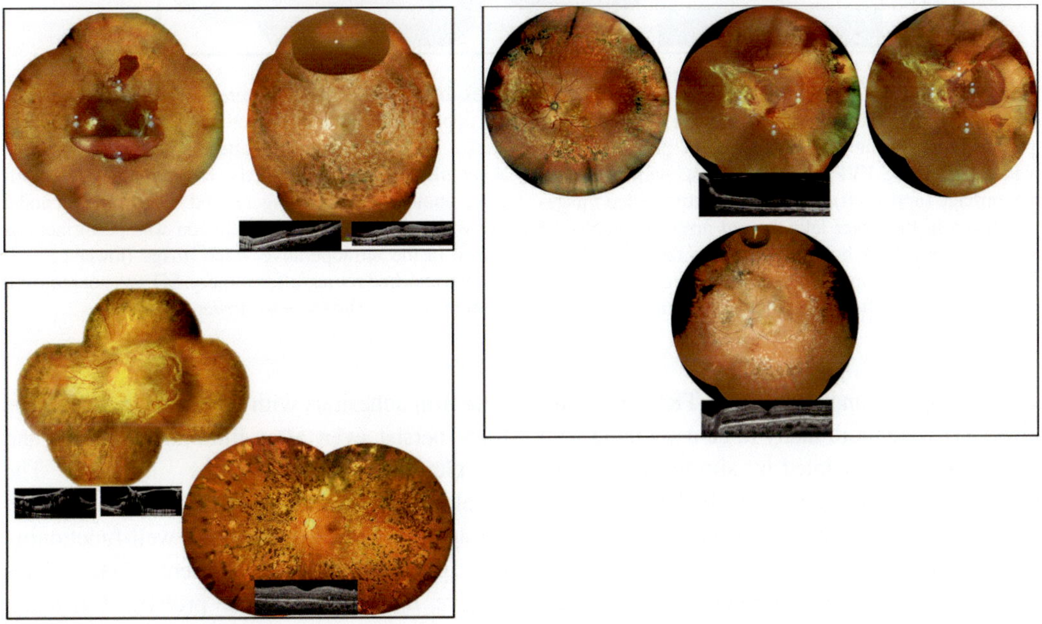

Fig. 24.2 Three sets of images showing different manifestations of active FVP in three patients. The left upper panel shows the active FVP with preretinal hemorrhage; the right upper panel shows the progression of FVP with VH (upper three wide angle color photos and OCT); the lower left panel shows the widespread FVP with minimal VH. All had attached retinas after surgery

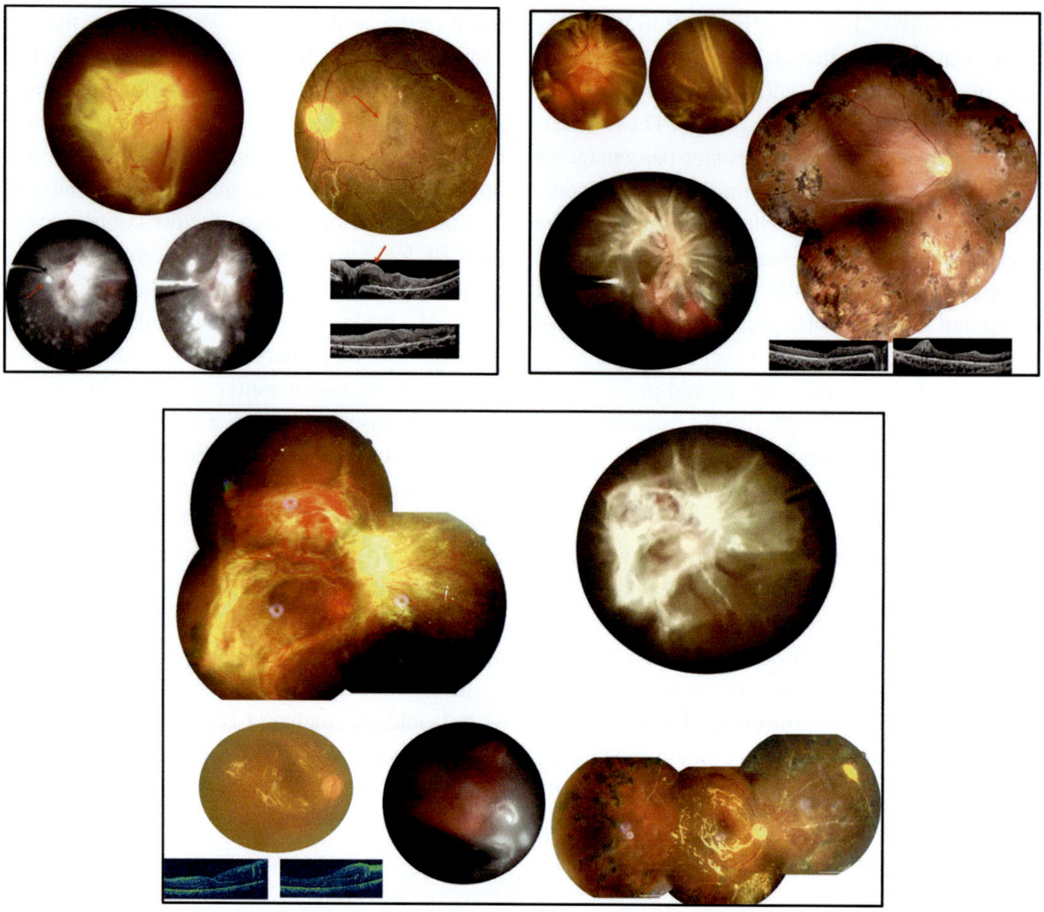

Fig. 24.3 Three sets of images showing different manifestations of active FVP with TRD in three patients. In the left upper panel, the preoperative color photo shows a plaque-like active FVP around the disc with preretinal hemorrhage (upper left); two intraoperative video images are shown in the lower left; the red arrow points to the endodiathermy mark before creating an iatrogenic break for drainage. In the upper right panel, pre- and intraoperative images show the TRD with prominent folding (left side). In the lower panel, severe active FVP is shown in the upper composite color photo (upper left) and intraoperative image (upper right); after surgery with SO, SRF accumulation was noted in the lower retina (lower left color photo and OCT images); and SRF drainage under SO with supplementary SO infusion was performed, as shown in the intraoperative video image (lower center). All had attached retinas after surgery. SO was not removed from the eye, as shown in the lower panel

Focusing on fundus changes, TRD and combined RD were more likely to be associated with active FVP accompanied by significant subretinal hemorrhage. Dissection of the adherent FVP from the detached retina was technically demanding and usually required bimanual manipulation. These factors contribute to poor vision in young patients with TRD. We also found (not presented in the study) that one of the unique features of fundus change in young patients with active FVP is the presence of prominent folds that have multiple firm adhesions with the overlying FVP. The folds persist even after fluid-air exchange and complete removal of the traction. The development of such folds is the net result of strong vitreoretinal traction and well-functioning RPE pumping in young patients. When folds involve the macular area, prolonged macular structure abnormalities may occur.

In the study group, the most significant risk factor for poor prognosis was the development of NVG, causing approximately three lines to decrease. NVG following vitrectomy may be the result of either the breakdown of the VEGF barrier between the posterior and anterior segments or increased inflammation caused by prolonged surgical procedures. In our study group, all of the patients who developed NVG had active FVP, which is known to be associated with high VEGF levels. Our analysis of fellow eye conditions indicated that younger-onset DM patients generally had a worse binocular visual prognosis than older-onset DM patients.

The subgroup analysis between NIDDM and IDDM in the study group revealed that the IDDM subgroup had earlier disease onset, longer disease duration, and younger operation age than the NIDDM subgroup. The two subgroups had similar clinical characteristics and visual prognoses. Nonetheless, there seemed to be a trend toward relatively favorable postoperative vision at 12 months and more visual improvement in NIDDM patients in our study.

In summary, we found that younger patients with DM, whether they had IDDM or NIDDM, presented with more extensive retinopathy when surgery was indicated. Although surgical intervention can achieve considerable anatomical and functional improvement, more patients with DM than older patients with DM have poor BCVA (HM or less) and worse fellow eye vision. The presence of NVG was associated with worse outcomes in the younger group. Finally, the IDDM and NIDDM subgroups in young-onset DM patients had similar clinical features and visual outcomes (Figs. 24.4 and 24.5).

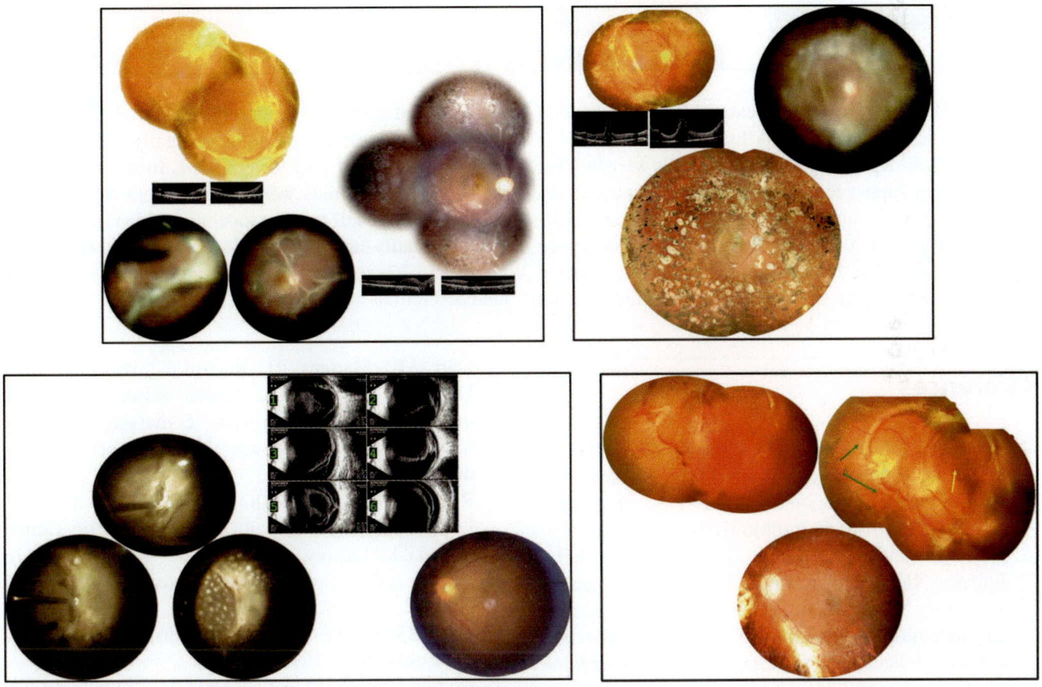

Fig. 24.4 Four sets of images showing prominent retinal folds in young patients with PDR and FVP. In the upper left and lower left panels, intraoperative images show persistent folds after traction had been released at the end of surgery. In the upper right and lower right panels, prominent retinal folds were noted before surgery. The folds gradually settled after surgery in all four patients

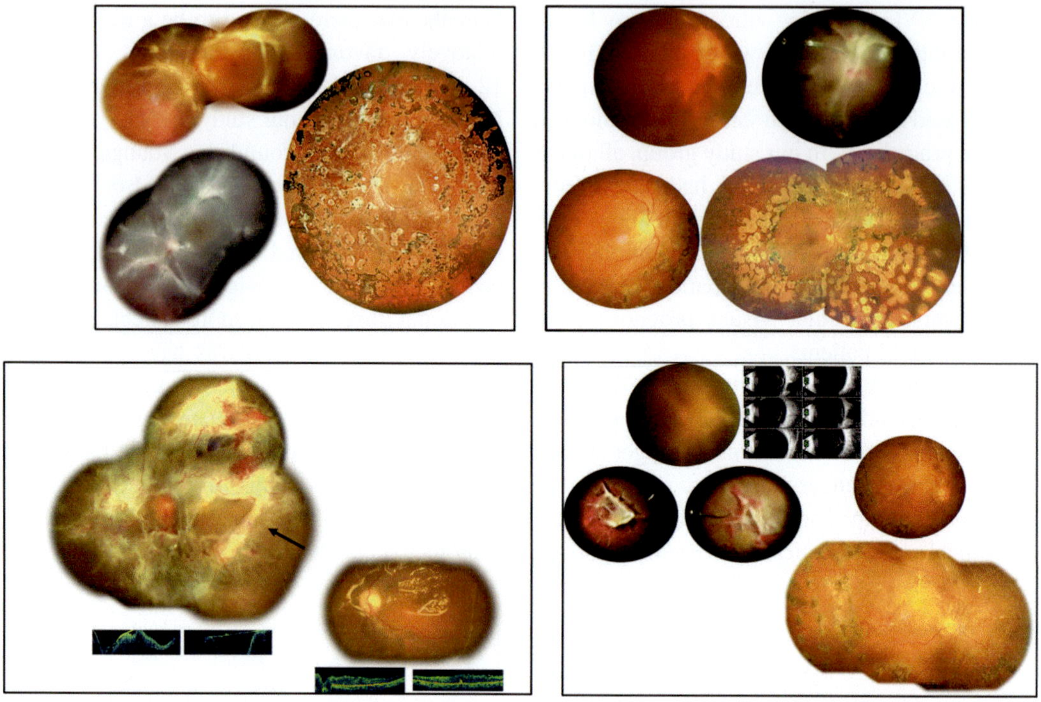

Fig. 24.5 Four sets of prominent folds in four young PDR patients. All four patients had active FVP. In the upper and lower left panels, prominent folds were evident before surgery (upper left composite color photos in the left two panels); the upper left panel also showed prominent folds at the end of surgery (lower left intraoperative video image). In the upper right panel, a preoperative color photo shows the FVP with VH; prominent folds were evident at the end of surgery (upper right intraoperative video image); and the folds gradually subsided after surgery (lower left and lower right). In the lower right panel, prominent folds were again evident at the end of surgery (middle left two intraoperative video images); the folds gradually subsided after surgery (middle right color photo and lower right composite color photos). All had attached retinas after surgery

References

1. Yoon KH, Lee JH, Kim JW, Cho JH, Choi YH, Ko SH, et al. Epidemic obesity and type 2 diabetes in Asia. Lancet. 2006;368(9548):1681–8. https://doi.org/10.1016/S0140-6736(06)69703-1.
2. Fagot-Campagna A, Pettitt DJ, Engelgau MM, Burrows NR, Geiss LS, Valdez R, et al. Type 2 diabetes among North American children and adolescents: an epidemiologic review and a public health perspective. J Pediatr. 2000;136(5):664–72. https://doi.org/10.1067/mpd.2000.105141.
3. Song SH. Complication characteristics between young-onset type 2 versus type 1 diabetes in a UK population. BMJ Open Diabetes Res Care. 2015;3(1):e000044. https://doi.org/10.1136/bmjdrc-2014-000044.
4. Dart AB, Martens PJ, Rigatto C, Brownell MD, Dean HJ, Sellers EA. Earlier onset of complications in youth with type 2 diabetes. Diabetes Care. 2014;37(2):436–43. https://doi.org/10.2337/dc13-0954.
5. Rajalakshmi R, Amutha A, Ranjani H, Ali MK, Unnikrishnan R, Anjana RM, et al. Prevalence and risk factors for diabetic retinopathy in Asian Indians with young onset type 1 and type 2 diabetes. J Diabetes Complications. 2014;28(3):291–7. https://doi.org/10.1016/j.jdiacomp.2013.12.008.
6. Huang CH, Hsieh YT, Yang CM. Vitrectomy for complications of proliferative diabetic retinopathy in young adults: clinical features and surgical outcomes. Graefes Arch Clin Exp Ophthalmol. 2017;255(5):863–71. https://doi.org/10.1007/s00417-016-3579-4.

25 Diabetic Vitrectomy in Both Eyes

Abstract

DR almost always affects both eyes. Despite recent rapid progress in the medical treatment of diabetic patients and advances in laser and pharmacological therapies for diabetic retinopathy (DR), particularly the wide application of anti-vascular endothelial growth factor (VEGF) agents, many DR patients still require surgery to preserve visual function. The severity of DR in both eyes may not be symmetric, and approximately 5–10% of DR patients have an asymmetric presentation and progression (Azad et al., Indian J Ophthalmol, 69(11): 3026–34, 2021, https://doi.org/10.4103/ijo.IJO_1525_21). It is not uncommon to perform surgery on one eye, but the patient's fellow eye is treated conservatively (Berrocal et al., J Clin Med, 11(18), 5399, https://doi.org/10.3390/jcm11185399). However, it is equally possible that both eyes develop severe DR either concurrently or sequentially, which requires surgery. Previous studies have demonstrated that approximately 20–38% of patients require vitrectomy in the fellow eye after surgery in the first eye (Sulak et al., Retina, 38(4): 698–707, https://doi.org/10.1097/IAE.0000000000001589, 2018; Hwang et al., Br J Ophthalmol, 97(3), 297–301. https://doi.org/10.1136/bjophthalmol-2012-302233, 2013; Vote et al., Clin Exp Ophthalmol, 32(4): 397–403. https://doi.org/10.1111/j.1442-9071.2004.00845.x, 2004; Smiddy et al., Ophthalmology, 102(11): 1688–95. https://doi.org/10.1016/s0161-6420(95)30808-1, 1995). In our study, the visual prognosis of patients who received bilateral vitrectomy, the potentially blinding condition, and the differences in disease severity and outcomes between the concurrent and sequential groups and between the first- and second-operated eyes will be presented and discussed.

25.1 Case Report

Patient 1 This 52-year-old man had underlying disease characterized by poorly controlled DM for more than 10 years. He also had HT, dyslipidemia, and chronic kidney disease. The patient was diagnosed with proliferative diabetic retinopathy (PDR) and underwent panretinal photocoagulation (PRP) in both eyes 3 years prior. He came to our clinic complaining of blurred vision in both eyes. On examination, best-corrected visual acuity (BCVA) was 0.3 in the right eye, and HM was 80 cm in the left eye. Fundus examinations revealed a broad fibrovascular proliferation (FVP) membrane in the temporal and temporal lower arcade and a tractional retinal detachment (TRD) involving the macula in the right eye, an active severe FVP around the temporal superior and inferior arcades with exten-

C.-M. Yang, *Surgery for Complications of Diabetic Retinopathy*,
https://doi.org/10.1007/978-981-96-2848-3_25

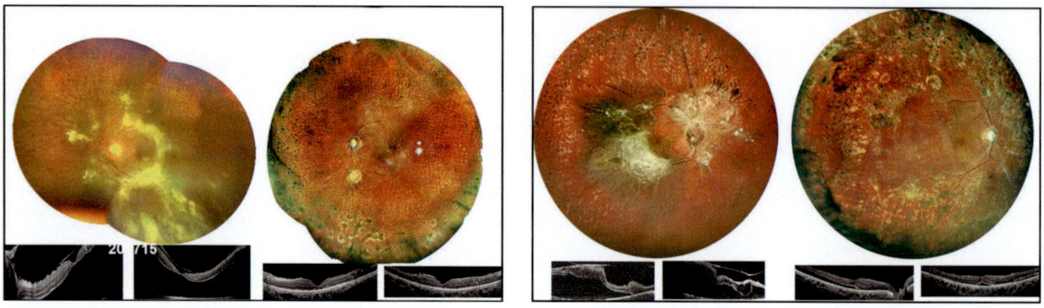

Fig. 25.1 Two sets of images showing pre- and postoperative retinal changes in bilateral TRD in a patient in the concurrent group. In the left panel, preoperative composite color photo and OCT images show severe FVP with TRD and VH (left); after surgery, the FVP was removed, and the retina was reattached (right). In the right panel, preoperative wide-angle color photo and OCT images show a broad FVP membrane in the temporal arcade spreading to the midperiphery and the TRD (left). Surgery was performed 3 months after surgery on the left eye. After surgery, the retinal structure greatly improved (right wide angle color photo and OCT images)

sion to the midperiphery, a macula-off TRD, and a VH in the inferior part of the left eye. Vitrectomy with membrane removal and internal limiting membrane (ILM) peeling was performed on the left eye. After surgery, the retina was reattached. However, the TRD in the right eye became more extensive, and 3 months later, the BCVA decreased to 0.1 in the right eye and improved to 0.1 in the left eye. Fundus examination revealed progression of TRD. He underwent vitrectomy with FVP tissue removal and ILM peeling in the right eye. Six months after surgery, the retina became reattached, and BCVA was 0.2 in the right eye and 0.1 in the left eye (Fig. 25.1).

Patient 2 This 60-year-old woman had DM for 15 or more years and had been treated with oral hyperglycemic agents. Her blood sugar had been poorly controlled for 3 years, but her recent HbA1c level was approximately 7%. She also had HT under medication. She had been treated with IVI anti-VEGF several times for ME and PRP for PDR in both eyes. During FU, posterior subcapsular cataracts and nonclearing VH were noted in the right eye. On examination, BCVA was HM at 1 M in the right eye and 0.05 in the left eye. A dense cataract was noted in the right eye. Findus examination revealed a dense VH obscuring the retina in the right eye and macular edema in the left eye. Phacoemulsification with posterior chamber intraocular lens (PCIOL) implantation and vitrectomy were performed on the right eye. During surgery, the LMH was noted, and the inverted ILM flap technique was used. After surgery, the vitreous was clear, and the retina was attached. During the FU, persistent VH for several months developed in the left eye, and VA decreased significantly. On examination, BCVA was 0.05 in the right eye and 0.01 in the left eye. Fundus examination revealed an attached and silent retina in the right eye but moderate VH in the left eye. Phacoemulsification with PCIOL implantation and vitrectomy were performed on the right eye 9 months after the operation. After surgery, the media became clear, and the retina was attached. Her BCVA was 0.1 in the right eye and 0.2 in the left eye 3 years later (Fig. 25.2).

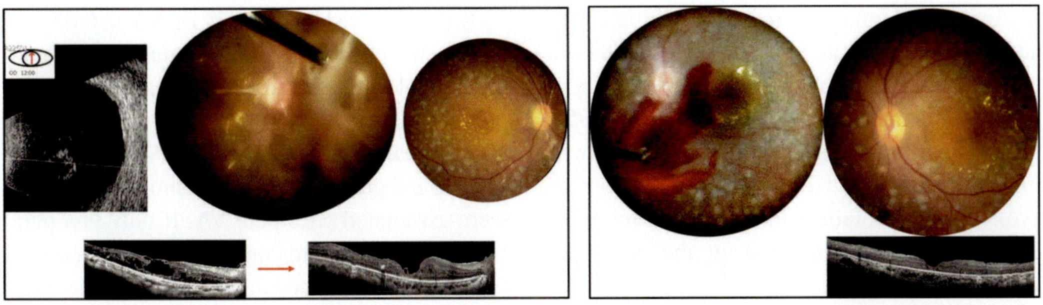

Fig. 25.2 Two sets of images showing sequential operations to treat complications of PDR in a 60-year-old patient. In the left panel, preoperative ultrasonography images and intraoperative video images show severe VH and FVP (upper left and upper center); after surgery, the FVP was removed, and the retina was reattached (upper right). Postoperative OCT images showed LMH evolution after the inverted ILM flap technique was performed during surgery (lower). In the right panel, 9 months after the right eye operation, an intraoperative video image of the left eye showed VH and paramacular hard exudates (left). After surgery, the vitreous cavity was clear, and no macular thickening or edema was noted (right side color photo and OCT image)

25.2 Diabetic Vitrectomy in Both Eyes

As noted in the beginning, some patients had complications of PDR requiring bilateral surgery concurrently, as in Patient 1, while others had the disease progressing to a severe condition necessitating surgery sequentially, as in Patient 2. It is clinically relevant to know whether specific features exist in these two groups of patients, including systemic conditions, DR severity, anatomical and functional results, and risk factors for poor VA. Furthermore, it is important to determine the differences in anatomical and functional prognoses between the two eyes in the concurrent and sequential operation subgroups.

In a retrospective study, we enrolled 117 patients with PDR who underwent vitrectomy of both eyes with postoperative FU for at least 6 months after surgery performed by a single experienced surgeon (the author) and analyzed the results to answer the above questions [1]. We separated the patients into two groups: concurrent and sequential. Concurrent patients were defined as patients who required surgery in both eyes at the same time, while sequential patients were defined as patients who required surgery in one eye at first but later required surgery in the other eye. Overall, 54 patients (108 eyes) were in the concurrent group, and 63 patients (126 eyes) were in the sequential group.

We found that there were no significant differences in HbA1c, blood pressure, renal function, hemoglobin, or BMI between the sequential and concurrent groups. Notably, the average age of the concurrent group (44.8 years) was significantly younger than that of the sequential group (50.3 years) ($p = 0.017$). The interval of operation between the two eyes was 4.6 months in the concurrent group and 27.3 months in the sequential group.

The severity grading of the first operated eyes, the second operated eyes, and the first operated eye in the sequential group was similar. The severity of the second operated eyes, including the FVP grade, percentage, and area of the TRD, in the sequential group was significantly lower than that of their earlier operated fellow eyes and lower than that of the two eyes in the concurrent group. More patients in the sequential group than in the concurrent group underwent PRP. There were more patients who received preoperative anti-VEGF therapy in the concurrent group.

The functional prognosis was better in the second operated eye in the sequential group than in the first operated eye in the sequential group and the two eyes in the concurrent group, including less postoperative IS/OS disruption in OCT, better postoperative BCVA, and a percentage of postoperative VA equal to or better than 0.05. This difference in prognosis between the two eyes was not found in the concurrent group.

Anatomical analysis revealed that the final anatomical failure rate was 8/108 eyes in the concurrent group, which was evenly distributed between the first and second operated eyes (4/54), and 8/126 eyes in the sequential group (6/63 in the first operated eye and 2/63 in the second operated eye). Anatomical failure in both eyes occurred in only one patient, who was in the concurrent group.

Functionally, if a cutoff point of 0.05 was used, 65% of the two eyes in the concurrent group had a BCVA equal to or better than 0.05, compared with 76% and 84% of the first and second operated eyes, respectively, in the sequential group.

When a cutoff point of the ND was used, 74% and 85% of the first and second operated eyes, respectively, in the concurrent group had a BCVA equal to or better than that of the ND, compared with 83% and 92% of the first and second operated eyes, respectively, in the sequential group.

Nine percent (five patients) of the patients in the concurrent group had a BCVA less than that of the ND in both eyes, while no patients had such poor BCVA in either eye in the sequential group ($P = 0.090$).

Among those with a BCVA equal to or less than that of the HM, 22 were in the concurrent group, and 15 were in the sequential group. The difference was not significant. Among those with BCVA equal to or less than the HM in both eyes, all four patients were in the concurrent group.

Among those with ambulatory vision (BCVA ≥ 0.05) in at least one eye, 36 were in the concurrent group, and 53 were in the sequential group. The difference was clinically significant.

Regarding risk factors, if BCVA < 0.05 was used as the cutoff for poor VA, multivariate analysis revealed that postoperative macular atrophy, postoperative IS/OS disruption, postoperative neovascular glaucoma (NVG), FVP outside the arcade, and preoperative use of anti-VEGF agents were associated with poor VA. If only preoperative risk factors were considered, combined tractional and rhegmatogenous retinal detachment (CTRRD), active FVP, FVP with broad adhesion, FVP outside the arcade, no preoperative use of anti-VEGF, concurrent group, and old age were associated with poor VA.

In the concurrent group, 34 patients were over 40 years old, and 20 patients were less than or equal to 40 years old; in the sequential group, 47 patients were over 40 years old, and 16 patients were less than or equal to 40 years old ($p = 0.246$). There were more patients whose postoperative VA was less than 0.05 in the older age group than in the younger age group.

Case examples of concurrent groups and sequential groups are shown in Figs. 25.3, 25.4, 25.5 and 25.6.

In summary, in patients who had both eyes operated on for complications of DR, those in the concurrent group were younger and generally had more eyes suffering from poor postoperative visual function (BCVA less than 0.05). The second eye in the sequential group had the best anatomical and functional results. The number of patients who eventually had very poor vision (BCVA equal to or less than HM), fortunately, was low, and all patients were in the concurrent group. Older age, severe vitreoretinal changes, and no previous use of anti-VEGF agents were associated with poor visual outcomes.

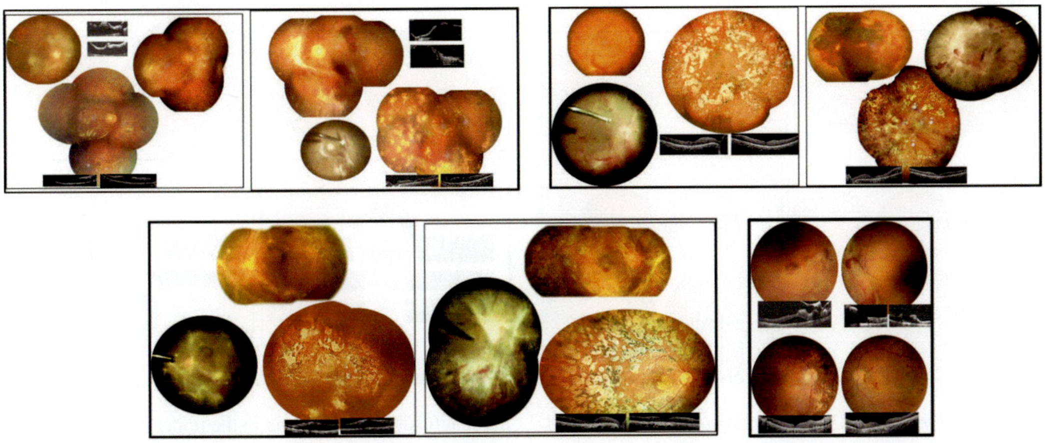

Fig. 25.3 Four sets of images showing pre- and postoperative changes in patients with mild to moderate concurrent PDR complications in both eyes of the same patient. In each panel, the images on the right side of the subset were obtained from the latter operated eye. Postoperative color photos and OCT images are shown in the lower panels, except for the upper right panel, in which the postoperative wide angle color photo and OCT images of the right eye are shown on the right side. In the upper left panel, both eyes had TRD; in the upper right panel, both eyes had active FVP with VH; in the lower left panel, both eyes had predominantly extramacular FVP; and in the lower right panel, both eyes had FVP around the disc, which caused TRD in the right eye (left upper color photo and OCT images) and LMH with schisis in the left eye (upper right color photo and OCT images)

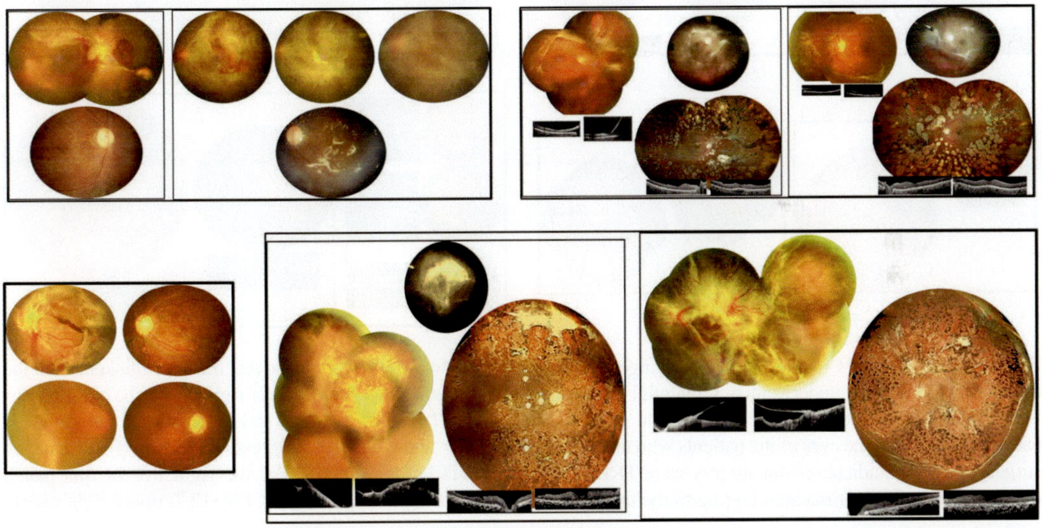

Fig. 25.4 Four sets of images showing pre- and postoperative changes in patients with severe concurrent PDR complications in both eyes. In each panel, the right or lower images are from the latter operated eye. All eyes had active FVP with TRD with or without macular involvement. In the upper left panel, the postoperative color photos are in the lower panels for both eyes. In all other panels, the postoperative images are on the right side. The two eyes in the lower right panel had the most severe FVP preoperatively. In this case, the left eye also had MH (not shown here; please refer to the images on the right side of Fig. 12.9, Chap. 12)

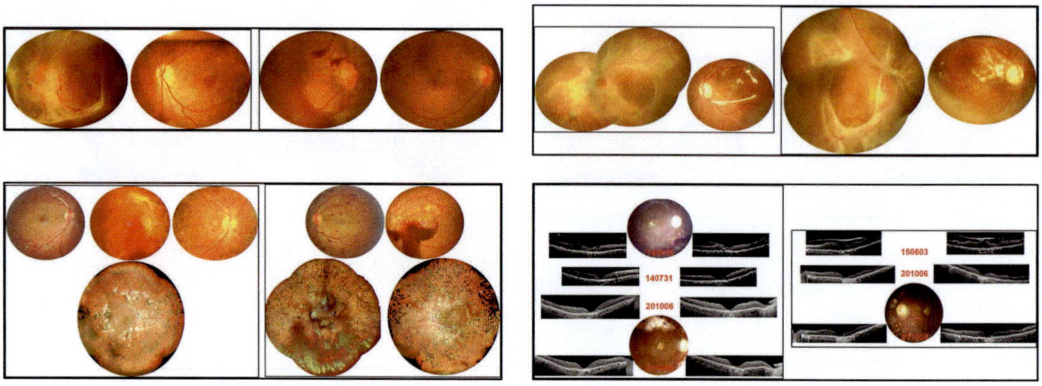

Fig. 25.5 Four sets of images showing pre- and postoperative changes in patients who underwent sequential surgery in both eyes with mild to moderate FVP. The right-side images in each panel are from the eyes of the patients who underwent surgery later. In the lower left panel, the progression of DR is shown in the two upper left color photos in the left subset images and in the upper two color photos and lower left wide angle color photo in the right subset images. Except for the lower right panel, which had a thick premacular membrane in both eyes, all the other patients had milder FVP in the latter operated eyes. The numbers in red indicate the date the images were obtained

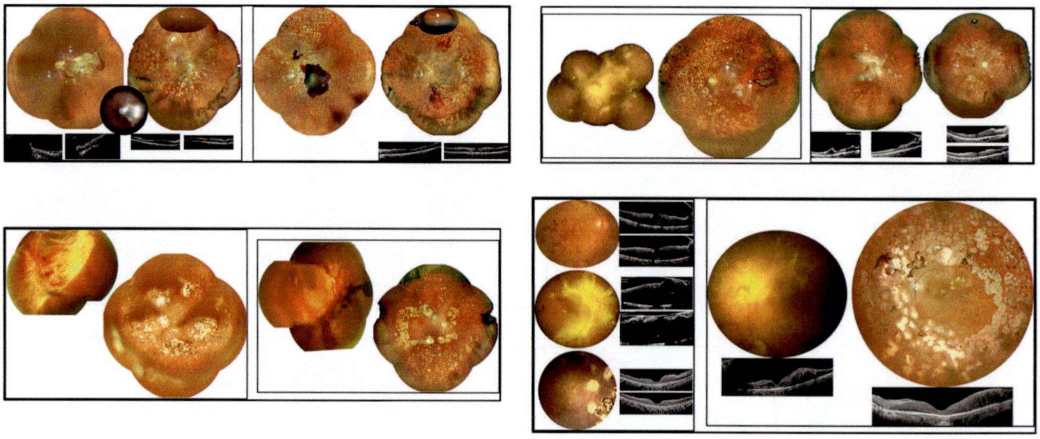

Fig. 25.6 Four sets of images showing changes in both eyes of patients who underwent a sequential operation with moderate to severe FVP. The right-side images in each panel are from the eyes of the patients who underwent surgery later. The indications for surgery were TRD in the left two panels, TRD or macular tenting in the upper right panel, and MHRD or parafoveal macular thickening in the lower right panel. In the lower right panel, the color photos and OCT images in the top and center rows of the right eye images show severe progression of the FVP causing MHRD before surgery. For the right eye in this panel, please also refer to Chap. 12, Fig. 12.7, upper right panel

Reference

1. Hsia Y, Yang CM. Bilateral vitrectomy in patients with proliferative diabetic retinopathy—characteristics and surgical outcomes. Graefes Arch Clin Exp Ophthalmol. 2024;262(9):2833–44. https://doi.org/10.1007/s00417-024-06462-5.

26 Preoperative Factors for Poor Vision After Vitrectomy in Severe Proliferative Diabetic Retinopathy

Abstract

Various pre- and postoperative factors associated with a poor visual outcome, including poor preoperative visual acuity (VA), older age, iris neovascularization, a history of lensectomy, the creation of iatrogenic breaks, and elevated intraocular pressure, have been reported in the literature (Thompson et al., Arch Ophthalmol, 105(4): 497–502, https://doi.org/10.1001/archopht.1987.01060040067035, 1987; Thompson et al., Ophthalmology, 93(3): 290–5, https://doi.org/10.1016/s0161-6420(86)33741-2, 1986; La Heij et al., Graefes Arch Clin Exp Ophthalmol, 242(3): 210–7. https://doi.org/10.1007/s00417-003-0815-5, 2004. Newman, Eye (Lond), 24(3): 441–9, https://doi.org/10.1038/eye.2009.325, 2010. Yorston et al., Br J Ophthalmol, 92(3): 365–8, https://doi.org/10.1136/bjo.2007.124495, 2008). However, few studies have specifically focused on the preoperative systemic and local factors that may be related to extremely poor visual function despite anatomical success and an uneventful postoperative course. The identification of these factors may be useful for predicting poor functional outcome and avoiding unnecessary surgical intervention. In this chapter, risk factors associated with anatomical success but functional failure after DV will be discussed.

26.1 Case Report

This 47-year-old female was a patient with DM under insulin control. She had no HT. Two years prior, she had blurred vision in her right eye, and diabetic retinopathy (DR) was diagnosed. She received bilateral eye panretinal photocoagulation (PRP) and right eye cataract surgery at an outside hospital. However, the vision of the right eye still worsened. She also suffered from progressive blurred vision in the left eye. She then visited our clinic for further evaluation. On examination, best-corrected visual acuity (BCVA) was 50 cm in HM in the right eye and 80 cm in counting fingers (CF) in the left eye. Fundus examinations revealed extensive predominantly fibrotic proliferation with tractional retinal detachment (TRD) in the right eye and extensive predominantly fibrotic proliferation in the posterior pole with TRD in the left eye. The laboratory data showed a BUN level of 23.2 mg/dL and a creatinine level of 1.5 mg/dL. She underwent vitrectomy, membrane removal, and SO infusion in the left eye. Cataract surgery was performed 10 months later. The retina was

C.-M. Yang, *Surgery for Complications of Diabetic Retinopathy*,
https://doi.org/10.1007/978-981-96-2848-3_26

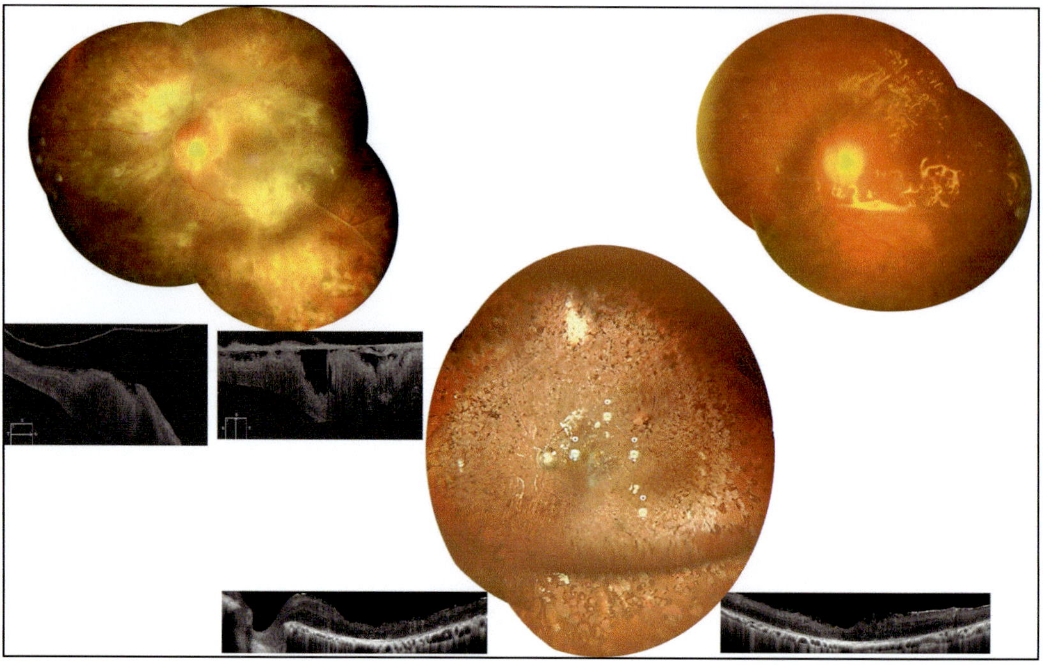

Fig. 26.1 Pre- and postoperative images of a patient with poor postoperative VA. Before surgery, the retina exhibited extensive fibrotic proliferation with vessel sheathing and TRD (upper left composite color photo and OCT images). After surgery with SO, the retina was reattached; diffuse EZ disruption was noted on OCT images (upper right composite color photo and lower wide angle color photo and OCT images)

attached under SO. Postop BCVA was HM/100 cm in the left eye (Fig. 26.1).

26.2 Preoperative Factors for Poor Vision After Vitrectomy in Severe PDR

To study the preoperative systemic and local factors that are associated with poor postoperative VA after an anatomically successful DV, we selected patients with poor initial vision who achieved a successful anatomical outcome after uneventful surgery and who experienced a smooth postoperative course. Patients with an extremely poor functional outcome (BCVA less than counting fingers) were compared with those who had a better visual outcome. Preoperative systemic and local factors were examined to identify possible preoperative risk factors associated with a poor visual outcome in severe proliferative diabetic retinopathy (PDR) patients [1].

Consecutive patients with poor preoperative BCVA (less than counting fingers) who underwent primary pars plana vitrectomy for complications of PDR were selected. All patients were followed up for more than 6 months postoperatively. Patients with retinal attachment at the end of the surgery, an uneventful postoperative course, regular postoperative FU, and postoperative retinal attachment for at least 6 months were enrolled. Patients who had elevated intraocular pressure greater than 35 mmHg for two consecutive postoperative days and patients who had significant vitreous hemorrhage and/or dense cataract before surgery were excluded. Thus, only those patients whose visual function reflected the severity of the anatomical changes were selected. The patients were separated into two groups according to postoperative VA. We defined the study group as patients whose postoperative VA was worse than the preoperative BCVA (hand motion, light perception, or no light perception) and the control group as patients whose postoperative BCVA was better than the preoperative VA (counting fingers or any Snellen acuity). The postoperative VA was measured at least 6 months postoperatively.

Certain parameters were defined. Chronic long-standing macular detachment was defined as 4-quadrant vessel sheathing, a pale disc, uniform fibrotic proliferation, and atrophic thinning of the detached macula if optical coherence tomography (OCT) data were available. Predominantly active neovascularization, predominantly fibrotic proliferation, the extent of fibrovascular proliferation (FVP), and the extent of RD were defined as described in the discussion of Chap. 1.

The results showed that the creatinine level was significantly greater in the study group than in the control group. In addition, univariate statistical analysis using fundus variables as risk factors revealed that chronic long-standing macular detachment, the extent of fibrovascular proliferation, and predominantly fibrotic proliferation were significantly associated with a poor prognosis. Multivariate analysis further revealed that chronic long-standing macular detachment and the extent of fibrovascular proliferation were the most important factors determining poor visual outcome.

Both DR and diabetic nephropathy are among the diabetic microvascular complications [2–4]. Microangiopathy in the kidney may indicate a similar microvascular environment in the retina. In addition, the presence of one preexisting complication (diabetic retinopathy, diabetic nephropathy, or diabetic neuropathy) may contribute to the development of another complication [2–4]. Our data showed that the patient's creatinine level and whether or not the patient was undergoing hemodialysis were significantly related to the outcome of surgery for PDR. We postulate that poor renal function reflects the general worsening of the microvascular environment. Surgery on a retina with extensively damaged microcirculation and preexisting poor visual function may result in a poor prognosis after surgery.

Regarding the severity of FVP, while none of the patients in the control group had FVP extending beyond the equator for more than two quadrants, this degree of severity was observed in 40% of the patients in the study group. Fibrovascular proliferation extending to the periphery not only indicates fulminant fibrovascular proliferation, which leads to a more distorted and detached macular, but also complicates surgery and prolongs the surgical duration, contributing to compromised postoperative circulation and functional recovery at the cellular level.

The PDR is no longer active when it has progressed to the burn-out stage, and a reduction in the caliber of the retinal vessels and sheathed vessels is often found in this stage. The quiescent neovascular activity may also reflect atrophy of the retina. Thus, a more advanced fibrotic stage indicates a more prolonged compromise of retinal conditions, which might be a factor for a poor prognosis. Although predominantly inactive neovascularization alone was not significantly correlated with a poor prognosis in our study ($P = 0.125$), 60% of the patients in the study group had predominantly inactive neovascularization compared to only 28% of patients in the control group. As PDR with macular detachment progresses to purely inactive fibrotic proliferation on the macula, it usually reaches the atrophic stage. An atrophic optic nerve can be a sign of chronic long-standing macular detachment or compromised disc circulation secondary to ischemia, vitreopapillary traction, or unstable intraocular pressure. Our study suggested that the necessity of surgery should be reconsidered when signs such as a pale disc, 4-quadrant vessel sheathing, pure fibrotic proliferation, and atrophic thinning of the detached macula are observed.

If poor renal function, especially on regular hemodialysis, also exists, the patient might not be a suitable candidate for surgery.

Another example of poor postoperative visual function after successful surgery is shown in Fig. 26.2.

Although our study may provide a general idea of risk factors for extremely poor postoperative vision, the actual decision to perform surgery on a specific patient remains an intriguing one. Factors such as the surgeon's capability, surgical

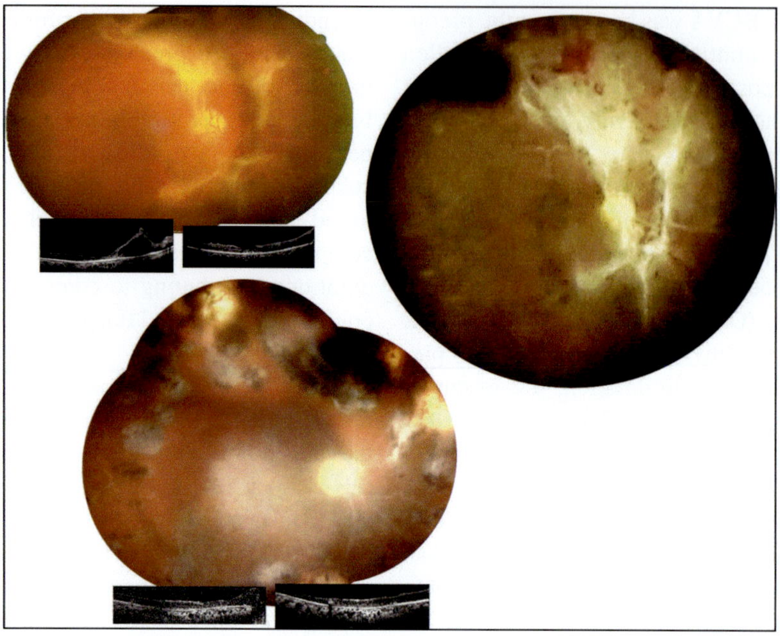

Fig. 26.2 Pre- and postoperative images of a patient with poor postoperative VA. Before surgery, the retina had fibrotic proliferation along the upper arcade and fibrotic bands nasal and lower to the disc; parafoveal macular tenting with schisis was noted. OCT revealed an extensive EZ defect, and the central foveal thickness was 172 μm (upper left composite color photo and OCT images, upper right intraoperative video image). The patient's BCVA was HM/100 cm. After vitreous surgery and subsequent cataract surgery, the retina was reattached; a pale disc, vessel sheathing, and diffuse macular thinning were noted on OCT images (upper right composite color photo and lower wide angle color photo and OCT images). The patient's BCVA was light perception

complexity, and condition of the patient's fellow eye should also be taken into consideration. Ultimately, the benefit to the patient should be prioritized first.

References

1. Lin S-J, Yeh P-T, Huang J-Y, Yang C-M. Preoperative prognostic factors in vitrectomy for severe proliferative diabetic retinopathy. Taiwan J Ophthalmol. 2014;4(4):174–8. https://doi.org/10.1016/j.tjo.2014.08.005.
2. Bloomgarden ZT. Diabetic retinopathy and neuropathy. Diabetes Care. 2005;28(4):963–70. https://doi.org/10.2337/diacare.28.4.963.
3. Girach A, Vignati L. Diabetic microvascular complications—can the presence of one predict the development of another? J Diabetes Complications. 2006;20(4):228–37. https://doi.org/10.1016/j.jdiacomp.2006.03.001.
4. Jeng CJ, Hsieh YT, Yang CM, Yang CH, Lin CL, Wang IJ. Diabetic retinopathy in patients with diabetic nephropathy: development and progression. PLoS One. 2016;11(8):e0161897. https://doi.org/10.1371/journal.pone.0161897.

MIX
Papier aus verantwortungsvollen Quellen
Paper from responsible sources
FSC® C105338

If you have any concerns about our products,
you can contact us on
ProductSafety@springernature.com

In case Publisher is established outside the EU,
the EU authorized representative is:
Springer Nature Customer Service Center GmbH
Europaplatz 3, 69115 Heidelberg, Germany

Printed by Libri Plureos GmbH
in Hamburg, Germany